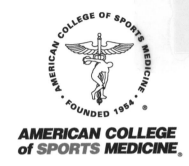

AMERICAN COLLEGE
of SPORTS MEDICINE®

Complete Guide to Fitness & Health

Second Edition

Barbara A. Bushman, PhD

Editor

D1439405

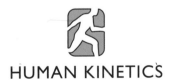

HUMAN KINETICS

Library of Congress Cataloging-in-Publication Data

Names: Bushman, Barbara Ann, editor. | American College of Sports Medicine.
Title: ACSM's complete guide to fitness & health / Barbara Bushman, PhD.,
  editor.
Other titles: Complete guide to fitness & health. | American College of
  Sports Medicine's complete guide to fitness and health
Description: Second edition. | Champaign, IL : Human Kinetics, [2017] |
  Revised edition of: Complete guide to fitness & health / Barbara Bushman,
  editor (Champaign, IL : Human Kinetics, c2011). | Includes bibliographical
  references and index.
Identifiers: LCCN 2016048914 (print) | LCCN 2017000135 (ebook) | ISBN
  9781492533672 (print) | ISBN 9781492548782 (ebook)
Subjects: LCSH: Exercise. | Physical fitness. | Health.
Classification: LCC RA781 .C575 2017 (print) | LCC RA781 (ebook) | DDC
  613.7--dc23
LC record available at https://lccn.loc.gov/2016048914

ISBN: 978-1-4925-3367-2 (print)

This publication is written and published to provide accurate and authoritative information relevant to the subject matter presented. Care has been taken to confirm the accuracy of the information presented and to describe generally accepted practices. However, the authors, editors, and publisher are not responsible for errors or omissions or for any consequences from application of the information in this publication and make no warranty, expressed or implied, with respect to the currency, completeness, or accuracy of the contents of the publication. It is published and sold with the understanding that the authors, editors, and publisher are not engaged in rendering legal, medical, or other professional services by reason of their authorship or publication of this work. If medical or other assistance is required, it is the responsibility of the reader or user to obtain the services of a doctor or other competent professional. Application of this information in an educational or any other situation remains the professional responsibility of the practitioner; the clinical treatments described and recommended may not be considered absolute and universal recommendations. THE AMERICAN COLLEGE OF SPORTS MEDICINE and the publisher disclaim responsibility for any injury to person or property resulting from any ideas or products referred to in this publication. If you do not agree to these limitations, do not buy this publication or employ the practices discussed in it.

The authors, editors, and publisher have exerted every effort to ensure that drug selection and dosage set forth in this text are in accordance with the current recommendations and practice at the time of publication. However, in view of ongoing research, changes in government regulations, and the constant flow of information relating to drug therapy and drug reactions, the reader is urged to check the package insert for each drug for any change in indications and dosage and for added warnings and precautions. This is particularly important when the recommended agent is a new or infrequently employed drug. Some drugs and medical devices presented in this publication have Food and Drug Administration (FDA) clearance for limited use in restricted research settings. It is the responsibility of the health care provider to ascertain the FDA status of each drug or device planned for use in their clinical practice, and it is the responsibility of the user or patient to ensure that he or she has obtained the advice of a doctor or other appropriate, competent medical professional before taking any drug or using any medical device.

The web addresses cited in this text were current as of October 2016, unless otherwise noted.

Acquisitions Editor: Michelle Maloney; **Developmental Editor:** Laura Pulliam; **Managing Editor:** Caitlin Husted; **Copyeditor:** Joyce Sexton; **Indexer:** Andrea Hepner; **Permissions Manager:** Martha Gullo; **Graphic Designers:** Dawn Sills and Nancy Rasmus; **Cover Designer:** Keith Blomberg; **Photographer (cover):** klenova/Getty Images/iStockphoto; **Photographs (interior):** Neil Bernstein, unless otherwise noted; **Photo Asset Manager:** Laura Fitch; **Visual Production Assistant:** Joyce Brumfield; **Photo Production Manager:** Jason Allen; **Senior Art Manager:** Kelly Hendren; **Illustrations:** © Human Kinetics, unless otherwise noted; **Printer:** Versa Press

Printed in the United States of America   10   9   8   7   6   5   4   3   2   1

The paper in this book is certified under a sustainable forestry program.

Human Kinetics
Website: www.HumanKinetics.com

United States: Human Kinetics, P.O. Box 5076, Champaign, IL 61825-5076, 800-747-4457, e-mail: info@hkusa.com

Canada: Human Kinetics, 475 Devonshire Road Unit 100, Windsor, ON N8Y 2L5, 800-465-7301 (in Canada only),
e-mail: info@hkcanada.com

Europe: Human Kinetics, 107 Bradford Road, Stanningley, Leeds LS28 6AT, United Kingdom, +44 (0) 113 255 5665,
e-mail: hk@hkeurope.com

Australia: Human Kinetics, 57A Price Avenue, Lower Mitcham, South Australia 5062, 08 8372 0999,
e-mail: info@hkaustralia.com

New Zealand: Human Kinetics, P.O. Box 80, Mitcham Shopping Centre, South Australia 5062, 0800 222 062,
e-mail: info@hknewzealand.com

To Tobin, my dear husband and partner in all life brings our way. Your encouragement and support are pivotal to completion of this project and all the other ventures (and adventures) that I "just can't pass up." We are, and always will be, Team Bushman.

BB

CONTENTS

PREFACE

Step one toward better health is already done! You have taken the first step by opening this book in order to see what additional steps you can take to promote your health and fitness. *ACSM's Complete Guide to Fitness & Health, Second Edition,* is unique in the merging of research-based, scientific information with practical and adaptable plans that you can use. Your choices related to physical activity and nutrition can have a major impact on your current and future health. The *Complete Guide* provides you with simple ways to assess your status and then, using insights gained, to enhance your exercise program as well as to make optimal nutrition decisions that fit with your personal goals.

The book is divided into four parts. Part I provides overviews and motivation to be more active and make positive dietary choices. Part II looks at the various fitness components and how you can include these elements in your exercise program. Part III gets specific with nutrition and physical activity recommendations for various age groups. Part IV expands discussion of diet and exercise to various medical and health conditions. The entire book has been refreshed and updated from the first edition.

More specifically, part I includes introductory chapters that set the stage for the following chapters, covering both physical activity and nutrition. These foundational chapters are packed with usable information plus encouragement to make healthy choices. Knowing what to do to improve health is nice, but, in order for this to be meaningful, you need to actually take action. The *Complete Guide* is focused on helping you link knowing and doing.

Part II focuses on the four elements of a complete exercise program: aerobic fitness, muscular fitness, flexibility, and neuromotor fitness. An entire chapter is devoted to each one of these fitness elements. The chapters clearly outline health and fitness benefits of various exercise components, offer simple fitness assessments, explain development of an effective exercise plan, and provide sample programs, pictures, and descriptions of exercises. You will understand both the *why* and the *how* of a complete exercise program after reading these chapters. Whether you are just starting or are looking for ways to progress your current exercise program, these chapters offer the guidance you need.

Part III includes nutrition and physical activity information specific to given age groups and provides sample programs for the age group covered. Chapters for each age group underscore the value of healthy choices over the lifespan. These chapters clearly illustrate how you can benefit from physical activity regardless of age, whether you are younger, older, or in between. Nutrition issues specific to the various age groups are included to help you make the best food selections.

Part IV includes nutrition and physical activity recommendations unique to various situations and conditions. Each chapter provides background related to a specific health or medical condition and then provides guidance in using nutrition and exercise to optimize health. For readers experiencing heart disease, diabetes, or cancer, there are chapters showing the benefits of physical activity and a healthy diet. Similarly, osteoporosis, Alzheimer's, arthritis, and depression can be affected by exercise and diet; entire chapters are devoted to each of these areas. In addition, chapters are dedicated to weight management and pregnancy.

The first edition of this book was an excellent resource, and with expanded topics and fresh content, this second edition is a tremendous new resource you can use to promote your personal health and fitness. The chapters are written by experts, providing scientifically-based guidance on optimizing health and fitness. You will continue to use this book as a resource for content as well as encouragement. Health and fitness are not destinations but a lifelong journey. You have many individual decisions every day that add up to influence your health and thus your life. With a solid foundation of health and fitness, you can live each day to the fullest. Embrace the journey and keep stepping forward!

ACKNOWLEDGMENTS

The first edition of this book provided readers from around the world with solid and research-based guidance on promoting personal health and fitness. This second edition continues in that effort with extensive updates and a number of new chapters. As with the first edition, specialists in various areas have generously contributed to this book. A heart-felt thank you to each of them for their willingness to be part of this project; the time and effort put forth have been significant. The level of knowledge these specialists have is coupled with a passion for their topic areas that comes through in their writing. In addition, I acknowledge the contribution of Drs. Peter Grandjean and Jeffrey Potteiger who contributed within the American College Sports Medicine review process, a key element of this publication to ensure that the material is based on the most current research. The chapter critiques were thorough, and as a result, this book is set apart from others that may rely on opinion or individual impressions.

I also acknowledge the contributions of the ACSM staff, Katie Feltman, and Angela Chastain. In addition, I appreciate all the work of the staff at Human Kinetics: acquisitions editor Michelle Maloney as well as developmental editor Laura Pulliam, managing editor Caitlin Husted, photographer Neil Bernstein, and graphic designers Dawn Sills and Nancy Rasmus. A project of this nature is a reflection of the dedicated efforts of *many* individuals, and I humbly thank each one, even if not named specifically, for making this second edition a tremendous resource.

Barbara Bushman

CREDITS

Photo Monkey Business/fotolia.com on page 14

Photo Doug Olson/fotolia.com on page 17

Photo © Human Kinetics on page 20

Photo © Human Kinetics on page 28

Photo Maria Teijeiro/Digital Vision/Getty Images on page 38

Photo Leonid Tit/fotolia.com on page 57

Photo Leonid Tit/fotolia.com on page 68

Photo ferrantraite/Getty Images on page 80

Photo Vasko Miokovic Photography/Getty Images on page 94

Photo Monkey Business/fotolia.com on page 104

Photo © Human Kinetics on page 155

Photo Monkey Business/fotolia.com on page 210

Photo Thomas Perkins/fotolia.com on page 219

Photo Maria Teijeiro/Digital Vision/Getty Images on page 221

Photo iStockphoto/Jacom Stephens on page 230

Photo Monkey Business/fotolia.com on page 248

Photo kali9/Getty Images on page 251

Photo falkjohann/fotolia.com on page 253

Photo yellowdog/Cultura RF/Getty Images on page 255

Photo Siri Stafford/Digital Vision/Getty Images on page 281

Photo Christopher Futcher/Getty Images on page 285

Photo Steve Debenport/Getty Images on page 331

Photo Christopher Futcher/Getty Images on page 344

Photo Steve Debenport/Getty Images on page 362

Photo kali9/Getty Images on page 367

Photo © Human Kinetics on page 373

Photo kali9/Getty Images on page 379

Photo Xavier Arnau/Getty Images on page 388

Figure 1.1—Source: U.S. Department of Health and Human Services and U.S. Department of Agriculture, 2015, *Scientific report of the 2015 Dietary Guidelines Advisory Committee.* [Online]. Available: http://health.gov/dietaryguidelines/2015-scientific-report/ [July 26, 2016].

Figure 1.2—Data from U.S Department of Health and Human Services Office of Disease Prevention and Health Promotion, 2016, *How to use data 2020.* [Online]. Available: https://www.healthypeople.gov/2020/How-to-Use-DATA2020 [July 26, 2016].

Figure 1.3—Data from U.S Department of Health and Human Services Office of Disease Prevention and Health Promotion, 2016, *How to use data 2020.* [Online]. Available: https://www.healthypeople.gov/2020/How-to-Use-DATA2020 [July 26, 2016].

Figure 1.4—Republished with permission of National Sleep Foundation, based on image available at http://sleepfoundation.org/sites/default/files/STREPchanges_1.png [September 16, 2016]. Permission conveyed through Copyright Clearance Center, Inc.

Figure 2.1—Reprinted with permission from the PAR-Q+ Collaboration and the authors of the PAR-Q+ (Dr. Darren Warburton, Dr. Norman Gledhill, Dr. Veronica Jamnik, and Dr. Shannon Bredin).

Figure 2.2—Adapted, by permission, from American College of Sports Medicine, 2018, *ACSM's guidelines for exercise testing and prescription,* 10th ed. (Philadelphia: Lippincott, Williams & Wilkins).

Table 3.1—Adapted, by permission, from M.H. Williams, 2007, *Nutrition for health, fitness, & sport,* 8th ed. (New York: McGraw-Hill), 404.

Table 6.1—Data provided by The Cooper Institute. Physical Fitness Assessments and Norms for Adults and Law Enforcement (2013). Used with permission.

Table 6.2—Data provided by The Cooper Institute, 1994. Used with permission. Study population for the data set was predominantly white and college educated. A Universal DVR machine was used to measure the 1RM.

Table 6.3—Source: Physical Activity Training for Health (CSEP-PATH) Resource Manual, © 2013. Adapted with permission from the Canadian Society for Exercise Physiology.

Table 6.4—Adapted, by permission, from The Cooper Institute, 2017, *FitnessGram administration manual: The journey to MyHealthyZone,* 5th ed. (Champaign, IL: Human Kinetics), 86, 87.

Table 6.5—Adapted, by permission, from R.E. Rikli and C.J. Jones, 2013, *Senior fitness test manual,* 2nd ed. (Champaign, IL: Human Kinetics), 89, 90.

Table 7.1—Adapted, by permission, from R.E. Rikli and C.J. Jones, 2013, *Senior fitness test manual,* 2nd ed. (Champaign, IL: Human Kinetics), 89, 90.

Table 7.2—Adapted, by permission, from R.E. Rikli and C.J. Jones, 2013, *Senior fitness test manual,* 2nd ed. (Champaign, IL: Human Kinetics), 89, 90.

Table 8.1—Adapted from B.A. Springer, R. Marin, T. Cyhan, H. Roberts, and N.W. Gill, 2007, "Normative values for the unipedal stance test with eyes open and closed," *Journal of Geriatric Physical Therapy* 30(1): 8-15.

Table 8.2—Adapted from P.W. Duncan, D.K. Weiner, J. Chandler, and S. Studenski, 1990, "Functional reach: A new clinical measure of balance," *Journal of Gerontology* 45(6): M192-M197.

Figure 8.3—Adapted from H. Edgren, 1932, "An experiment in the testing of agility and progress in basketball," *Research Quarterly* 3(1): 159-171.

Figure 8.4—Adapted from K. Pauole, K. Madole, J. Garhammer, M. Lacourse, and R. Rozenek, 2000, "Reliability and validity of the T-test as a measure of agility, leg power, and leg speed in college-aged men and women," *Journal of Strength and Conditioning Research* 14(4): 443-450.

Table 8.3—Adapted from K. Pauole, K. Madole, J. Garhammer, M. Lacourse, and R. Rozenek, 2000, "Reliability and validity of the T-test as a measure of agility, leg power, and leg speed in college-aged men and women," *Journal of Strength and Conditioning Research* 14(4): 443-450.

Table 8.4—Adapted, by permission, from R.E. Rikli and C.J. Jones, 2013, *Senior fitness test manual,* 2nd ed. (Champaign, IL: Human Kinetics), 89, 90.

Figure 9.1(a-b)—Developed by the National Center for Health Statistics in collaboration with the National Center for Chronic Disease Prevention and Health Promotion, 2000. Available: http://www.cdc.gov/healthyweight/assessing/bmi/childrens_bmi/about_childrens_bmi.html [August 9, 2016].

Table 9.1—Reprinted with permission, from S.G. Gidding et al., 2005, "Dietary recommendations for children and adolescents: A guide for practitioners," *Circulation* 112(13): 2061-2075. © American Heart Association, Inc.

Table 9.2—Data from USDA Center for Nutrition Policy and Promotion.

Table 9.3—Adapted from U.S. Department of Health and Human Services, 2008, *2008 physical activity guidelines for Americans.* [Online]. Available: www.health.gov/paguidelines [August 10, 2016].

Figure 9.2—© Human Kinetics

Table 9.4—Adapted from U.S. Department of Health and Human Services, 2008, *2008 physical activity guidelines for Americans.* [Online]. Available: www.health.gov/paguidelines [August 10, 2016].

Figure 9.4—Reprinted from *Journal of Pediatrics* 146(6), W.B. Strong, R.M. Malina, C.J.R. Blimkie, et al., "Evidence based physical activity for school-age youth," 732-737, Copyright 2005, with permission from Elsevier.

Figure 10.1—Source: U.S. Department of Health and Human Services Office of Disease Prevention and Health Promotion, n.d., Healthy people 2020. [Online]. Available: https://www.healthypeople.gov/2020/How-to-Use-DATA2020 [September 2, 2015].

Table 10.1—Sources: U.S. Department of Health and Human Services, National Institutes of Health, Office of Dietary Supplement, n.d., Vitamin and mineral supplement fact sheets. [Online]. Available: https://ods.od.nih.gov/factsheets/list-VitaminsMinerals/ [October 29, 2015]; and U.S. Department of Health and Human Services, Office of Disease Prevention and Health Promotion, n.d., Dietary guidelines. [Online]. Available: http://health.gov/dietaryguidelines/ [November 4, 2015].

Table 10.2—Source: U.S. Department of Health and Human Services and U.S. Department of Agriculture. 2015-2020 Dietary Guidelines for Americans. 8th Edition. December 2015. Available at http://health.gov/

dietaryguidelines/2015/guidelines/chapter-1/a-closer-look-inside-healthy-eating-patterns/#table-1-1 [August 10, 2016].

Table 12.1—Source: American Heart Association, n.d., Understand your risk of heart attack. [Online]. Available: http://www.heart.org/HEARTORG/Conditions/HeartAttack/UnderstandYourRiskstoPreventaHeartAttack/Understand-Your-Risks-to-Prevent-a-Heart-Attack_UCM_002040_Article.jsp# [November 15, 2015].

Table 12.2—Source: U.S. Department of Health and Human Services, National Heart, Lung, and Blood Institute, 2005, *Your guide to lowering your cholesterol with TLC.* [Online]. Available: https://www.nhlbi.nih.gov/files/docs/public/heart/chol_tlc.pdf [August 10, 2016].

Table 12.3—Source: U.S. Department of Health and Human Services, National Heart, Lung, and Blood Institute, n.d., Following the DASH eating plan. [Online]. Available: https://www.nhlbi.nih.gov/health/health-topics/topics/dash/followdash [August 10, 2016].

Figure 13.1—© Human Kinetics

Table 13.2—Adapted, by permission, from American College of Sports Medicine, 2018, *ACSM's guidelines for exercise testing and prescription,* 10th ed. (Philadelphia: Lippincott Williams & Wilkins.

Table 13.3—Adapted, by permission, from American College of Sports Medicine, 2018, *ACSM's guidelines for exercise testing and prescription,* 10th ed. (Philadelphia: Lippincott Williams & Wilkins.

Figure 15.1—Source: National Institutes of Health and Human Services, National Institute on Aging, n.d., Alzheimer's Disease fact sheet. [Online]. Available: https://www.nia.nih.gov/alzheimers/publication/alzheimers-disease-fact-sheet#changes [August 10, 2016].

Table 15.2—Adapted from M.C. Morris, C.C. Tangney, Y. Wang, F.M. Sacks, D.A. Bennett, and N.T. Aggarwal, 2015, "MIND diet associated with reduced incidence of Alzheimer's disease," *Alzheimer's & Dementia* 11(3): 1007-1014.

Table 16.1—Adapted from Institute of Medicine, 2011, *Dietary reference intakes for calcium and vitamin D* (Washington, DC: National Academies), 349.

Table 16.2—Source: National Osteoporosis Foundation, n.d., A guide to calcium-rich foods. [Online]. Available: https://www.nof.org/patients/treatment/calciumvitamin-d/ [September 16, 2016].

Table 16.3—Data from National Institutes of Health Office of Dietary Supplement, n.d., Vitamin D fact sheet for professionals. [Online.] Available: https://ods.od.nih.gov/factsheets/VitaminD-HealthProfessional/ [September 2, 2016].

Table 16.4—Adapted from Institute of Medicine, 2005, *Dietary reference intakes for energy, carbohydrate, fiber, fat, fatty acids, cholesterol, protein, and amino acids* (Washington, DC: National Academies), 621-649.

Table 16.5—Adapted, by permission, from American College of Sports Medicine, 2018, *ACSM's guidelines for exercise testing and prescription,* 10th ed. (Philadelphia: Lippincott Williams & Wilkins.

Figure 18.1—Adapted from U.S. Department of Health and Human Services, National Heart, Lung, and Blood Institute, 1998, *Clinical guidelines on the identification, evaluation, and treatment of overweight and obesity in adults: The evidence report.* [Online]. Available: http://www.nhlbi.nih.gov/health/educational/lose_wt/BMI/bmi_tbl.pdf

[September 22, 2016].

Table 18.2—Source: U.S. Department of Health and Human Services and U.S. Department of Agriculture. 2015-2020 Dietary Guidelines for Americans. 8th Edition. December 2015. Available at http://health.gov/dietaryguidelines/2015/guidelines/.

Table 19.1—From Institute of Medicine and National Research Council of the National Academies, Weight gain during pregnancy: Reexaminining the guidelines. Adapted with permission from the National Academies Press, Copyright 2009, National Academy of Sciences.

Table 19.2—Reprinted with permission from Physical activity and exercise during pregnancy and the postpartum period. Committee Opinion No. 650. American College of Obstetricians and Gynecologists. Obstet Gynecol 2015; 126: e135–e142.

Table 19.3—Adapted, by permission, from J.M. Pivarnik and L. Mudd, 2009, "Oh baby! Exercise during pregnancy and the postpartum period," *ACSM's Health & Fitness Journal* 13(3): 8-13.

Part I

Fit, Active, and Healthy

Although many aspects of life may feel out of one's control, *you* have choices each day that can affect your fitness and health. Physical activity and nutrition are two areas that have a major impact on many aspects of your life in regard to both disease risk and daily function. Chapters 1 to 4 will help you to place scientifically-based recommendations into the context of your life so you can tackle the challenge of establishing healthy habits for the long term.

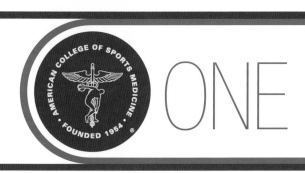

ONE

Making Healthy Lifestyle Choices: Physical Activity and Nutrition

What you do really does matter when it comes to your health. Your level of physical activity along with dietary choices affects day-to-day function as well as your risk of a number of diseases, including heart disease and some cancers. Healthy lifestyle choices are made within the context of individual and biological factors, as well as your home, work, and community environments (to help visualize this, see figure 1.1). You are an individual and, as such, need an individualized plan of action to achieve your health and fitness goals.

Rather than viewing healthy choices as distinct, unrelated activities, consider how various influences in your life interact to promote, or challenge, your efforts to make healthy choices. As you opened this book and started to peruse the pages, you have already taken the first step toward improving your health and wellness. In the upcoming pages, you will find research-based recommendations for exercise and dietary choices, with chapters on many specific topics written by experts in their fields. The value of these recommendations can be realized only when placed within the context of *your* life and *your* experiences. Armed with this perspective, you can develop your action plan to begin, or improve, your wellness journey. Time to jump on board!

You: Living Well

How do you define wellness? Your definition will reflect your personal experiences and perspectives. One way to consider the concept of wellness centers on engaging in activities in order to avoid negative consequences—for example, exercising in order to be free of disease and debilitating conditions, or substituting water for sweetened beverages to keep from gaining weight. To take a more positive viewpoint, contemporary approaches to wellness focus on balancing the many aspects, or dimensions, of life to promote health (8). Examples include exercising in order to develop a level of fitness that allows for full participation in recreational activities you enjoy, or consuming

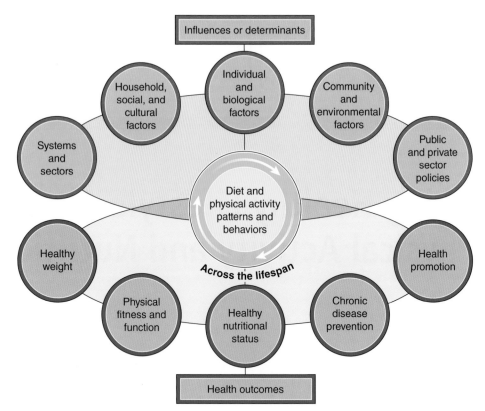

FIGURE 1.1   Diet and physical activity, health promotion, and disease prevention across the lifespan.

Source: U.S. Department of Health and Human Services and U.S. Department of Agriculture, 2015.

a balanced diet in order to provide your body with needed nutrients for optimal function. Outcomes may be similar, but the mindset is one of pursuing health rather than avoiding illness.

Wellness reflects physical, emotional, social, intellectual, spiritual, and occupational aspects (11). Wellness exists across a continuum between the presence and the absence of each dimension or aspect of life. Table 1.1 provides a brief definition and a pair of terms reflecting the presence or absence of each wellness dimension. Take a moment to consider where you fall on the continuum between two sample indicators listed for each dimension. Wellness isn't a static or all-or-none situation but rather is dynamic and changing. At any time, you may find some dimensions to be more present than others in your life. By adopting healthy behaviors, you can have greater balance in each dimension and therefore a greater sense of well-being and health.

Wellness touches all aspects of life, and fully discussing all areas is beyond the scope of this book. The focus of this book is physical wellness, and the following sections introduce the benefits of physical activity and a healthy diet. In addition, insights into two areas that can affect physical wellness—sleep and stress management—are discussed.

TABLE 1.1   **Dimensions of Wellness Indicators**

Dimension	Description	Indicator	
		Absent ....Present	
Physical	Ability to carry out daily activities with vigor and relative ease	Unfit..Fit	
Emotional	Ability to understand feelings, accept limitations, and achieve stability	Miserable............................Content	
Social	Ability to relate well to others within and outside the family unit	Disengaged................... Connected	
Intellectual	Ability to learn and use information for personal development	Mindless .... Aware	
Spiritual	Ability to find meaning and purpose in life and circumstances	Lost .... Secure	
Occupational	Ability to find personal satisfaction and enrichment through work	Frustrated .... Fulfilled	

Promoting Health and Wellness

Seeking better health involves many daily decisions and actions. This section explores the benefits of physical activity and exercise as well as dietary choices. In addition, taking steps to ensure adequate sleep and manage stress are integral to your pursuit of health and wellness.

Physical Activity and Exercise

Physical activity recommendations are not new, although the message has been clarified in recent years. In 1996, the U.S. Surgeon General's Report on Physical Activity and Health was described as "a passport to good health for all Americans," and the goal was to weave physical activity into the fabric of daily life as highlighted by these take-home points of the report (27):

- Americans can substantially improve their health and quality of life by including moderate amounts of physical activity in their daily lives.
- For those who are already achieving regular moderate physical activity, additional benefits may be gained by further increases in activity levels.
- Health benefits from physical activity are achievable for most Americans.

Armed with increased awareness of the value of physical activity provided by the Surgeon General's report, the U.S. Department of Health and Human Services provided clear recommendations on physical activity in its *Physical Activity Guidelines for Americans* (25). The *Physical Activity Guidelines for Americans* is based on hundreds of research studies conducted to examine the effects of physical activity on health. Following are some of the major findings:

- Regular physical activity reduces the risk of many unwanted health outcomes and diseases.

■ Q&A

What are current activity levels in the United States?

Although the Surgeon General's report gave high-level attention to the importance of physical activity, it did not ultimately spark the increase in physical activity desired and needed. Figure 1.2 shows the percentage of adults who engage in aerobic and muscular activity and also the percentage who are not active during leisure time (26). In a perfect scenario, 100 percent of people would exercise (aerobically and with resistance training), and no one would remain inactive during leisure time. The most active age group is the youngest; unfortunately, activity decreases and inactivity increases with age. Currently, the percentages are far from ideal. Now is the time for everyone to increase physical activity and find enjoyable ways to be more active.

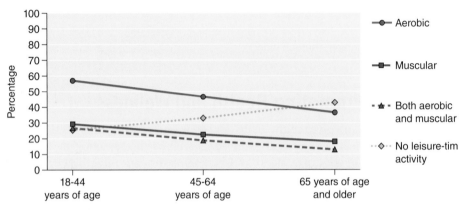

FIGURE 1.2   Percentages of Americans who engage in moderate aerobic activity and resistance training and those who are inactive in their leisure time.

Data from U.S. Department of Health and Human Services Office of Disease Prevention and Health Promotion, 2016.

- Some physical activity is better than none. The greatest health risk comes from being totally sedentary. Getting up and moving is important to start reducing disease risk and claiming benefits. Some health benefits have been identified with as little as 60 minutes of activity a week.

- A target of 150 minutes per week of moderate-intensity activity provides significant health benefits (additional benefits accrue to those who do more). An example of moderate-intensity activity is brisk walking.

- If you are already active, additional benefits are possible for most health outcomes if you increase the amount of physical activity by exercising at a higher intensity, more often, or for a longer period of time.

- When one considers risks versus benefits, the benefits of physical activity outweigh possible adverse outcomes.

- Regular exercise, week after week and year after year, is the goal. Maintaining such a program can produce both short-term and long-term benefits. Starting early in life and continuing throughout the lifespan is recommended.

Current recommendations from the American College of Sports Medicine (ACSM) continue to support the value of a comprehensive exercise program (1, 10). The upcoming chapters reflect these research-based guidelines, providing more detail on the components of a balanced exercise program and the role that activity and nutrition play in promoting health and fitness throughout the lifespan, as well as when people are faced with special health conditions.

Both physical activity and exercise are valuable. Although similar in some ways, there is a subtle difference between these two terms (1). "Physical activity" is the appropriate wording to use to refer to movement of the body that takes effort and requires energy above that required at rest. Day-to-day tasks such as light gardening, household chores, and taking the stairs at work are examples of baseline physical activity. Including activities like these in your daily routine is helpful, but adding exercise to your schedule provides additional health and fitness benefits. Exercise is a specific, planned type of physical activity that is done in a structured manner to promote physical fitness. Going for a brisk walk with the purpose of increasing your aerobic fitness or lifting weights to improve muscular fitness are both physical activity options that fall under the category of exercise. Thus physical activity is a broader, umbrella term, and exercise is one category of physical activity (i.e., all exercise is physical activity but not all physical activity is exercise). Over the past few years, the value of both physical activity (see Sit Less, Move More) and exercise has been supported. The focus of this book is exercise, but realize that exercise is a type of physical activity and that the terms are often used interchangeably.

Sit Less, Move More

Reflect on the amount of time you spend sitting over the course of the waking hours of the day: sitting while commuting, when working at the computer, during television watching, and at other times throughout the day. One study reported the following averages for nonsleeping activity levels (19):

- Moderate to vigorous physical activity = 0.3 hours
- Light physical activity = 4.1 hours
- Sedentary = 10.2 hours

These averages display a high amount of time spent each day in inactivity, with little time spent being physically active at moderate or vigorous levels.

Research supports the recommendation to sit less as a means to promote health. All-cause death rate is higher for those who sit more, and that association was found regardless of how active a person was otherwise (20). Sitting time has been associated with higher risk for heart- and metabolic-related issues such as increased waist circumference, poorer insulin resistance (how the body handles glucose), and changes in cholesterol (sitting is detrimental to "good" cholesterol levels) (23). Thus, finding ways to infuse more activity into the day appears to be key. Here are some examples:

- Stand or walk while talking on the phone.
- Get up and move during commercials when watching TV.
- Include some movement time every half hour when working on the computer or doing desk activities.
- Go for a short walk after meals.

Keep looking for additional ways to infuse activity into your day!

Being active is one of the most important habits people of all ages can develop to improve their health (1, 25). Why are physical activity and exercise so important to your well-being? Children who are active are more likely to be at a healthy body weight, perform better in school, and have higher self-esteem (22). They are also less likely to develop risk factors for heart disease, including obesity (25). Adults who exercise are better able to handle stress and avoid depression, perform daily tasks without physical limitation, and maintain a healthy body weight; they also lower their risk of developing a number of diseases (10, 25). Exercise continues to be important for older adults by ensuring quality of life and independence; regular exercise boosts immunity, combats bone loss, improves movement and balance, aids in psychological well-being, and lowers the risk of disease (9). Physical activity and nutrition information for children and adolescents is found in chapter 9, for adults in chapter 10, and for older adults in chapter 11.

Although disabilities may affect one's ability to be physically active, research supports the health benefits for avoiding inactivity and becoming as regularly active as possible within one's ability. An appropriate physical activity level can be determined in consultation with a health care provider (25). Similarly, people with chronic medical conditions should consult with their health care providers regarding the appropriate types and amounts of activity (25). Chronic medical conditions encompass a wide range of situations, including arthritis, type 2 diabetes, and cancer. Within the limitations of their ability, adults with chronic medical conditions can obtain health benefits from regular physical activity (25). Chapters 12 to 17 include nutrition and physical activity recommendations unique to a number of chronic conditions, including heart disease, high blood pressure, high cholesterol, diabetes, cancer, Alzheimer's disease, osteoporosis, and arthritis. In addition, the value of regular physical activity and healthy dietary choices is reviewed for weight management (chapter 18), pregnancy and postpartum (chapter 19), and depression (chapter 20).

The benefits of a regular exercise program extend into many areas of life. Improvements in body function as a result of exercise are well documented and are highlighted in this chapter. In addition to physiological benefits, psychological and mental health benefits can also be realized. Exercise appears to provide relief from symptoms of depression and anxiety; in addition, exercise enhances well-being and quality of life and is associated with a lower risk of dementia (10). Exercise also has the potential to enhance emotional well-being and improve mood (21). Researchers continue to explore why exercise promotes mental well-being. Potential reasons include offering a distraction, increasing self-confidence, providing physical relaxation, and promoting a positive body image (13).

Stated simply, exercise is the best prescription! No other "product" can provide so many positive changes with so few side effects. To underscore this, take a moment to review the impressive summary list of health benefits related to physical activity, for all age groups, in table 1.2. The scientists working with the U.S. Department of Health and Human Services rated available evidence as strong, moderate, or weak based on the type, number, and quality of the research studies (25). Only the health benefits with at least moderate evidence are included in this table.

As a reader of this book, you can claim these benefits for yourself. Be encouraged! Regardless of your current level of physical activity, the information provided in the upcoming chapters will help you create a realistic, workable exercise plan that has the potential to change your life for the better. Fitness is multifaceted, including health-

TABLE 1.2   Health Benefits Associated With Regular Physical Activity

Children and adolescents (ages 6 to 17)	
Strong evidence*	• Improved cardiorespiratory and muscular fitness • Improved bone health • Improved cardiovascular and metabolic health biomarkers • Favorable body composition
Moderate evidence*	• Reduced symptoms of depression
Adults and older adults (ages 18 and older)	
Strong evidence*	• Lower risk of early death • Lower risk of coronary heart disease • Lower risk of stroke • Lower risk of high blood pressure • Lower risk of adverse blood lipid profile • Lower risk of type 2 diabetes • Lower risk of metabolic syndrome • Lower risk of colon cancer • Lower risk of breast cancer • Prevention of weight gain • Weight loss, particularly when combined with reduced calorie intake • Improved cardiorespiratory and muscular fitness • Prevention of falls • Reduced depression • Better cognitive functioning (for older adults)
Moderate to strong evidence*	• Better functional health (for older adults) • Reduced abdominal obesity
Moderate evidence*	• Lower risk of hip fracture • Lower risk of lung cancer • Lower risk of endometrial cancer • Weight maintenance after weight loss • Increased bone density • Improved sleep quality

*The Advisory Committee (of the 2008 *Physical Activity Guidelines*) rated the evidence of health benefits of physical activity as strong, moderate, or weak based on an extensive review of the scientific literature including the type, number, and quality of studies available as well as the consistency of findings across the various studies.

related and skill-related components. Health-related components include aerobic fitness, muscular fitness, flexibility, and body composition; skill-related components include agility, coordination, balance, reaction time, power, and speed (1).

Although skill-related components of fitness are clearly important in sport and athletic competitions, they are also involved directly or indirectly in your day-to-day activities. Consider your ability to navigate around children's (or pets') toys scattered on the floor while carrying a full basket of laundry. You need to be able to physically handle the weight of the basket while maintaining a stable and upright body position. Within this book, individual chapters are dedicated to aerobic fitness, muscular fitness, flexibility, and neuromotor exercise training. This latter category encompasses many of the aspects of skill-related fitness. Each component contributes to ensuring that your body is operating at its optimal level. This influences your ability to engage in exercise and also in activities of daily living. The following sections offer insights on specific health benefits related to given components of fitness.

Aerobic Fitness

The word "aerobic" means "with oxygen." Your heart, lungs, and blood vessels work together to supply your muscles with needed oxygen during aerobic, or cardiorespiratory endurance, exercise. Examples of aerobic exercises are walking, jogging, running, cycling, swimming, dancing, hiking, and sports such as tennis and basketball.

Regular activity is associated with lowering risk factors related to heart disease such as high blood pressure and unhealthy cholesterol levels (10). If you are already somewhat active, you can further reduce your risk by engaging in additional physical activity. Cardiovascular health, including heart disease, high blood pressure, and high cholesterol, is discussed in more depth in chapter 12, and weight management is discussed in chapter 18. Aerobic activity also reduces the risk of type 2 diabetes (10). Progression from prediabetes (elevated blood glucose levels that increase the risk of developing diabetes in the future) to diabetes can be delayed or even prevented by losing weight and increasing physical activity (2). Lifestyle modifications can have a definite impact. In addition, physical activity can also help control blood glucose levels in people diagnosed with either type 1 or type 2 diabetes (see chapter 13 for details). Chapter 5 explains more fully the recommendations on aerobic activity as well as how you can progress over time.

Muscular Fitness

Muscular fitness refers to how your muscles contract to allow you to lift, pull, push, and hold objects. Muscular fitness can be improved with resistance training. As with aerobic fitness, many exercise options are available, including lifting weights, using resistance bands or cords, and performing body weight exercises such as push-ups and curl-ups. The key is to find activities that you enjoy and that are available to you. Chapter 6 provides details on various types and modes of activity that can help strengthen your muscles, as well as specific exercises and how-to photos to help you get started or improve your current resistance training program.

When you consider muscular fitness, the first picture in your mind might be a competitive athlete with large muscles. Although increases in muscle size are possible

■ Q&A

Why is it important to engage in aerobic exercise?

When you exercise so that your heart beats faster and you breathe at a quicker rate, you are providing a positive type of stress on your cardiorespiratory system as well as your entire body. This stress, or overload, is needed in order to improve fitness and health. An inactive lifestyle does not provide this positive stress and therefore leads to inactivity-related diseases such as heart disease. A sedentary lifestyle and obesity have been described as "parallel, interrelated epidemics in the United States" with reference to their contribution to the risk of heart disease (14). It is vital to find ways to fit physical activity into your daily life.

What typically happens to muscle mass over the course of adulthood?

Adults have a real need to maintain resistance training because typically, over the course of adulthood, the amount of muscle decreases while the amount of body fat increases (9). Declines in muscle mass begin around age 40, and the decline accelerates after around age 65 to 70 (9).

with resistance training, for most people a more relevant reason to include resistance training is to improve muscle function in order to handle activities of daily living with less stress. For example, sufficient muscular fitness will allow you to complete yard-work with less relative effort or climb stairs more easily. Of course, improved muscular fitness will also make recreational sport and athletic endeavors more enjoyable and give you a competitive edge.

Muscular fitness is important for everyone throughout the lifespan. Children benefit from activities that strengthen muscles such as climbing and jumping as well as calisthenics (e.g., jumping jacks, push-ups, or other activities in which the body is moved without needing any equipment) and more organized resistance training (25). For adults, resistance training improves quality of life and limits the muscle losses typically seen with aging.

In addition to promoting muscular strength, regular resistance training provides other health benefits, including improving body composition and blood pressure (10). Benefits of resistance training related to preventing or managing diabetes include improving glucose levels and the body's sensitivity to insulin (10).

Another aspect of your health that benefits from resistance training is bone strength (1, 9). As muscles contract to lift, push, or pull a heavy object, a stress is placed on the bone by way of connections between muscles and bones called tendons. When a bone is exposed to this force, it responds by increasing its mass. This makes bones stronger over time. Bone health is outlined in more detail in chapter 16.

Not to be ignored is the way resistance training can make you look and feel. Firm, toned muscles can inspire confidence. Stronger muscles can give you a real boost as you accomplish daily activities with greater ease and improve in competitive sport as well. For all these reasons, resistance training is an important part of your weekly activity plan.

Flexibility

Flexibility refers to the ability to move a joint through a full range of motion. Whether you are focusing on your golf swing or more practical aspects of daily life such as reaching for a high shelf in your closet, maintaining flexibility is important. Loss of flexibility as a result of injury, disuse, or aging can limit your ability to carry out daily activities. Flexibility can be maintained or even improved through a comprehensive stretching program (1). Chapter 7 outlines stretches for all the muscle groups in the body and discusses the benefits of including activities focused on improving range of motion.

Conditions such as arthritis and joint pain can result in having difficulty moving the joints through their normal range of motion. Although activity is beneficial in the treatment of arthritis, 38 percent of people with arthritis report no leisure-time activity (compared with about 27 percent of people without arthritis) (7). Full details on flexibility as well as muscular and cardiorespiratory exercises for people with arthritis and joint pain are provided in chapter 17.

Neuromotor Exercise

Neuromotor exercise training, also referred to as functional fitness training, includes activities that improve balance, coordination, gait, agility, and one's perception of physical location within space (i.e., proprioception) (1). Many activities include combinations of neuromotor, resistance, and flexibility, for example, yoga, tai ji (tai chi), and qigong (1).

Researchers have noted improvements in balance, agility, and muscular strength for older adults who engage in functional fitness training. In addition, older adults lower their risk of falling (1). Although most of the research studies have focused on older adults, younger adults likely can reap benefits as well. Regardless of your age, reflect on activities that occur over the normal course of the day when improved balance, coordination, or agility would be valuable—for example, sidestepping around a puddle on a busy sidewalk or juggling full bags of groceries when walking up stairs. Then, consider how all the facets of neuromotor exercise training can affect enjoyment in recreational activities or athletic endeavors. Examples are hiking with a loaded backpack, balancing on a surf- or skateboard, and playing basketball or soccer. It actually becomes hard to think of activities that are not affected by functional fitness! Chapter 8 unpacks this often overlooked aspect of fitness.

Body Composition

Body composition refers to the makeup of your body. The body is made up of lean tissue (including muscle) and fat tissue. Typically, the focus of body composition is the relative amounts of muscle versus fat. Although the bathroom scale can help you track your overall body weight, this measurement is general and does not reveal the amount of fat compared to muscle. Excessive amounts of body fat are related to poor health outcomes, and this is especially true for fat around the abdominal area (1). Chapter 18 discusses body weight management.

Whether you are looking to begin an exercise program or optimize the time you are already investing in exercise, the upcoming chapters show you what to include as well as how to track your progress. This book will help you balance the various fitness components so you can maximize the benefits from your personal exercise program.

Diet and Nutrition

Choices related to what to eat and drink are made over and over throughout the day. Determining what items to select can be a real challenge, even with the best of intentions. Unfortunately, many people associate good nutrition with a restrictive diet filled with unappealing options. This is unfortunate, as a healthy diet is one full of nutritious *and* delicious foods. Note that that the word "diet" in this context refers to what you eat, not a particular weight loss plan.

To help provide a foundation for nutritional choices, every five years the *Dietary Guidelines for Americans* is updated (28). Most recently, the 2015 Dietary Guidelines

■ Q&A ■

Considering a typical eating pattern in the United States, what are areas of concern?

In comparison with recommendations, about 75 percent of Americans do not consume adequate vegetables, fruits, dairy, and oils. In contrast, added sugars, saturated fats, and sodium are overconsumed. Overall calorie intake is another area of concern, as many eating patterns include too many calories (28). Consuming more calories than needed results in weight gain over time.

Advisory Committee reviewed the most current research and evidence in order to provide updates to the 2010 Guidelines. This review was guided by two realities (29). First, the committee noted that about two-thirds of American adults are overweight or obese and about half have at least one preventable chronic disease (see figure 1.3 for percentages of Americans who are obese [26], realizing that prevalence is even higher when one considers overweight in addition to obesity). Contributing factors include poor dietary patterns, calorie overconsumption, and physical inactivity. Second, the committee acknowledged the personal, social, organizational, and environmental context in which lifestyle choices—nutrition and physical activity—are made. Each person has a unique frame of reference, and, within that context, can develop optimal dietary patterns along with adequate physical activity to promote health (28).

Dietary patterns are linked to potential risk of obesity and chronic diseases, such as heart disease, high blood pressure, diabetes, and some cancers (29). Researchers are exploring potential relationships between dietary patterns and neurocognitive disorders and congenital anomalies (29). Thus, one's diet really does matter! The key question is, what does a healthy diet look like? A healthy eating pattern includes vegetables, fruits, grains (with at least half being whole grains), fat-free or low-fat dairy, and a variety of protein foods (e.g., seafood, lean meats and poultry, eggs, legumes, nuts, seeds, soy products) while limiting saturated and trans fats, added sugars, and sodium (28). Rather than dictating a single, stringent diet pattern, these strategies can be individualized to fit within one's health needs, dietary preferences, and cultural

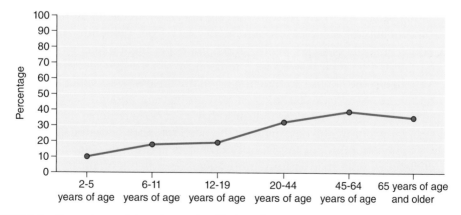

FIGURE 1.3   Percentage of Americans classified as obese.

Data from U.S. Department of Health and Human Services Office of Disease Prevention and Health Promotion, 2016.

traditions. The focus is on flexibility and combining foods in a variety of ways to promote healthy dietary patterns (29).

Understanding the various components of a healthy diet is helpful in developing nutritional patterns that meet your body's needs and promote optimal health. Chapter 3 provides an overview of the various nutrients and how each affects how your body functions.

Sleep and Stress Management

The previous sections have highlighted the myriad benefits that are possible when one embraces a physically active lifestyle and enjoys healthy food selections. In addition to these areas of physical wellness, sleep and stress influence health and, given the significant potential impact, are included here.

Influence of Sleep

If you struggle with getting a good night's sleep, you are not alone.

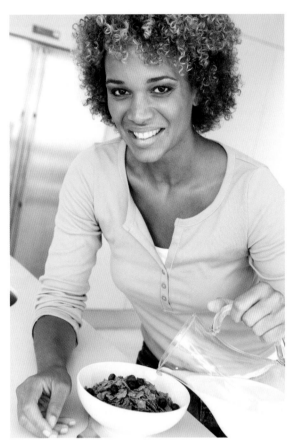

Good nutritional choices are part of physical wellness.

Chronic sleep loss or sleep disorders are estimated to affect up to 70 million people (15). Obtaining adequate sleep—in terms of both quantity and quality—contributes to how you feel and function. A restful night of sleep provides the energy and alertness necessary to handle daily challenges. In contrast, the lack of adequate sleep negatively affects productivity, relationships, and physical health.

Sleep is important for many reasons and significantly affects many dimensions of wellness and quality of life. Sleep requirements vary from person to person, but in general, adults typically need between 7 and 8 hours per night to feel well rested (15). For a helpful visual on typical sleep requirements across the age spectrum see figure 1.4 (18). Although some adults can function normally on less sleep, others may require significantly more. How can you know if you are getting enough sleep? Sleepiness during the day is a simple but clear indicator that your body requires more sleep. Significant sleepiness during the day suggests the need for more or better sleep, or both. You may also benefit from tracking your sleep habits and trends (18).

Lack of sleep is more than just an annoyance. Sleep is important for the body to function as intended; such functions include the following (15):

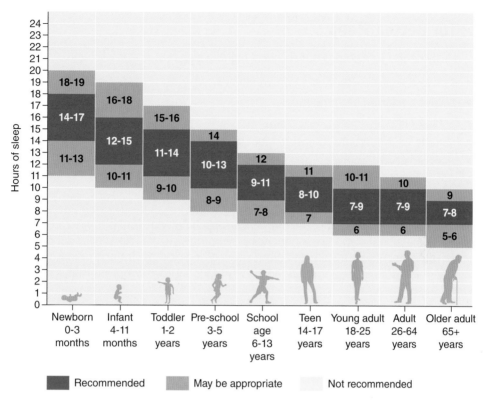

FIGURE 1.4 Sleep duration recommendations.
Republished with permission of National Sleep Foundation.

- Heart rate and blood pressure naturally fluctuate during sleep to promote cardiovascular health.
- Cells and tissues are repaired as growth hormone is released during deep sleep.
- Immune function is promoted with the creation of cytokines that target infections.
- Hormones related to appetite change (leptin, which suppresses appetite, increases while ghrelin, which stimulates appetite, decreases).

In addition, inadequate sleep can make daily tasks like learning, concentrating, and reacting more difficult (15).

Changing behavior to obtain the sleep you need requires making a conscious health choice. Implementing good sleep practices is key (see Tips for Better Sleep). One common recommendation to promote better sleep is exercise. The National Sleep Foundation has stated, simply, "Exercise is good for sleep" (17). Although some recommendations in the past have suggested that exercise near bedtime is detrimental, newer recommendations encourage healthy adults to exercise without any limitation related to time of day, other than ensuring that exercise time is not replacing time needed for sleep (18).

Tips for Better Sleep

Consider these tips to help promote a good night's sleep (18):

- Stick to a sleep schedule, even on weekends.
- Practice a relaxing bedtime ritual.
- Exercise daily.
- Evaluate your bedroom to ensure ideal temperature, sound, and light.
- Sleep on a comfortable mattress and pillows.
- Beware of hidden sleep stealers, like alcohol and caffeine.
- Turn off electronics before bed.

The National Sleep Foundation recommends consulting with your primary care physician or a sleep professional if you are experiencing symptoms such as sleepiness during the day or when you expect to be awake and alert; snoring; leg cramps or tingling; gasping or difficulty breathing during sleep; prolonged insomnia; or another symptom that is preventing you from sleeping well.

Influence of Stress

"I'm stressed out." Likely this statement has crossed your lips or you have heard another person utter these words. The reality is that everyone experiences stress at various points in life. So, what is stress? At the most basic level, stress is defined as the brain's response to demands (16). Not all stress is the same. Different types of stress have been identified, including acute stress, episodic acute stress, and chronic stress.

Acute stress stems from demands and pressures that result from recent events or even events anticipated in the near future (5). These stressors are short-term—for example, losing your car keys or handling a customer complaint at work. Common symptoms include irritability, anxiety, tension headache, muscular tensions, digestive system problems, and other physiological responses such as higher blood pressure, faster heart rate, sweating, and even shortness of breath or chest pain.

Episodic acute stress occurs when acute stress is experienced frequently (5). Picture the person who has taken on too many tasks, who is always late and rushing, who seems to move from one crisis directly into another, or who suffers from ongoing worry. Symptoms of episodic acute stress include persistent tension headaches, migraines, high blood pressure, chest pain, and heart disease.

Chronic stress is ongoing, grinding stress that is unrelenting for long periods of time (5). The health conditions that result from untreated chronic stress include anxiety, insomnia, muscle pain, high blood pressure, and a weakened immune system (6). In addition, stress can contribute to the development of heart disease, depression, and obesity (6).

Short-term stress reflects those situations in which you respond and then return back to a baseline state of relaxation. Long-term stress can be more troubling as the body has to continue in an alert state. This has been described as taking a "sprint" mechanism intended to occur for a brief time (see Fight-or-Flight Response) and forcing the body into a "marathon" or ongoing situation with resulting breakdown and system failure over time (12). Stress can affect almost every body system. Examples are muscular

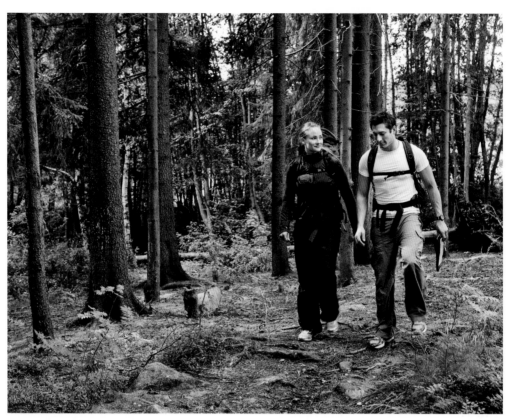

Exercising with a friend can be a great way to manage stress.

tension for the musculoskeletal system; diarrhea-constipation for the digestive system; elevated stress hormones and blood sugar levels for the endocrine system; and increased risk of high blood pressure, heart attack, or stroke for the cardiovascular system (3).

Chronic stress can bring feelings of being overloaded. Responses may be due to positive or negative changes, and can be real or perceived (16). Common sources of stress are money, work, the economy, family responsibilities, and personal health (4). Do any (or all) of these ring true? Symptoms of stress reported in a recent survey include feeling angry or irritated, feeling anxious or nervous, lacking motivation, feeling fatigued, being depressed or sad, or feeling overwhelmed (4). Can you picture yourself reacting in these ways?

Various approaches to dealing with stress have been proposed, including both prevention and management (12). Being prepared for life situations can be helpful in preventing stressors from having a negative impact. Of course, not all stressors can be avoided, so management of one's reaction is also important. One valuable tool used routinely to help handle stress is regular participation in exercise (24). The role of exercise in stress reduction is not yet clear, but active people appear to be able to buffer stress more effectively than sedentary people do. In addition, healthy diets facilitate a healthy state (see chapter 3 for current recommendations on healthy dietary patterns).

In addition to being active and eating well, other tools can be used to prevent or manage stress. As you consider some of the following tips, realize that no one tool works for all people, or even within all situations.

Fight-or-Flight Response

The fight-or-flight response is intended to be beneficial for survival when one is faced with a threat. The body gears up to act as needed, and in doing so, turns on some areas of the body while shutting down others that are not immediately needed. When confronted with an acute stress (e.g., being startled by a loud sound when walking on a darkened sidewalk), the body prepares to deal with the potential danger or to escape. The responses that prepare the body for action include these: the heart beats faster, blood pressure increases, breathing becomes heavy, pupils dilate, and muscles tense. At the same time the body increases the availability of glucose and fats to burn for fuel while shutting down areas not vital in the moment such as immune function, reproductive capacity, and digestion (12).

- *Plan your schedule.* Being aware of and in charge of your schedule provides an empowering feeling that helps to reduce the impact of stressful situations. Planning promotes effective time management.

- *Avoid procrastination.* Consider how stress can be prevented when a work-related project is completed in advance of a deadline compared with procrastination that brings on a hectic rush to beat the cutoff date.

- *Relax with deep breathing.* The process of consciously slowing your breathing rate as you increase the depth of each breath helps to counteract the fast and shallow breathing that is common when experiencing stress.

- *Limit alcohol consumption.* Although alcohol may reduce stress temporarily, relying on alcohol to cope with stress has the opposite effect and produces more bodily stress.

- *Talk to family and friends.* Discussing stressful events with others you trust can be beneficial both because it helps you "get it off your chest" and because you might receive helpful recommendations.

If faced with stress that cannot be managed with basic techniques, consider getting help from a psychologist or other licensed mental health professional (6).

Making healthy lifestyle choices can be a challenge, but developing healthy habits is well worth the effort. Although some benefits have a long-term focus, such as promoting heart health, others can be realized more immediately, such as stress reduction. Including regular physical activity along with healthy nutrition promotes physical wellness.

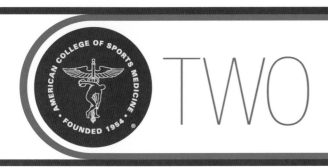

TWO

Embracing Physical Activity: A Complete Exercise Program

Getting started with an exercise program or finding ways to improve what you are already doing can seem like a daunting task. To simplify the process of developing a lifelong exercise habit, the *Complete Guide* proposes that you take two steps. The first is to examine your goals and consider how an exercise program can fit into your life (helpful pointers on goal setting and motivation are more fully explored in chapter 4). The second is to determine the specifics of what to include in your personal exercise program.

Rather than being an exact formula, an exercise prescription is more like an old family recipe handed down from generation to generation. Although instructions are given along with a list of ingredients, the actual cooking process gets interesting. One person might add more of a particular ingredient for a spicier dish, and someone else might use a substitution if short on an item. Exact measurements would ruin the cooking experience and would negate the opportunity to customize the dish. Individualizing the process personalizes the outcome. Similarly, your exercise program will be based on solid guidelines and a list of "ingredients," but then you will be presented with options to allow you to make the exercise program your own. You are unique in terms of your health status, your current level of activity, and your fitness goals. This chapter discusses some preliminary health screenings recommended before beginning, the basic guidelines and components of an exercise program (aerobic fitness, muscular fitness, flexibility, and functional [neuromotor] fitness), and some insights and considerations on personalizing that program.

Checking Your Status: Preparticipation Health Screenings

Physical activity provides many health and fitness benefits and is typically recommended for both prevention from and treatment for chronic diseases (e.g., heart disease, type 2 diabetes) (1). However, some may be hesitant to exercise for fear of injury or

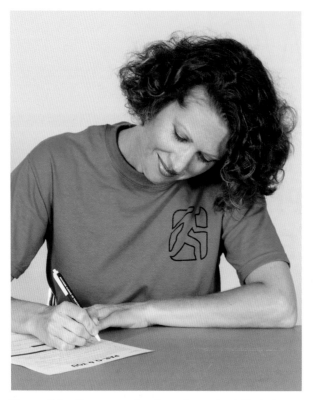

Preparticipation screening is an important first step in assessing your fitness.

even heart attack. The *Physical Activity Guidelines for Americans* suggests that although the risk of injury increases with one's total amount of physical activity, individuals who are more physically active may have fewer injuries from other causes (4). In addition, when doing the same activity, more fit individuals are less likely to be injured than those who are less fit. Cardiac events (e.g., heart attack) are rare, and the risk is greatest for those who suddenly engage in activity. This underscores the value of gradually progressing your exercise program (1). Regularly active individuals have a lower risk of cardiac events whether during exercise or at other times (4). Thus, the benefits outweigh the risks of adverse events for most people (4).

A key factor in maximizing safety during exercise is to consider your current level of activity as well as any health issues. A preparticipation screening is an important first step to maximize safety and to establish whether you are ready to start or advance your exercise program. The goals of screening are to determine if checking with your doctor is recommended before starting or progressing your program and—if you have a medical condition—if a medically supervised program or other intervention might be warranted (1).

Many self-screening tools are available. As an example, see the Physical Activity Readiness Questionnaire for Everyone in figure 2.1 (2). In addition, the American College of Sports Medicine has developed a step-by-step process designed to identify individuals who might be at a higher risk during or after exercise (1). Figure 2.2 reflects this screening process.

By answering a few questions, you can determine if checking with your health care provider is recommended or if you are ready to begin (or to continue) with your exercise program. The first question relates to your current level of physical activity. "Regular" exercise is defined as having performed planned, structured physical activity of at least 30 minutes at moderate intensity on at least three days each week for the past three months (i.e., both regular and established with your exercise program). The following two questions focus on current disease and then signs or symptoms of disease. The disease status items take account of cardiovascular disease, which includes cardiac (heart) disease, peripheral vascular disease, or cerebrovascular disease; metabolic disease, which includes type 1 and type 2 diabetes; and renal disease. Signs or symptoms reflect situations suggestive of disease (see footnote in figure 2.2 for signs and symptoms that should be considered).

PAR-Q+

The Physical Activity Readiness Questionnaire for Everyone

The health benefits of regular physical activity are clear; more people should engage in physical activity every day of the week. Participating in physical activity is very safe for MOST people. This questionnaire will tell you whether it is necessary for you to seek further advice from your doctor OR a qualified exercise professional before becoming more physically active.

GENERAL HEALTH QUESTIONS

Please read the 7 questions below carefully and answer each one honestly: check YES or NO.	YES	NO
1) Has your doctor ever said that you have a heart condition ☐ OR high blood pressure ☐?	☐	☐
2) Do you feel pain in your chest at rest, during your daily activities of living, **OR** when you do physical activity?	☐	☐
3) Do you lose balance because of dizziness **OR** have you lost consciousness in the last 12 months? Please answer **NO** if your dizziness was associated with over-breathing (including during vigorous exercise).	☐	☐
4) Have you ever been diagnosed with another chronic medical condition (other than heart disease or high blood pressure)? **PLEASE LIST CONDITION(S) HERE:** _____	☐	☐
5) Are you currently taking prescribed medications for a chronic medical condition? **PLEASE LIST CONDITION(S) AND MEDICATIONS HERE:** _____	☐	☐
6) Do you currently have (or have had within the past 12 months) a bone, joint, or soft tissue (muscle, ligament, or tendon) problem that could be made worse by becoming more physically active? Please answer **NO** if you had a problem in the past, but it *does not limit your current ability* to be physically active. **PLEASE LIST CONDITION(S) HERE:** _____	☐	☐
7) Has your doctor ever said that you should only do medically supervised physical activity?	☐	☐

✔ **If you answered NO to all of the questions above, you are cleared for physical activity.**
Go to Page 4 to sign the PARTICIPANT DECLARATION. You do not need to complete Pages 2 and 3.

- ▶ Start becoming much more physically active – start slowly and build up gradually.
- ▶ Follow International Physical Activity Guidelines for your age (www.who.int/dietphysicalactivity/en/).
- ▶ You may take part in a health and fitness appraisal.
- ▶ If you are over the age of 45 yr and **NOT** accustomed to regular vigorous to maximal effort exercise, consult a qualified exercise professional before engaging in this intensity of exercise.
- ▶ If you have any further questions, contact a qualified exercise professional.

⦿ **If you answered YES to one or more of the questions above, COMPLETE PAGES 2 AND 3.**

⚠ **Delay becoming more active if:**
- ✓ You have a temporary illness such as a cold or fever; it is best to wait until you feel better.
- ✓ You are pregnant - talk to your health care practitioner, your physician, a qualified exercise professional, and/or complete the ePARmed-X+ at **www.eparmedx.com** before becoming more physically active.
- ✓ Your health changes - answer the questions on Pages 2 and 3 of this document and/or talk to your doctor or a qualified exercise professional before continuing with any physical activity program.

✝OSHF
Ontario Society for Health and Fitness

Copyright 2016 PAR-Q+ Collaboration   1/4
01-01-2016

FIGURE 2.1   Physical Activity Readiness Questionnaire for Everyone.

Reprinted with permission from the PAR-Q+ Collaboration and the authors of the PAR-Q+ (Dr. Darren Warburton, Dr. Norman Gledhill, Dr. Veronica Jamnik, and Dr. Shannon Bredin).

> continued

PAR-Q+

FOLLOW-UP QUESTIONS ABOUT YOUR MEDICAL CONDITION(S)

1. Do you have Arthritis, Osteoporosis, or Back Problems?

If the above condition(s) is/are present, answer questions 1a-1c   If **NO** ☐ go to question 2

1a.	Do you have difficulty controlling your condition with medications or other physician-prescribed therapies? (Answer **NO** if you are not currently taking medications or other treatments)	YES☐ NO☐
1b.	Do you have joint problems causing pain, a recent fracture or fracture caused by osteoporosis or cancer, displaced vertebra (e.g., spondylolisthesis), and/or spondylolysis/pars defect (a crack in the bony ring on the back of the spinal column)?	YES☐ NO☐
1c.	Have you had steroid injections or taken steroid tablets regularly for more than 3 months?	YES☐ NO☐

2. Do you have Cancer of any kind?

If the above condition(s) is/are present, answer questions 2a-2b   If **NO** ☐ go to question 3

2a.	Does your cancer diagnosis include any of the following types: lung/bronchogenic, multiple myeloma (cancer of plasma cells), head, and neck?	YES☐ NO☐
2b.	Are you currently receiving cancer therapy (such as chemotherapy or radiotherapy)?	YES☐ NO☐

3. Do you have a Heart or Cardiovascular Condition? *This includes Coronary Artery Disease, Heart Failure, Diagnosed Abnormality of Heart Rhythm*

If the above condition(s) is/are present, answer questions 3a-3d   If **NO** ☐ go to question 4

3a.	Do you have difficulty controlling your condition with medications or other physician-prescribed therapies? (Answer **NO** if you are not currently taking medications or other treatments)	YES☐ NO☐
3b.	Do you have an irregular heart beat that requires medical management? (e.g., atrial fibrillation, premature ventricular contraction)	YES☐ NO☐
3c.	Do you have chronic heart failure?	YES☐ NO☐
3d.	Do you have diagnosed coronary artery (cardiovascular) disease and have not participated in regular physical activity in the last 2 months?	YES☐ NO☐

4. Do you have High Blood Pressure?

If the above condition(s) is/are present, answer questions 4a-4b   If **NO** ☐ go to question 5

4a.	Do you have difficulty controlling your condition with medications or other physician-prescribed therapies? (Answer **NO** if you are not currently taking medications or other treatments)	YES☐ NO☐
4b.	Do you have a resting blood pressure equal to or greater than 160/90 mmHg with or without medication? (Answer **YES** if you do not know your resting blood pressure)	YES☐ NO☐

5. Do you have any Metabolic Conditions? *This includes Type 1 Diabetes, Type 2 Diabetes, Pre-Diabetes*

If the above condition(s) is/are present, answer questions 5a-5e   If **NO** ☐ go to question 6

5a.	Do you often have difficulty controlling your blood sugar levels with foods, medications, or other physician-prescribed therapies?	YES☐ NO☐
5b.	Do you often suffer from signs and symptoms of low blood sugar (hypoglycemia) following exercise and/or during activities of daily living? Signs of hypoglycemia may include shakiness, nervousness, unusual irritability, abnormal sweating, dizziness or light-headedness, mental confusion, difficulty speaking, weakness, or sleepiness.	YES☐ NO☐
5c.	Do you have any signs or symptoms of diabetes complications such as heart or vascular disease and/or complications affecting your eyes, kidneys, **OR** the sensation in your toes and feet?	YES☐ NO☐
5d.	Do you have other metabolic conditions (such as current pregnancy-related diabetes, chronic kidney disease, or liver problems)?	YES☐ NO☐
5e.	Are you planning to engage in what for you is unusually high (or vigorous) intensity exercise in the near future?	YES☐ NO☐

FIGURE 2.1   *> continued*

PAR-Q+

6. **Do you have any Mental Health Problems or Learning Difficulties?** *This includes Alzheimer's, Dementia, Depression, Anxiety Disorder, Eating Disorder, Psychotic Disorder, Intellectual Disability, Down Syndrome*

If the above condition(s) is/are present, answer questions 6a-6b   If **NO** ☐ go to question 7

6a.	Do you have difficulty controlling your condition with medications or other physician-prescribed therapies? (Answer **NO** if you are not currently taking medications or other treatments)	YES☐ NO☐
6b.	Do you have Down Syndrome and back problems affecting nerves or muscles?	YES☐ NO☐

7. **Do you have a Respiratory Disease?** *This includes Chronic Obstructive Pulmonary Disease, Asthma, Pulmonary High Blood Pressure*

If the above condition(s) is/are present, answer questions 7a-7d   If **NO** ☐ go to question 8

7a.	Do you have difficulty controlling your condition with medications or other physician-prescribed therapies? (Answer **NO** if you are not currently taking medications or other treatments)	YES☐ NO☐
7b.	Has your doctor ever said your blood oxygen level is low at rest or during exercise and/or that you require supplemental oxygen therapy?	YES☐ NO☐
7c.	If asthmatic, do you currently have symptoms of chest tightness, wheezing, laboured breathing, consistent cough (more than 2 days/week), or have you used your rescue medication more than twice in the last week?	YES☐ NO☐
7d.	Has your doctor ever said you have high blood pressure in the blood vessels of your lungs?	YES☐ NO☐

8. **Do you have a Spinal Cord Injury?** *This includes Tetraplegia and Paraplegia*

If the above condition(s) is/are present, answer questions 8a-8c   If **NO** ☐ go to question 9

8a.	Do you have difficulty controlling your condition with medications or other physician-prescribed therapies? (Answer **NO** if you are not currently taking medications or other treatments)	YES☐ NO☐
8b.	Do you commonly exhibit low resting blood pressure significant enough to cause dizziness, light-headedness, and/or fainting?	YES☐ NO☐
8c.	Has your physician indicated that you exhibit sudden bouts of high blood pressure (known as Autonomic Dysreflexia)?	YES☐ NO☐

9. **Have you had a Stroke?** *This includes Transient Ischemic Attack (TIA) or Cerebrovascular Event*

If the above condition(s) is/are present, answer questions 9a-9c   If **NO** ☐ go to question 10

9a.	Do you have difficulty controlling your condition with medications or other physician-prescribed therapies? (Answer **NO** if you are not currently taking medications or other treatments)	YES☐ NO☐
9b.	Do you have any impairment in walking or mobility?	YES☐ NO☐
9c.	Have you experienced a stroke or impairment in nerves or muscles in the past 6 months?	YES☐ NO☐

10. **Do you have any other medical condition not listed above or do you have two or more medical conditions?**

If you have other medical conditions, answer questions 10a-10c   If **NO** ☐ read the Page 4 recommendations

10a.	Have you experienced a blackout, fainted, or lost consciousness as a result of a head injury within the last 12 months **OR** have you had a diagnosed concussion within the last 12 months?	YES☐ NO☐
10b.	Do you have a medical condition that is not listed (such as epilepsy, neurological conditions, kidney problems)?	YES☐ NO☐
10c.	Do you currently live with two or more medical conditions?	YES☐ NO☐

PLEASE LIST YOUR MEDICAL CONDITION(S) AND ANY RELATED MEDICATIONS HERE: _____

GO to Page 4 for recommendations about your current medical condition(s) and sign the PARTICIPANT DECLARATION.

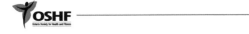

FIGURE 2.1   *> continued*

PAR-Q+

☑ **If you answered NO to all of the follow-up questions about your medical condition, you are ready to become more physically active - sign the PARTICIPANT DECLARATION below:**

▶ It is advised that you consult a qualified exercise professional to help you develop a safe and effective physical activity plan to meet your health needs.

▶ You are encouraged to start slowly and build up gradually - 20 to 60 minutes of low to moderate intensity exercise, 3-5 days per week including aerobic and muscle strengthening exercises.

▶ As you progress, you should aim to accumulate 150 minutes or more of moderate intensity physical activity per week.

▶ If you are over the age of 45 yr and **NOT** accustomed to regular vigorous to maximal effort exercise, consult a qualified exercise professional before engaging in this intensity of exercise.

⬤ **If you answered YES to one or more of the follow-up questions** about your medical condition:
You should seek further information before becoming more physically active or engaging in a fitness appraisal. You should complete the specially designed online screening and exercise recommendations program - the **ePARmed-X+ at www.eparmedx.com** and/or visit a qualified exercise professional to work through the ePARmed-X+ and for further information.

⚠ **Delay becoming more active if:**

✓ You have a temporary illness such as a cold or fever; it is best to wait until you feel better.

✓ You are pregnant - talk to your health care practitioner, your physician, a qualified exercise professional, and/or complete the ePARmed-X+ **at www.eparmedx.com** before becoming more physically active.

✓ Your health changes - talk to your doctor or qualified exercise professional before continuing with any physical activity program.

⬤ You are encouraged to photocopy the PAR-Q+. You must use the entire questionnaire and NO changes are permitted.
⬤ The authors, the PAR-Q+ Collaboration, partner organizations, and their agents assume no liability for persons who undertake physical activity and/or make use of the PAR-Q+ or ePARmed-X+. If in doubt after completing the questionnaire, consult your doctor prior to physical activity.

PARTICIPANT DECLARATION

⬤ All persons who have completed the PAR-Q+ please read and sign the declaration below.

⬤ If you are less than the legal age required for consent or require the assent of a care provider, your parent, guardian or care provider must also sign this form.

I, the undersigned, have read, understood to my full satisfaction and completed this questionnaire. I acknowledge that this physical activity clearance is valid for a maximum of 12 months from the date it is completed and becomes invalid if my condition changes. I also acknowledge that a Trustee (such as my employer, community/fitness centre, health care provider, or other designate) may retain a copy of this form for their records. In these instances, the Trustee will be required to adhere to local, national, and international guidelines regarding the storage of personal health information ensuring that the Trustee maintains the privacy of the information and does not misuse or wrongfully disclose such information.

NAME _____ DATE _____

SIGNATURE _____ WITNESS _____

SIGNATURE OF PARENT/GUARDIAN/CARE PROVIDER _____

───── **For more information, please contact** ─────
www.eparmedx.com
Email: eparmedx@gmail.com

Citation for PAR-Q+
Warburton DER, Jamnik VK, Bredin SSD, and Gledhill N on behalf of the PAR-Q+ Collaboration. The Physical Activity Readiness Questionnaire for Everyone (PAR-Q+) and Electronic Physical Activity Readiness Medical Examination (ePARmed-X+). Health & Fitness Journal of Canada 4(2):3-23, 2011.

Key References
1. Jamnik VK, Warburton DER, Makarski J, McKenzie DC, Shephard RJ, Stone J, and Gledhill N. Enhancing the effectiveness of clearance for physical activity participation; background and overall process. APNM 36(S1):S3-S13, 2011.
2. Warburton DER, Gledhill N, Jamnik VK, Bredin SSD, McKenzie DC, Stone J, Charlesworth S, and Shephard RJ. Evidence-based risk assessment and recommendations for physical activity clearance; Consensus Document. APNM 36(S1):S266-s298, 2011.

The PAR-Q+ was created using the evidence-based AGREE process (1) by the PAR-Q+ Collaboration chaired by Dr. Darren E. R. Warburton with Dr. Norman Gledhill, Dr. Veronica Jamnik, and Dr. Donald C. McKenzie (2). Production of this document has been made possible through financial contributions from the Public Health Agency of Canada and the BC Ministry of Health Services. The views expressed herein do not necessarily represent the views of the Public Health Agency of Canada or the BC Ministry of Health Services.

Copyright 2016 PAR-Q+ Collaboration   4/4
01-01-2016

FIGURE 2.1   *> continued*

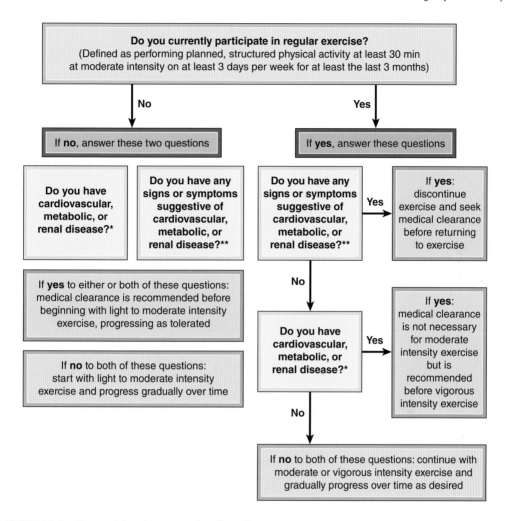

FIGURE 2.2   Preparticipation screening flowchart.

*The question on cardiovascular, metabolic, or renal disease includes cardiac, peripheral vascular, or cerebrovascular disease; type 1 and 2 diabetes; and renal diseases.

**The question on signs and symptoms includes concerns at rest or during activity and includes pain or discomfort in the chest, neck, jaw, arms, or other areas that may result from ischemia (impaired oxygen supply to the heart); shortness of breath at rest or with mild exertion; dizziness or syncope (fainting); orthopnea or paroxysmal nocturnal dyspnea (abnormally uncomfortable awareness of breathing when lying down that is relieved by sitting or standing); ankle edema (swelling); palpitations or tachycardia (rapid heart rate); intermittent claudication; known heart murmur; unusual fatigue or shortness of breath with usual activities.

Adapted by permission from American College of Sports Medicine, 2018.

If you do not currently engage in regular exercise, continue down the left side of the flowchart and answer the two questions related to diseases and signs or symptoms. If your answer is "no" to both of the questions, then you can begin with light to moderate activity (i.e., intensity that causes a slight increase in heart rate and breathing) and over time can continue to progress your exercise program as described in this book. However, if you do have a known disease (even if you don't have signs or symptoms currently) or if you have signs or symptoms (even if you have not been diagnosed with a disease), you should check with your health care provider before engaging in exercise. Once you have received clearance to exercise, exercise at a light to moderate level, with progression as appropriate given your health status.

If you do participate in regular exercise, continue down the right side of the flow-chart. If you are experiencing any signs or symptoms, as described previously, then you should stop exercising and check with your health care provider. After being cleared to exercise, gradually progress with your exercise program as appropriate based on your health status. If you do not have signs or symptoms but have been diagnosed with disease, then recommendations related to checking with your health care provider depend on the level of exercise you are doing. If your exercise program focuses on moderate-intensity activity (i.e., intensity that causes noticeable increases in heart rate and breathing), then medical clearance is not required. However, if your exercise program includes vigorous exercise (i.e., intensity that causes substantial increases in heart rate and breathing), then medical clearance within the prior 12 months is recommended (assuming no changes in signs or symptoms). If you have no known disease and no signs or symptoms, then continue with your moderate- or vigorous-intensity exercise program, or progress as appropriate.

Guidelines for selecting an appropriate level of activity and considerations for progressing your exercise program over time are introduced in the next section of this chapter and described in more detail in the chapters in part II of this book.

Components of a Complete Exercise Program

A balanced exercise program is like a sturdy, four-legged chair. If one leg of a chair is weak or too short, the chair isn't stable. In the same way, ignoring one of the exercise components will put your fitness program out of balance. Each component—aerobic, muscular, flexibility, and neuromotor exercise training—is important and should be considered (1, 3). Although you may have a slightly different focus than someone else, to meet your own personal health or fitness goals, you need to address each of these fitness components.

Aerobic Fitness

Aerobic fitness is also known as cardiorespiratory endurance. Aerobic activities are those that require oxygen to provide energy and are typically described as involving large-muscle groups used in a repeated or rhythmic fashion (1). One of the most popular aerobic exercises is walking. Other examples are jogging, running, bicycling, swimming, using aerobic equipment (e.g., elliptical machines, stair climbers), tennis, and team sports (e.g., basketball, soccer). When you are engaged in these activities, you can feel your breathing rate go up and your heart beat faster as your body strives to bring needed oxygen to your working muscles.

You should engage in aerobic exercise three to five days per week (1, 3). The intensity (i.e., how hard you are working) depends on your fitness level and your current level of activity. Some general guidelines are outlined in table 2.1, including aerobic activity targets for intensity and overall time spent in aerobic activities each week (for now, focus on the aerobic training column; resistance training is discussed in the next section).

Note the gradual progression of intensity listed in the table—starting with light to moderate (e.g., walking) and then progressing to moderate-intensity activity (e.g., brisk walking) or even to more vigorous activity for those who so desire (e.g., jogging). Intensity and duration are inversely related, meaning if one is higher the other will be

TABLE 2.1   **Aerobic and Resistance Training Targets Based on Activity Status**

Activity status	Aerobic training focus	Resistance training focus
Beginner (inactive with no or minimal physical activity and thus deconditioned)	*No prior activity:* Focus is on light- to moderate-level activity for 20 to 30 min over the course of the day. Accumulating time in 10-min bouts is an option. Overall, your target is 60 to 100 min per week. *Some prior activity* (i.e., once you have met the target level of 60 to 100 min per week): Focus is on light- to moderate-level activity for 30 to 45 min per day. Accumulating time in 10-min bouts is an option. Overall, your target is 100 to 150 min per week.	Select six exercises (one targeting each of the following muscle groups: hips and legs, chest, back, shoulders, low back, and abdominal muscles). Begin with one set of 10 to 15 repetitions twice per week. As you progress, your target is one or two sets of 8 to 12 repetitions done two to three days per week. (*Note:* For middle-age and older adults with limited resistance training experience, 10 to 15 repetitions per set is recommended.)
Intermediate (somewhat active but overall only moderately conditioned)	*Fair to average fitness:* Focus is on moderate activity for 30 to 60 min per day. Overall, your target is 150 to 250 min per week.	Select 10 exercises (one targeting each of the following muscle groups: hips and legs, quadriceps, hamstrings, chest, back, shoulders, biceps, triceps, low back, and abdominal muscles). Your target is two sets of 8 to 12 repetitions on two to three days per week. (*Note:* For middle-age and older adults with limited resistance training experience, 10 to 15 repetitions per set is recommended.)
Established (regularly engaging in moderate to vigorous exercise)	*Regular exerciser* (moderate to vigorous): Focus is on moderate- to vigorous-intensity activity for 30 to 90 min per day. Overall, your target is 150 to 300 min per week (duration depends on intensity; more information on this concept is given in chapter 5).	You can continue with the intermediate plan (but simply add more weight as you adapt), or you may want to consider splitting your workout and focusing more on specific muscle groups on a given day (more information on this option is given in chapter 6).

lower. For moderate-intensity activity, the target duration is greater (e.g., 150 to 300 minutes per week); for vigorous-intensity activity, the time spent is less (e.g., 75 to 150 minutes per week). One person may find walking 10 minutes before and after work, and during the lunch hour when at work, an effective way to reach 150 minutes per week of moderate aerobic activity. Another person may enjoy jogging for 20 to 25 minutes three days per week for a total of 75 minutes per week of vigorous-intensity activity. The options are almost unlimited. The point of examining these recommendations is to highlight the ranges with regard to frequency, intensity, and time, with the understanding that benefits continue to increase at higher levels of activity—although scientists have not identified the upper limit at which no additional benefits will be realized (4). Chapter 5 includes more details on aerobic exercise, including two basic fitness tests that can be used to help you estimate your level of aerobic fitness (the one-mile walking test and the 1.5-mile run test).

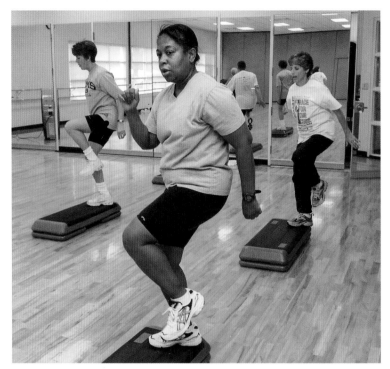

Group exercise classes are one way to build aerobic fitness.

Muscular Fitness

Muscular fitness training is typically referred to as resistance training and addresses muscular strength, muscular endurance, and power (1). Consider muscular strength and muscular endurance as the two ends of the muscular fitness continuum. Muscular strength is the maximum amount of force a muscle or muscle group can produce. Strength is focused on single-effort activity such as moving a heavy box or lifting a loaded barbell. Muscular endurance is the ability of a muscle or muscle group to exert a force repeatedly over time or to maintain a contraction for a period of time. Examples of muscular endurance are lifting a small child repeatedly or continuing to hold up a child so he can see over a crowd at a parade. Repeated or sustained contractions in other activities such as yoga or rock climbing also require muscular endurance. Muscular power incorporates the aspect of time. Power is greater when you are able to do the same movement in a shorter time or when more work can be done in the same time. Picture being able to rise quickly from a chair or move efficiently up a flight of stairs. Most activities involve aspects of muscular strength, endurance, and power; thus, in this book the term muscular fitness is generally used.

Table 2.1 offers guidance regarding resistance training for beginning, intermediate, and established exercisers. Note that you may be doing aerobic exercise regularly (and thus be in the "established" category) but may be a beginner when it comes to resistance training. For this reason, you should consider each component separately. Your muscular fitness training program should include exercises for the major muscle groups—chest, shoulders, arms, upper and lower back, abdomen, hips, and legs (1). You should also train opposing muscle groups to maintain muscle balance, which helps you avoid injury (e.g., include both low back exercises and abdominal exercises).

Your resistance training program consists of repetitions and sets. A repetition refers to the act of lifting a weight one time; lifting the weight multiple times in succession is called a set. Each muscle group should be trained in sets. You can repeat a given exercise, or you can select different exercises that target the same muscle group. The number of repetitions and sets depends on your goals. In general, individuals should perform 8 to 15 repetitions and complete two to four sets of each exercise (1, 3). For resistance training focused more specifically on muscular endurance, the repetition number is typically higher (e.g., 15 to 25 repetitions) (1). For example, consider using a body weight exercise like push-ups in which multiple sets of 25 could be performed.

To improve muscular fitness, you have to apply an overload, or stress beyond typical use, to the muscle or muscle group. This concept of relative intensity of the resistance training session is related to the number of repetitions and sets. If you cannot complete eight repetitions, then the weight or resistance is too heavy. If you can exceed 15 repetitions, the weight or resistance is too light. When starting out, you may find the need to make more frequent adjustments.

Including rest is key in order for the muscle to be able to adapt. When scheduling resistance training sessions, do not train a given muscle group on two consecutive days (1, 3). Some soreness may be experienced, but with gradual progression this can be minimized. Consulting a fitness professional may be appropriate, especially if you are unfamiliar with the various types of exercises or equipment. Muscular fitness can be improved with resistance training, and examples of specific exercises are provided in chapter 6, along with some simple muscular fitness assessments.

Flexibility

Flexibility is the ability to move a joint through its full range of motion, or in other words, the amount of movement possible given the anatomical structure of the joint. Many people consider flexibility a characteristic that either you have or you don't. Although some people naturally have a higher level of flexibility than others do, everyone has the potential to improve flexibility even if gymnast-type flexibility isn't a possibility. The value of flexibility can be clearly seen in daily activities such as bending to tie your shoes, looking over your shoulder to check for cars in traffic, securing a back zipper, or engaging in recreational activities such as swimming or golfing.

Flexibility can vary greatly not only among people but also among the various joints in the body. The ability to have full movement at the joint, also referred to as a full range of motion, can be influenced by injury, disuse, and age. When a joint is not used throughout its normal or potential range of motion, full movement of the joint is lost over time. To improve flexibility, you need to include stretching exercises in your exercise program (1, 3).

Stretching refers to exercises that move joints, along with the related muscles, tendons, and ligaments, through their range of motion. Include stretching in your exercise program at least two to three days per week, although daily time spent stretching provides greater potential benefits (1, 3). Typically, about 10 minutes allows you to stretch the major muscle groups (neck, shoulders, back, pelvis, hips, and legs) (1). Chapter 7 includes more information about stretching, along with specific examples of stretches.

Neuromotor Exercise Training

Most exercise programs should also address functional fitness with neuromotor exercise training (1). Your nervous system interacts with your muscles to move your body as well as to optimize agility and balance. Aging can result in a loss of balance and agility, thus leading to an increased risk of falling. Balance-enhancing activities, often referred to as neuromuscular exercises (because of the brain–nerve and muscle connection), are recommended for adults in the form of activities such as tai chi, Pilates, and yoga, and for older adults who are at risk of falling or who have impairments in mobility (1, 3). Chapter 8 includes a number of activities that can be included as part of a neuromotor exercise training program.

Creating an Individualized Program

Creating an exercise program is not difficult, but it requires some thought and planning. The first step is often the hardest. If you have been reading from the beginning of this book, you have seen compelling evidence regarding the health-related benefits of physical activity. Knowledge is good, but now it is time to develop an action plan by assessing where you are in your life and how you can find the motivation to move forward. Consider the following list of questions and take a moment to reflect on your answers:

- What aspect of my body or my current health situation makes me unhappy but could be positively affected by a regular exercise program?
- What do I want to change and why?
- Am I willing to give up my current routine to make that change?
- Do I have the motivation to make that change?
- What has been my previous experience with personal health behavior change? What worked? What didn't? How can reflecting on my previous experience help me this time?

Your exercise program should be developed within the framework of your answers to these questions. An honest review of your current status can help to identify areas of high fitness as well as areas that might need some improvement. With this in mind, you then can consider the various program options and how they may work for you. These areas are covered in the remainder of this chapter.

Reviewing Your Fitness Assessments

Self-analysis of your current activity level along with fitness testing results (various assessments are found in chapters 5-8) provides helpful baseline information. Reflecting on your current status is a good starting point. If you are already active, be encouraged to continue and to find additional ways to maintain or improve your fitness. If you have realized shortcomings or are unhappy with some of your fitness assessment results, do not be discouraged. No matter what your current level of fitness is, you can always improve. This is true whether you are currently inactive or already active.

Fitness assessments are helpful to provide evidence of improvement over time (1). Repeating the assessments periodically can provide objective evidence of your improvement, or can show you areas that may need some extra attention. If you are a beginner, you may want to include assessments more frequently (every two to four months) because the feedback can be used to help you adjust your program. If you are a more established exerciser, you will not experience substantial changes and thus may need or want to conduct assessments only a couple of times per year. Charting your scores along with the ranking for each assessment lets you watch for progress over time. If you aren't seeing improvement in a particular area, you may need to increase your focus on that fitness component. If you are already at a good level of fitness, then seek to maintain your fitness in that area.

Although the scores and rankings from fitness assessments are useful in establishing a baseline as well as in marking your progress, your reasons for becoming active are not likely linked to a number on a chart. More likely, your wake-up call was realizing that lack of fitness prevents you from engaging fully in life activities. Consider the following examples:

Aerobic Fitness

- Do you find yourself breathless going up a short flight of stairs?
- Do you avoid social or recreational situations that may involve physical activity?
- Are you unable to keep up with peers in recreational activities or sport competitions?

Muscular Fitness

- Are you unable to lift a full bag of groceries from your vehicle?
- Do you struggle to hold your child or grandchild?
- Are you limited in your recreational pursuits by a lack of strength?

Flexibility

- Are you unable to reach over your shoulder to fasten a zipper?
- Do you find it difficult to look behind you to check for traffic when driving?
- Do you have to modify your movements (e.g., a golf swing) to compensate for limited joint mobility?

Functional Fitness

- Do you find yourself unsteady when moving quickly from one position to another?
- Are you prone to falling?

Body Composition

- Are your clothes tighter than they were last year?
- Do you feel unhappy with your appearance because of weight gain?
- Does added body fat limit your enjoyment of recreational activities such as jogging or cycling?

Although assessing each of the components of fitness is encouraged, acknowledge that you are more than a score! Your quest for improved health and fitness relates to how you function on a daily basis. Make the changes you need to fulfill your potential. The scores or rankings provided by the fitness assessments are simply intended to help you monitor your progress.

Activity Program Options

As you look to initiate or add to your existing exercise program, you face a multitude of decisions that may affect your adherence and the benefits you receive from the exercise program. For example, should you exercise alone or participate with a partner or in a larger group? Would it be best to join a community-based fitness facility or a large commercial health club? What types of equipment should you buy? The sections that follow provide assistance in navigating some of these decisions.

Should I Exercise Alone or in a Group?

Exercising alone is a viable option for many people. Unless you have health issues that need to be professionally monitored, going solo with an exercise program can be very satisfying. Exercising alone can be done at home, outdoors, or even at a health club (many are now open 24 hours a day). If your schedule is busy, you may appreciate the freedom of not having to coordinate your schedule with anyone else. The time you spend exercising can be a chance to turn off your mind from the stress of the day and focus on your exercise experience.

An important consideration when exercising alone at home or outdoors is safety. Staying within a level of intensity appropriate to your current fitness level enhances the safety of a home-based program. Exercising outdoors brings up safety issues in terms of people, traffic, and weather conditions. When exercising outdoors, always walk or run on a sidewalk, if available, and face traffic at the edge of the road when a sidewalk is not available. When cycling, ride with traffic in a designated bike lane, or as far to the right as possible in the outside lane when bike lanes are absent. Avoid exercising in high heat and humidity, and always wear appropriate clothing and shoes in cold, snowy, and inclement weather. Although listening to portable music devices is enjoyable, use caution when exercising in places where you will encounter motor traffic because these devices reduce the ability to attend to sounds that may be important for safety. To help prevent accidents and injuries, never assume that others around you are being diligent with respect to your safety. If you exercise in and around traffic, wear bright and reflective clothing and be vigilant and careful in every way possible.

Although exercising alone is a great choice for some, many people prefer exercising with others. By involving your family members, friends, and coworkers in your activity program, you can help each other make exercise a regular habit. In doing so, you claim health and well-being benefits for yourself while also helping those around you to do the same. You may also find opportunities to expand your social network with others already involved in activities of interest to you.

Exercising in groups can take the form of organized classes in aerobics, spinning, or kickboxing at fitness facilities, or of more informal situations such as mall-walking groups. Most commercial health clubs and community fitness facilities offer a variety of group exercise classes as part of the regular membership package. These classes can be a great way to meet people with similar interests. Be sure to check what is available when deciding where to join.

Community-based programs foster group dynamics that offer support and encouragement, which can be highly beneficial regardless of your level of experience. Examples include cycling clubs, running clubs, and ballroom dance groups. Such groups form within communities either spontaneously, through the grassroots efforts of a group of individuals, or by way of local agencies hoping to promote physical activity and healthy living. Along with fitness benefits, such groups also typically provide a great social outlet.

Should I Join a Fitness Facility or Exercise at Home?

Although there are many ways to participate in exercise and focus on health, one of the most popular is membership at a fitness facility. Options include large commercial health clubs, community fitness centers, and small storefront centers. Issues to consider when making your choice are the services that are most important to you and the cost of membership.

A great advantage of fitness facilities is the variety of options available for aerobic and muscular fitness training. Most facilities have a number of treadmills, stationary bikes, and elliptical machines, and many also include a swimming pool and areas to play basketball and court-based sports. Likewise, many facilities offer a wide range of weights and resistance machines for muscular fitness training. These options, along with any number of group exercise classes and child care, make joining a fitness facility an attractive choice for many individuals and families.

When deciding whether to join a fitness facility, consider location, hours of operation, equipment, supervision, shower facilities, member services, and cost (see table 2.2). One other important part of your decision relates to the environment of the facility. Some exercisers are drawn to facilities that are family focused and more relaxed, whereas others prefer a more serious athletic environment. Before joining, tour the facility at the time of day you plan to exercise to get a clear picture. Many facilities offer short-term memberships at very low cost, allowing you to see if the facility is a good match for you. Careful consideration of each of these issues and others unique to your circumstances can help you make your decision.

Rather than joining a health club or fitness facility, you may prefer to exercise in the comfort and convenience of your own home. You can develop a very effective fitness program at home with little to no equipment, or you may choose to look into purchasing some exercise equipment. Examples of no-cost, equipment-free options include calisthenics (such as push-ups, curl-ups, jumping jacks), walking or jogging in place, flexibility exercises that require only a space on the floor, fitness-based programming on public television, exercise DVDs from the local public library, or videos available from reputable sources on YouTube and the Internet. With regard to the last

TABLE 2.2   Considerations in Selecting a Fitness Facility

Location	• Is the facility located in a safe area? • Is the facility easily accessible from work or home?
Hours of operation	• Can you access the facility during the time of day that you plan to exercise? • How busy is the facility during this time? • Will the pool be available for open swim when you want to swim?
Equipment	• Is the equipment clean and in good repair? • Does the facility have enough equipment to accommodate members?
Shower facilities	• Are the shower and changing facilities clean and well-maintained? • Does the facility provide a towel service?
Supervision	• Are the employees properly trained and certified for their positions? • Does the facility have an emergency action plan?
Member services	• Does the facility have special incentive programs to enhance participation and motivation? • Is the cost reasonable and affordable? • Are staff members friendly and knowledgeable? • Is child care available?

two options, it is beyond the scope of this book to evaluate all of the available fitness programs, videos, and DVDs. If you choose these options, consider the credentials of the people associated with the materials. In addition, take into account your own personal style and follow the guidelines outlined in this book when choosing a home-based program.

Although no-cost options present viable opportunities for physical activity, you may want more variety in your home-based program. Purchasing some rather inexpensive items can broaden the scope of activities you can do—for example, an exercise mat for stretching or doing yoga, elastic tubing or medicine balls for resistance training, or a stability ball to work on balance and coordination.

Exercise equipment is another consideration, depending on your budget and the space you have available. The starting cost for exercise equipment likely is more than a yearly membership to a local fitness facility or health club, but this may be a worthwhile investment when you consider the long-term use and convenience. If you decide to purchase your own equipment for use at home, the challenge will be to meet your personal fitness needs while simultaneously finding a good blend of price and quality. The following list of questions will help you purchase equipment that will provide years of use rather than turning into a garage sale casualty:

- *What are your fitness goals?* If you plan to focus on a walking program, you don't need a treadmill with capabilities for an Olympian! However, if you have some competitive goals in mind, be sure the equipment can withstand the rigors of your training. Match your use with the construction and purpose of the equipment and also the activities you most enjoy.

- *How much space do you have available?* Take time to measure your floor space. A piece of equipment always looks much smaller in a showroom than it will in your home. You will need some space around the equipment to allow for safe usage, so calculate that into your plans. Some resistance training equipment has a significant vertical component, so knowing ceiling height is also important.

- *How much money do you want to spend?* Home exercise equipment varies greatly in price. Cost is always a consideration, but keep the first question in mind, too. If a simple piece of equipment will fulfill your fitness goals, don't be pulled into purchasing more expensive equipment with options you will never use. Quality should be a major consideration. One or two high-quality pieces of equipment are better than a number of poor-quality items that do not provide the enjoyment you anticipated.

- *How does the equipment feel?* You should try out any piece of equipment you plan to purchase. You are not likely to buy a car based on viewing a picture in a magazine. In the same way, you should take exercise equipment on a "test drive" to ensure that it matches your needs. All moving parts should be smooth and fluid, not jerky or rubbing. Also make sure the equipment fits—treadmill belts should be long enough for your stride; stationary bikes should be adjustable to allow about a 10-degree bend at your knee at the bottom of the pedal stroke; and resistance training equipment should adjust to your limb lengths.

- *Is assembly provided?* When it comes to any home-based purchase, there are three dreaded words: "to be assembled." Some items may be simple to assemble, but for others you may want to ensure that professional assembly is included in the purchase price.

If you start out with this list of questions, you will maximize the benefits of home-based exercise equipment and realize years of enjoyment.

Should I Hire a Fitness Specialist or Personal Trainer?

One other important variable you may want to consider when planning a new or revised exercise program is hiring a fitness professional to help with assessment and prescribe appropriate exercise. Though titles vary considerably within the fitness industry, this kind of professional has typically been known as a personal trainer, health fitness specialist, or exercise physiologist. Unlike the situation in the medical field, mandated standards are not in place for personal trainers or fitness specialists, so you should ask some specific questions to determine whether the person has appropriate qualifications. A list of questions you can ask is presented in figure 2.3; several "no" responses indicate that you may need to look elsewhere.

Until more uniform and rigorous hiring standards are in place within the fitness industry, a "buyer beware" mindset seems to be appropriate and prudent. Your interview should help you determine whether the prospective trainer is a good match for you in terms of style and general approach to health and fitness. Some people prefer a very nurturing and encouraging style, whereas others tend to respond more positively to a trainer who has a lot of energy and is more demanding. Your task is to determine what motivational style and approach best suits your personality.

One last question is whether hiring a fitness professional is a necessity or a luxury. Most experts agree that meeting recommendations for physical activity does not require a trainer, but having someone who is focused on helping you reach your health and fitness goals can be very useful. Also, with some activities (e.g., resistance training), guidance provided by a trainer not only enhances the experience but also promotes

---

FIGURE 2.3

Checklist for selecting a qualified personal trainer.

Do you have a certification from a nationally recognized organization such as the American College of Sports Medicine* or the National Strength and Conditioning Association?   ____ Yes ____ No

Do you have a college degree in the health and fitness field?   ____ Yes ____ No

Do you participate in continuing education to stay current in the field?   ____ Yes ____ No

Do you have certifications in CPR and first aid?   ____ Yes ____ No

Do you have liability insurance?   ____ Yes ____ No

Do you have experience working with people similar to me in terms of age, sex, and goals?   ____ Yes ____ No

Do you use preactivity screenings and fitness assessments?   ____ Yes ____ No

Do you include cardiorespiratory, muscular, and flexibility training in your program?   ____ Yes ____ No

*You can find ACSM-certified professionals in your area by looking at ACSM's Pro Finder (see www.acsm.org).
From ACSM, 2017, *ACSM's complete guide to fitness & health,* 2nd ed. (Champaign, IL: Human Kinetics).

safety. One reasonable option is to hire a trainer to conduct fitness assessments, develop a comprehensive fitness program, and provide instruction and feedback in the early stages of the program. Thereafter you may be able to consult with the trainer periodically for updates.

Do I Need Special Apparel to Exercise?

Whatever your preference—solo exercise or in a group, home-based, or fitness facility—common considerations for safety and comfort are shoes and clothing. Attention to these basic items can optimize your enjoyment and help you avoid injury that could derail your exercise plans.

Before selecting a pair of shoes, determine your primary activity and the surface (e.g., pavement, exercise facility floor). Spend some time in an athletic shoe store consulting with an expert regarding the type of shoe that will best serve your purpose. For example, running shoes are constructed for forward motion rather than side-to-side, so if you are taking an aerobic dance class or playing tennis, you want a shoe that is constructed to handle lateral movements. Don't fall into the trap of believing that the most expensive shoe is the best. The most important factor when selecting a shoe is good support and proper fit.

Clothing doesn't have to be high priced to provide comfort during exercise. Select clothing appropriate for the temperature and environmental conditions in which you will be exercising. Clothing that is appropriate for exercise and the season can improve your exercise experience. In warm environments, clothes that have a wicking capacity are helpful in dissipating heat from the body. In contrast, it is best to face cold environments with layers so you can adjust your body temperature to avoid sweating and remain comfortable.

Deciding to take charge of your health and to improve your fitness is a powerful resolution. Before getting started, a health status check is recommended to identify any current concerns (including follow-up with your health care provider as needed) in order to maximize safety when you are active. The benefits of physical activity are so great that being active is recommended for most people. A complete exercise program includes aerobic activity, resistance training, flexibility, and neuromotor exercise training. With these tools in hand, reflect on your reasons for exercising and your goals. Your exercise program will not be static but will likely change over time as you continue to reflect on fitness assessments and develop new and more challenging goals.

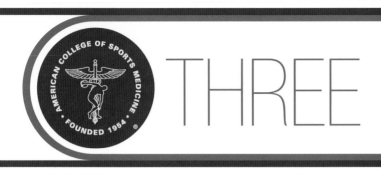

THREE

Balancing Nutrition: Recommended Dietary Guidelines

Eating well, in combination with participating in a regular exercise program, is a positive step you can take to prevent and even reverse some diseases. Though nutrition is a broad science, this chapter focuses on some of the basics, along with how to make healthy choices in your daily food intake and how those choices can influence your ability to be active.

Too often, people associate nutrition and diet with restriction and unappealing options (note that the word "diet" refers to what you eat, not a particular weight loss plan). This chapter presents a positive view of nutrition and offers suggestions for taking control of your diet to improve how you feel. By providing your body with needed calories and nutrients, you will fully fuel your body for physical activity and exercise, as well as for competition if you are so inclined. Just as a car needs quality fuel to run smoothly, your body needs a balance of nutrients to function optimally.

The *Dietary Guidelines for Americans,* published jointly by the U.S. Department of Health and Human Services and the U.S. Department of Agriculture, provides general guidance regarding nutrition for people 2 years of age and older. The *Dietary Guidelines* provides advice about how good dietary practices can promote health and prevent chronic disease.

The *Dietary Guidelines for Americans* includes the following five guidelines to promote healthy eating (32):

1. Follow a healthy eating pattern across the lifespan.
2. Focus on variety, nutrient density, and amount.
3. Limit calories from added sugars and saturated fats and reduce sodium intake.
4. Shift to healthier food and beverage choices.
5. Support healthy eating patterns for all.

Key recommendations from these Guidelines include following a healthy eating pattern that accounts for all foods and beverages within an appropriate calorie level (32).

A healthy eating pattern includes the following:

- A variety of vegetables from all of the subgroups—dark green, red and orange, legumes (beans and peas), starchy, and other
- Fruits, especially whole fruits
- Grains, at least half of which are whole grains
- Fat-free or low-fat dairy, including milk, yogurt, cheese, and fortified soy beverages
- A variety of protein foods, including seafood, lean meats and poultry, eggs, legumes (beans and peas), nuts, seeds, and soy products
- Oils

A healthy eating pattern limits the following:

- Saturated fats and *trans* fats, added sugars, and sodium.
  - Consume less than 10 percent of calories per day from added sugars.
  - Consume less than 10 percent of calories per day from saturated fats.
  - Consume less than 2,300 milligrams (mg) per day of sodium.
- If alcohol is consumed, it should be consumed in moderation—up to one drink per day for women and up to two drinks per day for men—and only by adults of legal drinking age.

These Guidelines are an excellent place to start on the path to a healthier diet. The next step is to look at the nutrients and distribution you require to meet your energy needs.

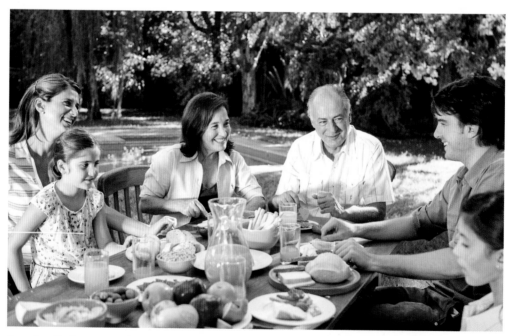

People of all ages can benefit from healthy foods.

Nutrition and Overall Health

Researchers of nearly all chronic diseases have studied the role of nutrition. (The term *chronic* is used to refer to diseases that often begin at a younger age and develop over time.) Six of the top 13 causes of death are related to poor nutrition and inactivity. By rank, these are heart disease (number 1), cancer (2), stroke (4), type 2 diabetes (6), chronic liver disease or cirrhosis (12), and high blood pressure (13) (20). Obesity is related to many of these causes of death; and although some have a genetic component, most are related to poor nutrition and lack of exercise, both of which are lifestyle habits.

Chronic diseases resulting from poor nutrition also lead to other disabilities, resulting in further loss of independence. For example, type 2 diabetes is one of the leading causes of blindness and amputation (22). Hip fractures are typically a result of osteoporosis, and people who suffer from a hip fracture are more likely to die within one year of their fracture or require long-term care than people who do not suffer a hip fracture (23). Approximately 69 percent of people who have a first heart attack, 77 percent of those who have a first stroke, and 74 percent of those with congestive heart failure have blood pressure higher than 140/90 mmHg (i.e., hypertension) (4). Obesity is an epidemic, with about a third of adults in the United States considered obese (8). Furthermore, about 17 percent of American children and teenagers (2 to 19 years of age) are considered obese (24).

Researchers have reported that unhealthy eating and sedentary behavior cause around 400,000 deaths per year in the United States (21). Because most Americans consume diets too high in total fat, trans fat, saturated fat, sodium, and sugar, and too low in whole grains, fruits, vegetables, and fiber, poor health and death are often related to poor nutrition. The combination of unhealthy diets and inactivity is the leading cause of death in the United States, above tobacco and alcohol use, and far above drug use and motor vehicle accidents (18). In addition, the health care costs of poor nutrition and inactivity are astronomical. Healthier diets could save billions of dollars in medical costs per year and also prevent lost productivity and, most important, loss of life.

Good nutrition and physical activity are the two most beneficial "medicines" you can use to prevent disease and live a good-quality life. Take control! You owe it to yourself to treat your body well.

Determining Calorie Needs

Because total calorie requirements are addressed throughout this chapter, this section explains the factors that influence your daily caloric needs and shows you how to estimate the number of calories you need. Total energy expenditure (TEE) is the total number of calories your body needs on a daily basis and is determined by the following:

- Your basal metabolic rate (BMR)
- The thermic effect of food (also known as dietary-induced thermogenesis)
- The thermic effect of your physical activity

Basal metabolic rate is defined as the energy required to maintain your body at rest (e.g., breathing, circulation). To precisely determine your BMR, you would need to fast from 8 to 12 hours and then undergo a laboratory test in which you sit quietly for about 30 minutes while the air you exhale is analyzed. This test determines how many calories you are burning at rest. Basal metabolic rate is 60 to 75 percent of TEE. Typically, the larger and more muscular a person is, the higher the BMR is.

The thermic effect of food is the energy required to digest and absorb food. The thermic effect of food is measured similarly to BMR, although the measurement time is usually about 4 hours after you have consumed a meal. The thermic effect of food is 10 to 15 percent of your TEE.

The thermic effect of activity is the amount of energy required for physical activity. It can be measured in a laboratory when you are exercising on a stationary bike or treadmill. The thermic effect of activity is the most variable of the three major components of TEE because it can be as low as 15 percent for sedentary people and as high as 80 percent for athletes who train 6 to 8 hours per day.

One other component of TEE that plays a role is nonexercise activity thermogenesis (NEAT), which is energy expended in unplanned physical activity. Nonexercise activity thermogenesis is characterized by any unplanned physical activity that is not exercise but is more than just sitting still. This can include taking the stairs instead of the elevator, sitting on a balance ball at your desk, parking farther from your destination in a parking lot, fidgeting, and other calorie-burning activities. By figuring out BMR, thermic effect of food, thermic effect of physical activity, and NEAT, an estimate can be made of how many total calories a person would need in a single day, or the individual's TEE.

Although determining your energy needs in a laboratory is precise, you do not need to go to that expense to estimate the number of calories you use. Simpler yet less precise methods of estimation require first calculating your BMR based on your age, sex, height, and weight (13, 19) and then adding in the thermic effects of food and of activity, but this method can be rather time-consuming. For general purposes, the easiest way requires some simple math that allows you to quickly estimate your energy needs. Keep in mind that this method, although the simplest, is the least accurate and should be used only as a rough estimation. See table 3.1 for the estimated daily caloric intake needed to maintain your current weight (34). To calculate your needed daily calorie intake, look at the first column, then find the activity level that best represents your current status. If you know your body weight in pounds, multiply that number by the estimated number of calories per pound in the second column; if you know your weight in kilograms, look at the third column in the table.

Take a moment to do this calculation based on your body weight and activity level. Keep in mind that your final estimate is just that—an estimate. Your actual daily calorie needs may vary somewhat, but this provides an approximate starting point. To maintain your body weight, this is about how many calories you should consume. To lose or gain weight, you will need to adjust your food intake accordingly.

■ Q&A ■

What is a calorie?

A calorie is defined as the heat required to raise the temperature of 1 gram of water 1 degree Celsius. Because this is a relatively small amount, scientists use the larger unit Calories (uppercase C), also called a kilocalorie (abbreviated as kcal). The Calorie, or kilocalorie, is equal to 1,000 calories. Food labels in the United States display Calories, or kilocalories. This is all pretty technical and does not reflect typical usage in everyday language. In this book, the word "calories" refers to Calories, or kilocalories (i.e., 1,000 calories), which is common usage.

TABLE 3.1   **Approximate Daily Caloric Intake per Unit of Body Weight Needed for Maintaining Desirable Body Weight**

Activity level	Calories per pound of body weight	Calories per kilogram of body weight
Very sedentary (restricted movement, e.g., as for a patient confined to home)	13	29
Sedentary (most Americans, office job, light work)	14	31
Moderate activity (weekend recreation)	15	33
Very active (meets ACSM standards for vigorous exercise three times per week)	16	35
Competitive athlete (daily vigorous activity in high-energy sport)	17 or more	38 or more

Adapted by permission from M.H. Williams, 2007, p. 404.

Determining Nutrient Needs

Nutrients include carbohydrates, proteins, fats, vitamins, minerals, and water. The first three—carbohydrates, proteins, and fats—are found in larger ("macro") quantities in the body and thus are referred to as macronutrients. Vitamins and minerals are found in smaller ("micro") amounts and are referred to as micronutrients.

Macronutrients

Macronutrients (carbohydrates, proteins, and fats) provide energy for daily activities and during exercise, recreational activity, and sport training. They provide slightly different numbers of calories per gram, as follows:

- Carbohydrates provide about 4 calories per gram.
- Proteins provide about 4 calories per gram.
- Fats provide about 9 calories per gram.

These values show clearly that on a gram per gram basis, fat is much denser with regard to calories than carbohydrate or protein. This is the reason a food high in fat provides more calories than a food lower in fat. Chapter 18 provides additional information on the macronutrients as they pertain to weight management. Although alcohol is not a required nutrient, it has its own unique calorie content of 7 calories per gram.

Carbohydrates

Although some diets (e.g., the Atkins diet) seem to suggest that carbohydrates are the villain when it comes to weight management, carbohydrates are actually vital for the optimal functioning of your body. For example, your brain and central nervous system rely on carbohydrate or glucose in the blood for energy. Carbohydrates are also an important source of energy during physical activity. Without sufficient carbohydrate in your diet, you will not be able to fully enjoy a vigorous workout or competition because your body will not have the fuel it needs to perform.

Carbohydrates exist in the form of sugars, starches, and fiber. Sugars are naturally found in items such as fruit and milk products. Sugar is also added to various products for flavor and taste. Cutting down on products with added sugar is recommended (e.g., candy, nondiet soda, and fruit drinks). These are rather obvious, but checking food labels can reveal added sugars that aren't as obvious. When searching for added sugars in foods, first check the ingredients list. Added sugars can be identified by many different names, including brown sugar, corn sweetener, corn syrup, dextrose, high-fructose corn syrup, glucose, honey, lactose, maltose, malt syrup, molasses, and sucrose. Be especially careful when these items are listed among the first few ingredients on the food label because components are listed in the order of predominance by weight (31). Based on the 2015 *Dietary Guidelines for Americans,* the recommendation is to limit calories from added sugars to 10 percent per day (30, 32).

Focusing on fruits, vegetables, and whole-grain products maximizes the health benefits of carbohydrates. Starches are a more complex form of carbohydrate that the body can use for energy and are found in products such as vegetables, dried beans, and grains. Starches are different from sugars because they are chemically composed of long chains of sugars linked together. Consumption of whole grains can help prevent cardiovascular disease, type 2 diabetes, and other chronic diseases mainly because they are high in vitamins and minerals, as well as antioxidants (15, 25). More information on disease prevention appears in part IV of this book.

The third category of carbohydrate—fiber—includes parts of food that the body cannot break down and absorb. Sources of fiber include vegetables, fruits, and whole grains. Consuming higher-fiber foods promotes greater feelings of fullness as well as bowel health. Higher-fiber diets have been found to reduce the risk of diabetes, colon cancer, and obesity (32). Table 3.2 provides examples of good sources of carbohydrates, including the contribution made by fiber (29).

Approximately 45 to 65 percent of your calorie intake should be from carbohydrates (10). This is a relatively wide range to account for the variety of nutritional approaches while avoiding deficiencies or adverse health consequences. Out of this 45 to 65 percent, strive to consume a variety of these types of carbohydrates. Typical diets tend to over consume the simple sugars and under consume starches and fiber. The Daily Value listed on food labels (see the full discussion later in this chapter) is based on 60 percent of the calorie intake. If you are active, or if you are a competitive athlete, keeping your carbohydrate intake near the upper end of this range provides sufficient fuel for your working muscles. Now that you know about how many calories you need per day, as figured from table 3.1, you can determine how much carbohydrate is recommended. For example, for someone who needs 2,500 calories per day, approximately 1,125 to 1,625 calories should be from carbohydrate. This would be calculated as follows:

2,500 calories per day × 0.45 (45%) = 1,125 calories from carbohydrate

2,500 calories per day × 0.65 (65%) = 1,625 calories from carbohydrate

To determine the number of grams of carbohydrate you need, recall that each gram of carbohydrate supplies 4 calories. Simply take the number of calories from carbohydrate and divide by 4 to determine how many grams you need:

TABLE 3.2   **Sources of Carbohydrates and Fiber**

Food	Serving size	Carbohydrate per serving (g)	Fiber per serving (g)
Grains			
Raisin bagel	1 whole	36	2
Whole-grain bread	1 slice	13	2
Raisin bran cereal	1 oz (30 g)	46	7
Brown rice	1 cup	46	4
Spaghetti	1 cup	43	3
Fruits			
Banana, mashed	1 cup	51	6
Blueberries	1 cup	21	4
Figs, dried	2 figs	24	4
Grapefruit juice	6 fl oz (180 mL)	72	<1
Vegetables			
Beans (dry), cooked	1 cup	45 to 55	13 to 19
Baked beans, canned	1 cup	47	18
Carrots, cooked	1 cup	12	5
Sweet potato	1 cup	54	5
Dairy			
Milk, low or nonfat	1 cup	12	0
Yogurt, plain, skim milk	8 oz (240 g)	13	0
Cottage cheese, nonfat	1 cup	10	0

Source: U.S. Department of Agriculture, Agricultural Research Service, Nutrient Data Laboratory.

1,125 calories / 4 calories per gram = 281 grams from carbohydrate

1,625 calories / 4 calories per gram = 406 grams from carbohydrate

Proteins

Proteins are made of small units called amino acids, which are considered the building blocks of the body. Proteins promote muscle growth and are required for many body functions, including assistance with chemical reactions and hormones. Even though proteins can provide 4 calories per gram, you typically do not use protein for energy unless you are deficient in your intake of carbohydrate or fat. This is so the protein you consume can be used to promote growth and for normal body functions. See table 3.3 for the protein content of various foods (29).

Proteins should account for about 10 to 15 percent of total calories (AMDR is 10 to 35 percent for adults—see What Do All the Abbreviations Mean later in this chapter for a definition of AMDR) (10). As with carbohydrates, a range is provided to account for differences in diet and to suggest a safe upper limit. Depending on your total calorie intake, you may be near the low or high end of this range. Your personal protein

Reading Food Labels

Food labels are important windows of information for products that have them (fresh produce does not). Because there is not enough room to place all the nutrient information on a food label, the label provides only a quick look at the nutrient content. Reading labels, however, can be confusing; the following clarifies the information that labels provide. See figure 3.1 for an example of a food label (33).

Serving Size

Serving size is usually the first item listed on a food label. Serving sizes are standardized for similar foods. Pay close attention to the serving size, because in some cases, food companies package items in a set of two or more (i.e., the serving size is half of the total amount in the package). Consider a regular-size bag of microwave popcorn. If you eat the whole bag, you have consumed two or three servings of popcorn! Some products list values per serving as well as per package. Paying attention to the serving size helps you track your calorie intake and avoid overeating and gaining weight over time.

Calories and Calories From Fat

You should always check the total number of calories provided in a food item, as well as

Nutrition Facts
8 servings per container
Serving size　　　　**2/3 cup (55g)**

Amount per serving	
Calories	**230**

	% Daily Value*
Total Fat 8g	**10%**
Saturated Fat 1g	**5%**
Trans Fat 0g	
Cholesterol 0mg	**0%**
Sodium 160mg	**7%**
Total Carbohydrate 37g	**13%**
Dietary Fiber 4g	**14%**
Total Sugars 12g	
Includes 10g Added Sugars	**20%**
Protein 3g	
Vitamin D 2mcg	10%
Calcium 260mg	20%
Iron 8mg	45%
Potassium 235mg	6%

*The % Daily Value (DV) tells you how much a nutrient in a serving of food contributes to a daily diet. 2,000 calories a day is used for general nutrition advice.

FIGURE 3.1　Sample food label.
Source: U.S. Department of Health and Human Services.

requirement is based on your body weight; you should consume approximately 0.36 grams of protein for each pound of body weight. Simply multiply your body weight in pounds by 0.36 to determine approximately how many grams of protein you need to consume each day. If you know your body weight in kilograms, multiply that value by 0.8 (3). For example, for a 150-pound or a 68-kilogram person, this would be figured as shown:

150 pounds × 0.36 = 54 grams protein × 4 calories/gram = 216 calories from protein

68 kilograms × 0.8 = 54 grams protein × 4 calories/gram = 216 calories from protein

Note that protein requirements are increased for athletes and are different depending on the sport, the intensity and frequency of the workout, and how experienced

the total number of calories from fat. Paying attention to serving size is key to determining your overall calorie intake of each food item. As a quick guide to calorie intake, consider the following (31):

- A food item providing 40 calories per serving is considered "low calorie."
- A food item providing 100 calories per serving is considered "moderate calorie."
- A food item providing 400 calories or more per serving is considered "high calorie."

Throughout the course of a typical day, you will likely consume food items in various categories. As long as you keep an eye on the total calories you consume over the course of the day, you will be able to remain in energy balance (i.e., your consumed calories will match the number of calories you expend).

Percent Daily Value

Another item to pay attention to on a food label is the "% Daily Value" (%DV) listed for certain nutrients on all food labels. These values are based on a 2,000-calorie diet. Although this caloric intake might not be a direct match of the calories you need on a daily basis, it does provide general guidance and covers a wide range of people. Daily value reflect recommended levels of intake. For some nutrients (e.g., total fat, saturated fat, cholesterol, and sodium), it is better to aim to consume less than the recommended amount; however, for others, such as total carbohydrate and dietary fiber, it is important to try to consume at least the recommended amount. In general, a %DV of less than 5 percent is considered low, and 20 percent or greater is considered high (31).

When looking at the section of the label focused on fat, note that both saturated and trans fats are listed. You should restrict trans fats as much as possible from your diet and consume no more than 10 percent of total calorie intake in the form of saturated fat. Similarly, keeping cholesterol and sodium levels in check is important. For carbohydrate, the subcategories of dietary fiber, sugars, and added sugars are listed. Limit amounts of added sugars. You should try to increase, rather than limit, your intake of dietary fiber.

the athlete is. Typical recommendations for strength-trained athletes (e.g., American football players, bodybuilders) and endurance athletes (e.g., marathon runners) are between 0.55 and 0.77 grams of protein per pound of body weight (or 1.2 to 1.7 grams

■ Q&A

Do protein requirements change with age?

It is often believed that as individuals age, protein needs change. This is not necessarily true for the average healthy adult. The Dietary Reference Intakes recommend that adult males consume 56 grams of protein per day and adult females consume 46 grams of protein per day, regardless of their age (29). It is important to remember that these numbers are general guidelines for the average individual. Protein needs always vary depending upon the individual.

TABLE 3.3 **Protein Content of Various Foods**

Food	Serving size	Protein per serving (g)
Meat (including turkey, pork)	3 oz (85 g)	24
Fish (including trout, perch, haddock, flounder, tuna)	3 oz (90 g)	20 to 22
Beans (including pinto, kidney, black, navy)	1 cup	13 to 15
Yogurt, plain, skim milk	8 oz (226 g)	13
Cinnamon–raisin bagel	4-in. (10 cm)	9
Peanuts	1 oz (28 g)	8
Hard-boiled egg	1 large	6
Raisin bran cereal	1 cup	5
Whole wheat bread	1 slice	4
Sweet potato	1 potato	3
Squash	1 cup	2
Orange	1 cup	2
Banana	1 banana	1

Source: U.S. Department of Agriculture, Agricultural Research Service, Nutrient Data Laboratory.

of protein per kilogram of body weight) (3). Because many Americans already consume more than the Recommended Dietary Allowance for protein, athletes or other highly active people may already be consuming adequate protein. For those with inadequate intake, increased focus on consuming a variety of protein foods is recommended (30).

Fats

Fats, also called lipids, are provided in the diet from such sources as animal protein, butter, oils, nuts, and many refined products. Fats are often thought of as bad, a myth perpetuated by the many fat-free products flooding store shelves. However, fats are needed in appropriate amounts for normal functioning in the body (3). For example, lipids are the main component of each cell in your body. In addition, fat is a major source of energy, especially when you are at rest or performing low- to moderate-intensity physical activity. Excessive consumption of fat is unhealthy, but concerns also arise when fat intake is too low. A balanced approach to fat intake provides the necessary amount of fat for optimal health.

Fats are present in a number of forms, including saturated fats, monounsaturated fats, and polyunsaturated fats. These designations have to do with the chemical structure of the fat. Trans fats are found naturally in some animal products (mainly meat and dairy products), but also are a result of a manufacturing process called hydrogenation. Hydrogenation changes the structure of a fat to make it more stable and as a result more like saturated fats (which are solid at room temperature). Food companies hydro-genate fat to increase the shelf life of the product, to make it taste more like butter, and to save money because it is less expensive to hydrogenate oil than it is to use butter.

In general, health concerns result from consuming too much saturated and trans fats. Trans fats have been shown to increase the "bad" cholesterol in blood (low-density lipoprotein cholesterol, or LDL-C), even more so than saturated fats. Sources of trans fats include animal products, margarine, and snack foods. The good news is that as a result of health concerns, the food industry is reformulating many products to remove or at least reduce the amount of trans fat. Many restaurants have also now gone "trans

Determining Calorie Needs and Nutrient Ranges

Determining the number of required calories and target amounts from carbohydrates, fats, and proteins requires some simple calculations. As an example, consider a very active female (body weight is 135 pounds or 61.4 kg) who is in training for a marathon and includes resistance training a couple days per week as well. The first step is to determine how many calories are needed and then what targets she should have for various nutrients.

To provide an estimate of her calorie needs, check table 3.1 for the number of calories she needs per unit of her body weight. She is in the "very active" category given her running and resistance training activities. Thus, to determine calories needed, her body weight (135 pounds) is multiplied by 16.

$$135 \times 16 = 2,160 \text{ calories}$$

To keep things simple for calculating, round this off to 2,100 calories needed per day. Next the amount of calories she needs to consume from carbohydrates, fats, and proteins is determined. Starting with protein is easiest because this is based on her body weight. Because of her higher level of endurance training, an appropriate target is 0.55 grams per pound of body weight. Thus, body weight is multiplied by 0.55:

$$135 \times 0.55 = 74.25 \text{ grams of protein}$$

To check the percentage of calories from protein, multiply the grams by 4 (because there are 4 calories per gram of protein):

$$74.25 \times 4 = 297 \text{ calories from protein}$$

Thus, about 14 percent of her calories should be from protein (297 calories from protein divided by 2,100 total calories = 0.14, which is the decimal representation of 14 percent). For carbohydrate, an appropriate amount for someone with her high level of aerobic training is 60 percent of calories, so the remaining 26 percent should come from fat. The calculations are as follows:

$$2,100 \times 0.60 = 1,260 \text{ calories from carbohydrate}$$
$$2,100 \times 0.26 = 546 \text{ calories from fat}$$

These calculations provide some general targets to help create balance in her diet. Not every meal has to fall precisely within these percentages; rather, this is more appropriate to consider over the course of the entire day. Some meals may be higher in protein, whereas others may have more fat or carbohydrate. She needs to reflect on the foods and beverages consumed over the course of the day rather than becoming too focused on each food item or meal.

Now it's your turn! Take this time to calculate your estimated calories from carbohydrate, protein, and fat. You can start with your daily caloric needs that you calculated earlier in this chapter. Remember that when calculating your calories you should choose the appropriate percentages for your lifestyle based on the ranges for each category. The ranges are 45 to 65 percent for carbohydrate, 10 to 15 percent for protein, and 20 to 35 percent for fat.

fat free." Companies that make processed food products are required to list the amount of trans fat in their products. Although some products have labels that state they are "trans fat free," this actually means that they contain no more than 0.5 percent trans fat.

Monounsaturated fats, such as olive oil, canola oil, avocados, walnuts, and flaxseeds, have been shown to be protective against heart disease and type 2 diabetes mellitus.

That is not to say that you can consume as much monounsaturated fat as you want; however, selecting monounsaturated fats instead of saturated fats may lead to better health (e.g., healthier blood cholesterol levels). Polyunsaturated fats, such as safflower oil, corn oil, and fish oils, have also been shown to be protective against many diseases. Fish oils (eicosapentaenoic [EPA] and docosahexaenoic [DHA]) have been shown to decrease inflammation within the body and may protect against heart disease, type 2 diabetes, and arthritis. This does not mean that EPA and DHA are protective against everything, but they are important to overall health. Therefore, you should try to consume 2 to 3 ounces (56 to 85 g) of fatty fish (e.g., tuna, salmon, and sardines) at least two days per week (30). Fish oil supplements may also be warranted (consult with your health care provider to see if this is appropriate for you).

Saturated fats are found in products such as butter, cheese, meat, palm oil, and whole milk. Because of the increased risk of disease associated with saturated fats, less than 10 percent of your calories should come from saturated fats (30, 32), with an even better target of less than 7 percent (32). Trans fats also should be limited to as little as possible (30). Because of the focus on saturated and trans fats, the nutrition labels on food products include total fat as well as the amount of saturated and trans fats (see figure 3.1).

Although not technically a fat, cholesterol is in the lipid family and is found in animal products. Your body needs a certain amount of cholesterol; thus, even if your diet contained none, the liver would produce what your body needs. The problem arises when cholesterol levels in the blood become too high. Total blood cholesterol levels, as well as LDL-C levels, are predictors of heart disease (for more information, see chapter 12). Although you consume cholesterol in your diet, a major factor influencing your blood cholesterol levels is the amount of saturated and trans fats you consume. Thus, limiting saturated fat intake to no more than 10 percent of your calories is recommended (no more than 7 percent is even better) (30, 32).

Total fat intake should be between 20 and 35 percent of calories (30). Most of these calories should come from monounsaturated and polyunsaturated fats (e.g., fish, nuts, vegetable oils), and your consumption of saturated fat should be limited. For example, for someone with a target of 2,500 calories per day, total fat intake should be between 20 and 35 percent of total calories. In this example, a target of 28 percent is selected (middle of the range). This would be approximately 700 calories from fat and would be calculated as follows:

$$2,500 \times 0.28 = 700 \text{ calories}$$

To keep saturated fat at no more than 10 percent of total calories, the calories from saturated fat would total only 250, determined as follows:

$$2,500 \times 0.10 = 250 \text{ calories from saturated fat}$$

To determine how many grams this represents, the calories from fat can be divided by 9 (recall that each gram of fat provides 9 calories). Thus, in this example, total fat would be around 78 grams (700 / 9 = 78), and saturated fat would be no more than around 28 grams (250 / 9 = 28).

Some of the food groups contributing to saturated fat intake are cheese, beef, milk products, frozen desserts, snack foods (e.g., cookies, cakes, doughnuts, potato chips), butter, salad dressings, and eggs. Making small changes in the foods you select could result in meaningful decreases in the saturated fat and calories you consume. See table 3.4 for some comparisons between higher- and lower-fat food selections (30).

TABLE 3.4   **Food Selection Alternatives for Lower Saturated Fat Consumption**

Food	Higher-fat option	Lower-fat option
Cheddar cheese (1 oz or 28 g)	Regular cheddar cheese (6 g saturated fat; 114 calories)	Low-fat cheddar cheese (1.2 g saturated fat; 49 calories)
Milk (1 cup)	Whole milk, 3.24% (4.6 g saturated fat; 146 calories)	Low-fat milk, 1%* (1.5 g saturated fat; 102 calories)
Frozen desserts (1/2 cup)	Regular ice cream (4.9 g saturated fat; 145 calories)	Low-fat frozen yogurt (2.0 g saturated fat; 110 calories)
Ground beef (3 oz or 85 g, cooked)	Regular ground beef, 25% fat (6.1 g saturated fat; 236 calories)	Extra-lean ground beef, 5% fat (2.6 g saturated fat; 148 calories)
Chicken (3 oz or 85 g, cooked)	Fried chicken, leg with skin (3.3 g saturated fat; 212 calories)	Roasted chicken, breast, no skin (0.9 g saturated fat; 140 calories)
Fish (3 oz or 85 g)	Fried fish (2.8 g saturated fat; 195 calories)	Baked fish (1.5 g saturated fat; 129 calories)
Ranch dressing (2 Tbsp or 30 mL)	Regular ranch dressing (2.5 g saturated fat; 140 calories)	Light ranch dressing (1.0 g saturated fat; 80 calories)
Mayonnaise (1 Tbsp or 13 g)	Regular mayonnaise (1.5 g saturated fat; 90 calories)	Light mayonnaise (0.5 g saturated fat; 35 calories)

*Skim milk would decrease the saturated fat to 0 grams and only 80 calories.

Source: U.S. Department of Health and Human Services and U.S. Department of Agriculture, 2015.

Micronutrients

Micronutrients include vitamins and minerals. Minerals and vitamins, although part of energy-yielding reactions in your body, cannot provide energy directly. Many have antioxidant, or cell-protecting, functions (e.g., vitamins A, C, and E; copper; iron; selenium; and zinc). It is important to consume the DRI amounts for vitamins and minerals (or at least obtain 70 percent of the DRI) to maintain overall health (9, 10). It is beyond the scope of this chapter to discuss all the vitamins and minerals in detail; however, table 3.5 provides a listing of the major vitamins and minerals, including common sources as well as concerns with consuming too much or too little (11, 34).

You may be feeling overwhelmed thinking about consuming each of the macro-nutrients and the micronutrients (all the vitamins and minerals) each day. However, if you consume a diet that is varied, includes five to eight servings of fruits and vegetables per day, and is composed mostly of whole foods and less of processed foods, you will be doing your body good. You may also feel daunted by the idea of consuming five to eight servings of fruits and vegetables per day, but remember that these servings include fruits and vegetables (not five to eight servings of each!), and that a serving can be a medium banana, 4 ounces (118 mL) of 100 percent fruit juice, 1/2 cup of broccoli, and the like. The website ChooseMyPlate.gov can help you better understand serving sizes, as well as your particular requirements. See figure 3.3 for a peek at the premise behind the plate (28). When making food choices, consider the following simple guidelines:

- Whole grain is better than processed or white grain.
- More color is better than less color (e.g., dark green leafy vegetables, deep red vegetables and fruits, and dark blue or purple fruits have more vitamins and minerals than those with less color).
- Less-processed foods are best.

Often, contemplating how to improve your diet is difficult because it is hard to know where to start. As with any change it is important to focus on short-term and long-term goals. Consider a long-term goal of cutting down on fat intake as well as improving the nutrient content of your diet (e.g., increasing consumption of whole grains, fruits,

What Do All the Abbreviations Mean?

Understanding what you need in your diet can be difficult. You can gain clarity by examining the Dietary Reference Intakes (DRIs) and Acceptable Macronutrient Distribution Range (AMDR), which are reference values and ranges for the amounts of nutrients your body needs. This looks like alphabet soup; however, each set of standards is helpful (9, 10).

DRI

DRI is an umbrella term. It includes the Estimated Average Requirement (EAR), the Recommended Dietary Allowance (RDA), the Adequate Intake (AI), and the Tolerable Upper Intake Level (UL). The DRIs are focused on the nutrition requirements of nearly all healthy people (i.e., they focus on 97 percent of that population). The DRIs are set by a committee established by the Food and Nutrition Board of the National Academy of Sciences.

- EAR—The nutrient values established when there is enough scientific information. Once an EAR is established, an RDA can be established for that particular nutrient.
- RDA—Target values established by scientists with a focus on preventing nutrition-related diseases.
- AI—Values set for nutrients when there is not enough scientific evidence to support establishing the RDA.
- UL—The upper limits established for nutrients to prevent toxic consumption levels (11). These were set because so many people take vitamin and mineral supplements.

AMDR

The AMDR is not under the main umbrella of DRIs but rather provides ranges for the amount of carbohydrates, fats, and proteins (i.e., macronutrients) you should consume. The macronutrients are given in a range because the requirements vary among people more than those of the micronutrients (i.e., vitamins and minerals, which are covered by the DRI).

It is not necessary to obtain 100 percent of the established DRI for every nutrient every day; however, it is good to strive for at least 70 percent of the established DRI per day for each nutrient (9, 10). As you will see later in this chapter, the AMDR also provides guidance for dietary choices. All of the nutritional choices you make on a daily basis can make a difference for your health.

TABLE 3.5 Vitamins and Minerals

Vitamins					
Vitamin	Requirement (adults under 50)*	Functions	Deficiency	Toxicity	Food sources
Thiamin (vitamin B₁)	Males: 1.2 mg/day Females: 1.1 mg/day	Needed for carbohydrate and protein metabolism and functioning of the heart, muscles, and nervous system	Weakness, fatigue, psychosis, nerve damage	Not identified	Fortified breads and cereals, whole grains, lean meats (e.g., pork), fish, soybeans
Riboflavin (vitamin B₂)	Males: 1.3 mg/day Females: 1.1 mg/day	Needed for energy production and red blood cell production	(Rare) Fatigue, sore throat, and swollen tongue	Not identified	Lean meats, eggs, nuts, green leafy vegetables, milk and milk-based products, fortified cereals
Niacin (vitamin B₃)	Males: 16 mg/day Females: 14 mg/day	Needed for energy production and health of digestive system, skin, and nerves	Pellagra (symptoms include diarrhea, dementia, and dermatitis)	Liver damage, peptic ulcers, skin rashes, skin flushing	Poultry, dairy products, fish, lean meats, nuts, eggs
Pantothenic acid (vitamin B₅)	Males and females: 5 mg/day	Needed for energy production	Rare	Typically no toxicity	Eggs, fish, milk and milk products, lean beef, legumes, broccoli
Biotin	Males and females: 30 µg/day	Needed for energy production	Rare	Typically no toxicity	Eggs, fish, milk and milk products, lean beef, legumes, broccoli
Vitamin B₆	Males: 1.3 to 1.7 mg/day Females: 1.3 to 1.5 mg/day	Needed for protein metabolism, immune and nervous system functions	Dermatitis, sore tongue, depression, confusion	Neurological disorders and numbness	Beans, nuts, legumes, eggs, meats, fish, whole grains, fortified breads and cereals
Folate	Males and females: 400 µg/day	Needed for cellular growth, replication, regulation, and maintenance	Diarrhea, fatigue, headaches, sore tongue, poor growth	Not identified	Beans and legumes, citrus fruits, whole grains, dark green leafy vegetables, poultry, shellfish

> continued

Table 3.5 > *continued*

Vitamins					
Vitamin	**Requirement (adults under 50)***	**Functions**	**Deficiency**	**Toxicity**	**Food sources**
Vitamin B$_{12}$	Males and females: 2.4 µg/day	Needed in red blood cell formation, neurological function; role in metabolism	Anemia, numbness, weakness, loss of balance	Not identified	Eggs, meat, poultry, shellfish, milk and milk products
Vitamin C	Males: 90 mg/day Females: 75 mg/day	Needed for its antioxidant properties, iron absorption, and role in connective tissues (skin, bones, and cartilage)	Dry–splitting hair, gingivitis, dry skin, depressed immune function, slow wound healing	Gastrointestinal disturbances (cramps and diarrhea)	Citrus fruits, red and green peppers, tomatoes, broccoli, greens
Vitamin A	Males: 900 µg/day Females: 700 µg/day	Important role in vision, as well as maintenance of healthy teeth, bones, and skin	Night blindness, decreased immune function	Toxic at higher doses, birth defects	Eggs, milk, cheese, liver, kidney (beta-carotene, which can be converted into a form of vitamin A, is found in orange and dark green vegetables)
Vitamin D	Males and females: 5 mg/day	Needed for calcium absorption and for bone growth and remodeling	Rickets (in children) and osteoporosis, osteomalacia, or both (in adults)	Kidney stones; calcium deposits in heart and lungs	Skin exposure to sunlight; fish, fortified milk
Vitamin E	Males and females: 15 mg/day	Needed for its antioxidant properties and has an important role in immune function	Rare	Increased risk of death at higher doses (400 IU or higher)	Wheat germ, nuts, seeds, vegetable oils
Vitamin K	Males: 120 µg/day Females: 90 µg/day	Major role in blood clotting	Excessive bleeding due to clotting impairment, more likely to bruise	Not identified	Green vegetables and dark-colored berries

Minerals					
Mineral	**Requirement (adults under 50)**	**Functions**	**Deficiency**	**Toxicity**	**Food sources**
Calcium	Males and females: 1,000 to 1,200 mg/day	Needed for bone growth and maintenance, muscular contractions, cardiovascular and nervous system functions, hormone and enzyme secretions	Numbness, muscle cramps, convulsions, lethargy, abnormal heart rhythms, low bone mineral density	High amounts for a long time can increase risk of kidney stones	Milk, cheese, yogurt, leafy green vegetables
Iron	Males: 8 mg/day Females: 18 mg/day (8 mg/day if >51 years of age)	Major role in oxygen transport in the blood	Iron deficiency anemia, lack of energy, headache, dizziness, weight loss	Fatigue, dizziness, nausea, vomiting, weight loss, shortness of breath	Dried beans, eggs, liver, lean red meat, oysters, salmon, whole grains
Zinc	Males: 11 mg/day Females: 8 mg/day	Major role in energy production, immune function, and wound healing	Slow growth, impaired immune function, hair loss, delayed healing of wounds, problems with sense of taste and smell	Vomiting, abdominal cramps, diarrhea, and headaches can occur with large amount of supplements	Oysters, beef, pork, lamb, peanuts, peanut butter, legumes
Chromium	Males: 35 µg/day Females: 25 µg/day	Enhances the function of insulin and involved with metabolism of fat and carbohydrate	Impaired glucose tolerance	Not identified from dietary sources	Beef, liver, eggs, chicken, bananas, spinach, apples, green peppers
Magnesium	Males: 400 to 410 mg/day Females: 310 to 320 mg/day	Major role in proper muscle and nerve function	(Rare) Muscle weakness, sleepiness	No established upper limit for dietary intake	Dark green leafy vegetables, nuts, whole grains, soy products
Selenium	Males and females: 55 µg/day	Helps with antioxidant function to prevent cellular damage	(Rare) Joint, bone disease, mental retardation	(Rare) Selenosis (gastrointestinal upset, hair loss, fatigue, irritability, some nerve damage)	Vegetables, fish, shellfish, grains, eggs, chicken, liver

> continued

Table 3.5   > *continued*

		Minerals			
Mineral	**Requirement (adults under 50)**	**Functions**	**Deficiency**	**Toxicity**	**Food sources**
Copper	Males and females: 900 µg/day	Role in the formation of red blood cells as well as healthy blood vessels, nerves, immune system, and bones	Anemia and osteoporosis	Poisonous in large amounts	Organ meats (kidneys, liver), oysters and other shellfish, whole grains, beans, nuts, potatoes, dark leafy greens
Iodine	Males and females: 150 µg/day	Major role in the metabolism of cells and in normal thyroid function	Goiter or hypothyroidism	(Rare) Reduced functioning of the thyroid gland	Iodized salt, seafood (e.g., cod, sea bass), kelp
Phosphorus	Males and females: 700 mg/day	Major role in the formation of bones and teeth; involved in the utilization of fats, carbohydrate, and protein for growth and maintenance of cells, and for energy production	(Rare) Available widely in the food supply	(Rare) Can form deposits in muscle	Milk and milk products, meat

*Requirements vary for different ages and status (e.g., pregnancy, lactation). Values given here represent average adults under 50 years of age. For more information on specific requirements, see http://fnic.nal.usda.gov/dietary-guidance/dietary-reference-intakes and then find the DRI under "Topics A-Z" on the top navigation bar.

Sources: Food and Nutrition Board of the Institute of Medicine and U.S. National Library of Medicine.

and vegetables). A short-term goal might be, *I will pack my lunch (including vegetable sticks, lean meat sandwich on whole-wheat bread, piece of fruit, and a yogurt cup) rather than stopping at fast-food restaurants each day for the upcoming week.* This is a SMARTS goal (see chapter 4 for more on SMARTS goals) (1). It is *specific* in terms of the activity as well as the time frame. At the end of the week, you can reflect on whether you packed a lunch *(measurable)*. The goal provides for specific action to be taken (i.e., it is *action-oriented*) and is an activity that can be accomplished without excessive difficulty (i.e., it is *realistic*). A specific time frame is provided so that the action starts now rather than being too open-ended (i.e., it is *timely*). And finally, as you set goals, each will be *self-determined*. Following are other examples of short-term goals:

- To stop at a local farmer's market each weekend for the next month to select enough fruit to provide at least two selections each day
- To include a salad with romaine lettuce, tomatoes, onions, peppers, and carrots, topped with low-fat vinaigrette dressing, for dinner on at least two days during the upcoming week

Maximize Nutrient Density

Nutrient density reflects foods and beverages that provide vitamins and minerals with little or no added fats, sugars, refined starches, or sodium (30, 32). For example, dairy products are excellent sources of calcium, but many milk options are available. Consider 2 percent milk or nonfat (skim) milk. Which one would be preferred to optimize calcium intake while minimizing caloric intake? A 1-cup serving of each provides the same amount of calcium, vitamins, carbohydrate, and protein, but the 2 percent milk has a third more calories than the nonfat milk, all coming from added fat. See figure 3.2 for a comparison of the food labels for the two (31). Thus, the nonfat milk might be a better option since it provides the same amount of calcium at a lower number of calories.

Reduced-fat milk (2% Milkfat)

Nutrition Facts

1 serving per container
Serving size   1 cup (236ml)

Amount per serving
Calories   120

	% Daily Value*
Total Fat 5g	**8%**
Saturated Fat 3g	**15%**
Trans Fat 0g	
Cholesterol 20mg	**7%**
Sodium 120mg	**5%**
Total Carbohydrate 31g	**10%**
Dietary Fiber 0g	**0%**
Total Sugars 11g	
Includes 0g Added Sugars	
Protein 9g	
Vitamin D 0mcg	25%
Calcium 0mg	30%
Iron 0mg	0%
Potassium 0mg	0%

*The % Daily Value (DV) tells you how much a nutrient in a serving of food contributes to a daily diet. 2,000 calories a day is used for general nutrition advice.

Nonfat milk

Nutrition Facts

1 serving per container
Serving size   1 cup (236ml)

Amount per serving
Calories   80

	% Daily Value*
Total Fat 0g	**0%**
Saturated Fat 0g	**0%**
Trans Fat 0g	
Cholesterol 5mg	**7%**
Sodium 120mg	**5%**
Total Carbohydrate 11g	**4%**
Dietary Fiber 0g	**0%**
Total Sugars 11g	
Includes 0g Added Sugars	
Protein 9g	
Vitamin D 0mcg	25%
Calcium 0mg	30%
Iron 0mg	0%
Potassium 0mg	0%

*The % Daily Value (DV) tells you how much a nutrient in a serving of food contributes to a daily diet. 2,000 calories a day is used for general nutrition advice.

FIGURE 3.2   Comparison of two milk products.
Source: U.S. Department of Health and Human Services.

- To replace an afternoon candy bar from the vending machine with a piece of fruit and some almonds

Another, more in-depth way to monitor eating is to use an online tracking tool. Online tracking tools allow you to enter in the foods you eat in a given day and give

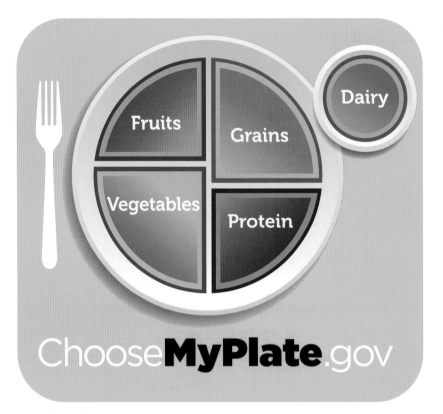

FIGURE 3.3   Illustration for MyPlate.
USDA Center for Nutrition Policy and Promotion.

you a breakdown of all your nutrients and the food groups you consumed within that day. Although there are many online tools to use, SuperTracker (www.supertracker. usda.gov), developed by the U.S. Department of Agriculture (USDA), has an extensive in-depth database (28). SuperTracker works by allowing you to track your meals by entering them into a personal profile. After meals are entered, the online tool is able to give an extensive breakdown of calories, carbohydrates, proteins, fats, and micronutrients. This can help you identify changes that you may need to make in your diet, whether it be increasing or reducing the intake of a certain food group or nutrient or increasing or changing your exercise routine (SuperTracker also allows for tracking of physical activity).

Although many tools are available for use, it is important that you focus on your own unique lifestyle and behaviors. Building on short-term goals and maintaining those healthy behaviors will ultimately result in success at reaching your long-term goal.

Water

Water is a required nutrient for all living beings. Water is important for hydration; however, it may be valuable for disease prevention as well. For example, researchers have found a relationship between water intake and reduction of gallstones and kidney stones, as well as between water intake and colon cancer (6, 7, 16, 27). Similarly, maintaining a sufficient intake of water during flying may help reduce the risk of blood clots (12).

With respect to physical activity, water is important for hydration. When you are active, you need to remain in a euhydrated (balanced) state (26). The DRI for water is 2.7 liters (91 oz or 11 cups) per day for women and 3.7 liters (125 oz or 16 cups) per day for men (9). Water balance means that you are replacing the fluid you lose through sweating and urine production.

This may sound daunting, but remember, hydration does not occur just from drinking water. Water intake can be obtained from food, which makes up about 20 percent of total water intake, and as well as from other beverages. Thus, although water is an excellent source of fluid, other beverages, such as tea, milk, coffee, and 100 percent juice, can also fulfill your fluid needs (9).

Sweating during exercise is one way the body tries to cool you (2). Sweat is composed of water as well as other substances such as electrolytes (sodium, potassium, and chloride) (17). The amount of electrolytes in sweat varies among people depending on sweat rate, fitness level, and electrolyte intake, as well as the temperature of the environment. Sodium (salt) is one electrolyte you may have noticed dried on your skin after prolonged sweating. Replacement of sodium lost in the sweat is not an issue for most people, considering that, in general, Americans consume far more salt than their bodies need (see chapter 12 for insight into how sodium intake can influence blood pressure).

You should start focusing on water balance before you are active by consuming fluids in advance of your exercise bout. While you are exercising, your goal should be to avoid excessive dehydration. For shorter workouts (less than an hour), consuming water is fine (26). For longer workouts, consider using a sport performance beverage that provides fluids as well as some carbohydrate and sodium (14). Ideally, by consuming adequate fluids, you can avoid dehydration. One simple way to check your

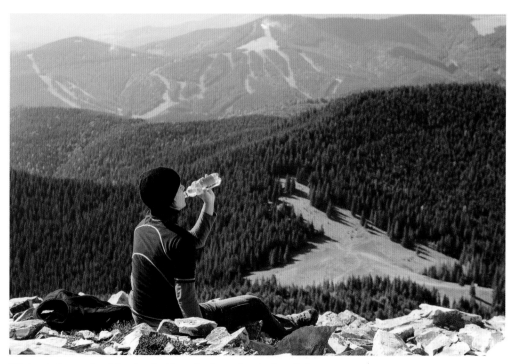

Water is important for hydration during physical activity.

Nutrition and Weight

When you consume basically the same number of calories as you expend, your body weight remains relatively stable. If you want to gain or lose weight, you must manipulate this balance between calories consumed and calories expended.

Gaining Weight

Some people have a difficult time gaining weight. This can be a result of a higher than normal BMR or a high physical activity level. When weight gain is a goal, the focus is on gaining muscle and not fat weight. To do this in a healthy way, you should consume more frequent meals with healthy snacks. For example, in addition to three main meals, consume three snacks per day. Consuming about 300 to 500 calories more per day would result in about a 1-pound (0.45 kg) per week weight gain. Healthy snacks include yogurt, peanut butter and jelly sandwiches, cereal with milk, fruit smoothies, and turkey sandwiches. It is also important to continue to exercise to ensure that the weight gain is mostly muscle. In particular, resistance training is an important factor for building muscle (see chapter 6 of this book for more information on resistance training). Although it will take some time, the slower the weight gain, the more likely it will be to consist of muscle gain and not fat or water gain.

Losing Weight

Weight loss is a more common goal than gaining weight. Losing weight involves a negative energy balance. This can be achieved by increasing exercise and decreasing caloric intake. See chapter 18, "Weight Management," for more details on weight loss.

hydration status is to look at the color of your urine; it should be a clear, pale yellow color (5). The darker the color of your urine the less hydrated you are. Another way to track fluid lost during exercise is to check your body weight before and after your workout. For each pound (0.45 kg) lost during exercise, you should consume about 16 to 20 ounces (475 to 600 mL) of water or sport performance beverage (26).

Supplements

There are a number of supplements on the market today, resulting in a multibillion dollar industry. It is beyond the scope of this chapter to discuss all of the nutritional supplements that are sold. If you are thinking about taking a multivitamin–mineral supplement, you should analyze your diet first to assess if a supplement is required. The best way to obtain nutrients is through whole foods (e.g., fruits, vegetables, whole grains; foods that are not processed). An analogy that can serve is this: If a bucket is already full, there is no need to continue to fill it. If you are interested in taking a supplement, you should first check with your primary health care provider. If you do decide to take a multivitamin–mineral supplement, consider taking it every other day to enhance your ability to digest and absorb it and to save money.

When considering a supplement, be cautious, as dietary supplements are not regulated by the Food and Drug Administration (FDA). Reports have been made of supplements being contaminated or not containing what is stated on the label (i.e., either more or less). One way to check the safety of supplements is to look for third-party testers (e.g., NSF Certified for Sport, http://nsfsport.com/). These testers take common supplements and test them to see if their labels accurately represent what is actually in them, check that no adulteration has occurred, and report on their safety.

The best way to know if a supplement is harmful, helpful, or neutral is to meet with a Registered Dietitian, especially one who specializes in sports nutrition. In addition, some supplements interact or interfere with medications. A Registered Dietitian will be able to guide you on safe and correct choices. A reliable website that can also help you to know if a supplement is beneficial or harmful is from the National Institutes of Health (34): www.nlm.nih.gov/medlineplus (and see the Drugs and Supplements section).

Understanding the importance of macronutrients, micronutrients, water, and the *Dietary Guidelines for Americans* provides a framework for improving your diet. Knowing how to read labels and how to calculate your energy needs helps you make healthy choices regarding your diet. A healthy diet should include a wide variety of foods that you enjoy. Following the *Dietary Guidelines for Americans* is a good start to working toward consuming a healthy, varied, and nutrient-dense diet that will help prevent disease and give you more energy each day.

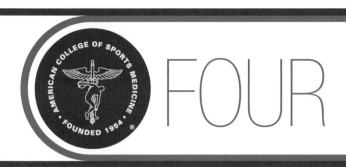

Promoting Healthy Habits: Getting Started and Staying Motivated

Knowing about the many benefits of a physically active life and nutritious dietary choices provides a foundation for action. However, knowing does not always translate into making healthy choices; the difficulty comes in actually acting on your knowledge of healthy behaviors. This chapter focuses on helping you advance from just knowing to doing. Whether you desire to start being more physically active, expand your current exercise program, make some nutritious substitutions, or improve your overall diet, you need to reflect on how *you* can make changes that work for *you*. Each person is unique with regard to health status, fitness level, work and family responsibilities, ethnic and social environments, and many other facets of life. Given the complexity of each individual, the chapter provides various methods and suggestions to allow you to find what works for you.

Motivation to Change

Developing and maintaining a physically active lifestyle involves attention to the issue of motivation. Motivation is the determination, drive, or desire with which you approach or avoid a behavior. Although this may seem to be a simple concept, many different forces make up your motivation to embrace or withdraw from a given behavior. In addition, behaviors tend to be ingrained over time and therefore are often difficult to modify. This may be a positive characteristic for healthy behaviors already in place, but may be an obstacle for change in those areas in need of improvement. However, change *is* possible, especially with the use of basic principles of behavior modification.

Self-Determination and Motivation

The idea of self-determination suggests that you develop your motivation for an activity based on both your psychological energy and the goal to which that energy or focus is directed. Rather than being an on-and-off switch, motivation slides across a continuum ranging from no or low extrinsic motivation to intrinsic motivation (1). Figure 4.1 provides an overview of the various levels of motivation: amotivation, extrinsic motivation (including external regulation, introjected regulation, identified regulation, and integrated regulation), and intrinsic motivation (1).

Amotivation

Amotivation represents the absence of motivation (1). For example, if you are at this level, you don't expect exercise to meet your needs and thus you have absolutely no interest in or intention to exercise. Amotivation often includes a "Why bother?" or "What difference can exercise make?" mindset. This level of motivation may be the result of negative experiences in the past that affect your beliefs about the purpose and benefits of exercise. The same is true in relation to nutrition. If you don't believe dietary changes can benefit your health, you will have little desire to alter your eating habits. To move beyond this level of motivation, consider the overwhelming evidence provided throughout this book on the positive potential impact of exercise and diet.

Extrinsic Motivation

Extrinsic motivation results in engaging in a behavior for a particular outcome or is based on outside factors (1). Levels of extrinsic motivation vary as to the degree to which they are internalized. The least internalized form is external regulation (1). Exercising in order to earn a T-shirt has an external focus. Selecting a side dish of fruit rather than french fries to avoid negative comments from health-focused coworkers is another example of external regulation. Motivation is based on seeking to gain

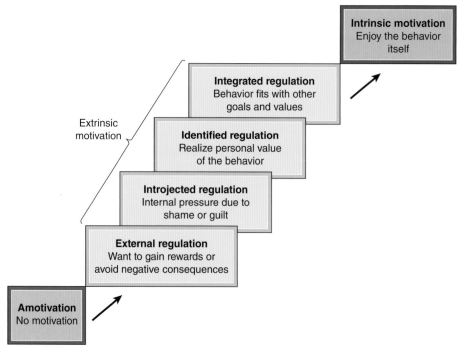

FIGURE 4.1   Motivation continuum.

Adapted by permission from American College of Sports Medicine, 2014, p. 284.

rewards or avoid negative consequences. Pressure to make healthy choices can also come internally due to shame or guilt; this is referred to as introjected regulation (1). An example is feeling guilty about not exercising after investing in a home treadmill. Although these types of external motivation have the potential to stimulate exercise initially or promote healthy dietary choices, because the behavior is not freely chosen, the changes are often short-lived and the chances of dropping out are higher.

Shifting toward finding personal importance in a given behavior provides a greater likelihood for sticking with the behavior for the long term. Acting on motivations to exercise that are free of pressure and evaluation by others gives you the best chance of sticking with your exercise plan. Identified regulation refers to believing in the value or importance of a given behavior (1). An example is making nutritious dietary choices because of your belief that eating well promotes health. The most internalized form of extrinsic motivation is integrated regulation and involves engaging in behaviors that are consistent with other goals and values (1). An example is exercising regularly as a habit consistent with goals of losing weight and improving fitness.

Intrinsic Motivation

Intrinsic motivation exists when the reason for exercise is the fun and satisfaction received from the exercise itself and when the reason for healthy food selections is the enjoyment of the meal itself. Intrinsic motivation has the highest degree of self-determination. This type of motivation is difficult to achieve because, in many ways, it is less of an achievement and more of an experience.

Understanding the levels of motivation can help you develop healthy habits that you will continue in the future. Moving from amotivation toward intrinsic motivation is possible through education, positive encouragement, and successful experiences. Although you may not always attain an intrinsic motivation, by adopting a positive approach to exercise and nutrition you can advance to motives known to increase participation and adherence. The following sections highlight some of the effective strategies for increasing healthy behaviors (1, 2).

Enhancing Self-Efficacy

Self-efficacy is the confidence you have in your ability and is a key factor in making changes in behavior. For example, do you believe you have the ability to be physically active? What and how you think about exercise affects the likelihood that you will begin or continue being physically active. Some ways to increase self-efficacy are included in this section (1, 2).

■ Q&A

Are there different types of self-efficacy?

With regard to exercise behavior, two types of self-efficacy have been identified: task self-efficacy and barriers self-efficacy (2). Task self-efficacy reflects your belief that you can do a particular activity. Barriers self-efficacy represents your belief that you can do that activity when faced with a barrier (e.g., limited time). Having belief in your ability both to do an activity and to continue with an exercise program when challenges arise is important when you are seeking to change a behavior.

Mastery Experiences

Mastery experiences involve selecting activities that you are able to successfully complete. This supports the premise "start low and go slow" when beginning with an exercise program or a new activity (2). By starting with activities that you are able to carry out, you can build your confidence to continue to exercise. Realize that the body takes time to adapt when you are beginning to be physically active or advancing in your current exercise program. Progression needs to start from where you are now rather than where you want to be. This could also apply to changes in diet. Rather than attempting a complete, abrupt overhaul of what you eat, consider some substitutions that increase the healthfulness of your diet. You can build on this success over time.

Vicarious Experiences

Vicarious experiences involve observing peers who are having positive experiences. For example, observing someone your age completing a 10K run may be inspiring to you—suggesting that you can train and do the same in the future. Reading of someone's successful weight loss using sound nutritional practices and regular physical activity could promote confidence in your ability to lose weight, if needed, with healthy choices. Seeing others like yourself realize success can promote your own confidence in doing the same.

Verbal Persuasion

Verbal persuasion involves receiving encouragement from others. Receiving encouraging feedback promotes confidence. Seek those who can provide that type of support and consider how you can provide support to someone else as well. A buddy system benefits both yourself and your health buddy! Feedback and support can even come from social media through connections maintained with online support groups or forums such as Facebook or Twitter (1).

Physiological Feedback

Physiological feedback includes many aspects such as enjoyment and positive mood. Reflect on the improvements in your fitness that are realized with a regular physical activity program and how these affect your ability to function in routine day-to-day activities. With regard to nutrition, you can enjoy healthy food choices, realizing the nutrients consumed provide energy for your daily activities.

Creating a Decisional Balance Sheet

Increasing your level of exercise and making better nutritional choices are major decisions. As with any big decision, creating a list of the pros and cons can be very productive. Consider the factors that support your decision to change while also acknowledging the factors that may inhibit that change. This is called a decisional balance sheet (1). See figure 4.2 for an example of a balance sheet related to exercise.

As you examine your own list of factors impeding your commitment to regular exercise, consider how you might modify them to move them to the pro side of the list, or at least how you might address them. For example, the extra time that a regular exercise program takes cannot be denied. However, you can modify your perspective on the time spent. You can think of your exercise time as a time to clear your mind and unwind from the stresses of school, work, or home responsibilities. You may select

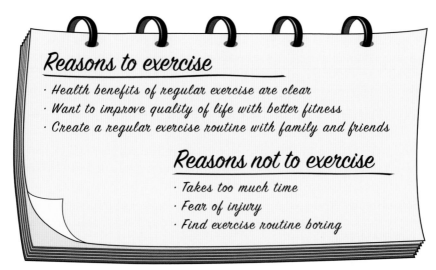

FIGURE 4.2   Sample decisional balance sheet.

aerobic activities such as treadmill walking or stationary biking that allow you to read or watch television—activities you find rewarding but typically don't take time to enjoy.

If you have a jam-packed schedule, consider breaking your exercise routine into multiple shorter bouts. You may be able to take advantage of your lunch break to add extra activity to your day. Another option many people use is an early morning exercise routine. Although you may need to adjust your bedtime, morning workouts ensure that you exercise before the hectic schedule of the day takes over. The key is to reflect on your schedule and find an option that fits the best into your daily routine.

Another common concern is the fear of injury or even death with increased physical activity. As discussed in chapter 2, certain health-related situations may require you to meet with your health care provider to increase the safety of your exercise program. This is the reason for completing the preparticipation screening process outlined in chapter 2. For most apparently healthy people, starting with light to moderate intensity and progressing slowly minimizes the likelihood of injury as well as heart attack or death (2). The health benefits of a regular physical activity program are greater than the risk of adverse events for almost everyone (9).

Finally, if you find your current exercise routine boring—find other options! Your exercise program should include activities you enjoy. Consider adding more variety or joining a group exercise class. Listening to music or downloading an audio book can provide mental variety even if you keep your activity the same. Remember, when using a headset, be sure to be indoors or in a controlled environment so you do not become distracted and fail to observe traffic or others around you.

Setting Goals

Goal setting is one of the most important aspects of successful behavior change (1, 2). Without goals, you cannot develop a plan because you don't know where you want to go. That would be like going on a trip but never identifying the geographic location of your final destination. To succeed, you need to develop both long-term and short-term goals. Long-term goals are like your final destination; short-term goals are the individual routes that will get you there.

Short-term goals are those that can be realistically accomplished within a brief period of time such as this week or this month. For example, if you have been totally inactive, a short-term goal might be to walk around your neighborhood for 10 minutes each night after work for the upcoming week. This short-term goal has some valuable characteristics that you can remember with the acronym SMARTS, as follows (2):

- **S**pecific: The activity has been clearly defined in terms of both length and location. The goal is unambiguous with respect to what is desired.
- **M**easurable: At the end of the week, you can reflect back on whether you walked each day after work. This is better than having a goal such as "I want to get in better shape," which would be hard to measure.
- **A**ction-oriented: The goal includes an activity rather than generalities or an outcome, such as improving fitness or losing weight. It is focused on what you will actually be doing.
- **R**ealistic: The location for the activity is convenient, and the length of the walk is not excessive. Too often, goals are so far out of reach that they become a source of discouragement rather than encouragement. Your goals should be relevant to you and firmly based in the reality of what you can accomplish.
- **T**imely: This goal is linked with a specific time frame. Rather than being too open-ended, the goal specifies the upcoming week. Without a time-centered approach, you might be tempted to procrastinate starting or moving forward with an exercise program.
- **S**elf-determined: Rather than having someone else set your course of action, you need to be the one to define your goals (and this will promote your self-efficacy as well).

SMARTS short-term goals can provide wonderful encouragement and focus. In addition, they can instill a sense of self-confidence that you can perform the activity. By creating a series of short-term goals, you can build toward your long-term goals.

Long-term goals are those that you can achieve in the future—three months to a year from now. With careful planning, meeting your short-term goals should lead to accomplishing your long-term goals. For example, a long-term goal for a person who is currently jogging only a mile at a time might be to complete a 5K (3.1 miles) race three months from now without having to walk. To prepare for this race, the time spent jogging needs to increase in order to progress from being able to run only about one-third of the target distance to being able to run continuously for the entire 5K distance. Short-term goals could be set weekly with increased distance (e.g., adding an extra lap or two when running on the track). By mapping out short-term goals, an effective plan can be established, leading to successfully meeting the long-term goal (1).

Continuing to set new goals or revising prior goals keeps you moving forward in your journey toward improved fitness and health. Setting both short-term and long-term goals in each of the fitness areas allows you to individualize your exercise program. You may already be walking on a regular basis but see that you have neglected your muscular fitness or flexibility. By including goals in all areas, you can create a balanced exercise program. The same can be done with the various dietary components. For example, are you consuming adequate amounts of fruits and vegetables? Are you consistently replacing refined grains with whole grains? Is your sodium intake in the recommended range? As you identify your own strengths and weaknesses, you can

■ Q&A

How can I turn my goal from a dream into a reality?

Writing down your goals is helpful. Whether you put pen on paper or use technology to document your goals, this process of clearly identifying your goals can give you an opportunity to reflect on what you really want to accomplish with your exercise program and with your nutritional plan, providing you with a clear reference point. Keep your short-term goals prominently visible. Some people write their goals in their schedule books or post them on a note board, mirror, or even the refrigerator. Smartphone apps are also available for documenting and tracking goals. Find a method that works for you, one that allows you to see your goals as a reminder of the actions you want to take. You can check off completed short-term goals and add new ones as you progress toward your long-term goals.

focus additional attention on the areas in which you struggle, and you can seek to maintain your status in the areas in which you already have a solid foundation.

Reinforcing Behavior

Using rewards is another way to promote positive behavior change (2). External rewards may be tangible (for example, purchasing a new pair of running shoes) or even social (for example, praise and encouragement from a family member or friend). Internal rewards come from within you. An example is the feeling of accomplishment when you try a new activity or when you complete a workout that was challenging. Although all rewards are beneficial, doing activities for internal rewards, or intrinsic reasons, tends to be related to one's ability to stick with a program for the long term.

Finding Social Support

Social support is a very strong motivator (2). Consider the encouragement provided by a friend who supervises a young child so that a parent can head outside for a run or attend a group exercise session at a local health club. In addition, parents who model an active lifestyle are providing a wonderful example for their children. It is even better to be active together as a family. A family outing to a local park can be a great stress reliever as well as an opportunity for everyone to be active. Physical activity is important throughout the lifespan. Developing active habits early in life will have lifelong benefits.

Social support skills allow you to reach out to others. Establishing a network of people you trust can help facilitate healthy lifestyle changes. Beyond the family unit, consider coworkers and neighbors, as well as fitness and health care professionals, as sources of support. Others in your personal network can provide encouragement, assistance, and guidance as needed (2).

Participating in group activities—with family members, friends, or local groups—can also be a strong motivator to stay active. Most communities have clubs or associations of people with similar interests (e.g., cycling, running, mall walking, ballroom dancing). These are wonderful opportunities to meet new people and find real enjoyment in your exercise program.

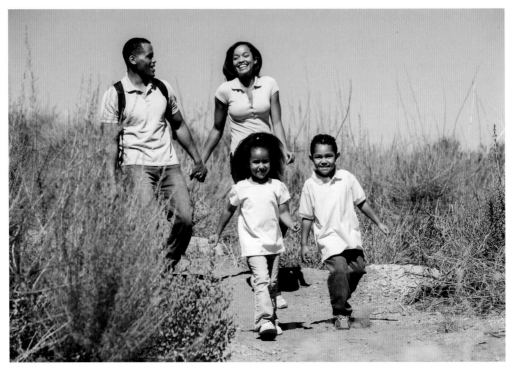

Exercising as a family is a great way to build fitness together.

If your family members or close friends do not support your desire to be active or to improve your diet, seek out other support systems. Some people, when facing their own health problems, may feel threatened by your resolution to move forward to better health. Don't let others sabotage your plans. Find people who have goals for activity and nutrition similar to yours. By encouraging each other, you can generate the motivation to continue. Hopefully, over time, your example will persuade your family members and friends to also join you in making healthy lifestyle choices.

Sticking With Your Plan

With your goals for both physical activity and nutrition written down, you now need to plan for success. To reap health and fitness benefits, your plan needs to become a regular part of your life—for your life. This section outlines a number of skills and strategies that experts have identified as helpful for promoting lasting behavior change.

Promoting Change

Resolving to change is the first step, but actually changing the behavior is key to realizing health and fitness benefits. Various tactics can be included to promote behavior change (6).

Counterconditioning

Counterconditioning involves using a behavior that circumvents the problem (5). For example, if you want to cut down on time spent sitting and watching TV, you instead make an appointment to meet a friend for a walk at a nearby park. On the nutritional front, you may want to avoid the draw of the vending machine, so you plan ahead by bringing an appealing and nutritious snack.

Fading

Rather than attempting abrupt changes, fading reflects a more gradual reduction in an undesired behavior as you increase the desired behavior (5). Extreme changes in diet or in exercise can be overwhelming. Instead, make a series of smaller changes. Reducing time spent sitting while gradually increasing the time spent exercising would be manageable. Dietary changes also can be promoted with fading. As you shift your food and beverage choices to healthier options, you will promote new habits that can be continued.

Stimulus Control

Surround yourself with reminders to make healthy choices (5). Having a bowl of fresh fruit on the kitchen counter and hanging a picture of a favorite hiking trail on your wall are ways to keep a focus on healthy behaviors. Stimulus control provides a positive and uplifting framework that can promote development of healthy habits.

Overcoming Barriers

Breaking down barriers often requires creativity, assistance from others, and careful planning (2). What factors are getting in your way when it comes to exercise or good nutritional choices? Table 4.1 explores some physical activity barriers and includes helpful suggestions on how to overcome those barriers (8). Frequent barriers to making good nutritional choices and tips on overcoming the barriers are included in table 4.2 (4, 7).

TABLE 4.1   **Suggestions for Overcoming Physical Activity Barriers**

Lack of time	• Identify available time slots. Monitor your daily activities for one week. Identify at least three 30-min time slots you could use for physical activity. • Add physical activity to your daily routine. For example, walk or ride your bike to work or shopping, organize school activities around physical activity, walk the dog, exercise while you watch TV, park farther away from your destination. • Select activities requiring minimal time, such as walking, jogging, or stair climbing.
Social influence	• Explain your interest in physical activity to friends and family. Ask them to support your efforts. • Invite friends and family members to exercise with you. Plan social activities involving exercise. • Develop new friendships with physically active people. Join a group, such as the YMCA or a hiking club.
Lack of energy	• Schedule physical activity for times in the day or week when you feel energetic. • Convince yourself that if you give it a chance, physical activity will increase your energy level; then try it.

> *continued*

Table 4.1 > *continued*

Lack of motivation	• Plan ahead. Make physical activity a regular part of your daily or weekly schedule and write it on your calendar. • Invite a friend to exercise with you on a regular basis; both of you write it on your calendars. • Join an exercise group or class.
Fear of injury	• Learn how to warm up and cool down to prevent injury. • Learn how to exercise appropriately considering your age, fitness level, skill level, and health status. • Choose activities involving minimal risk.
Lack of skill	• Select activities requiring no new skills, such as walking, climbing stairs, or jogging. • Take a class to develop new skills.
Lack of resources	• Select activities that require minimal facilities or equipment, such as walking, jogging, jumping rope, or calisthenics. • Identify inexpensive, convenient resources available in your community (community education programs, park and recreation programs, work-site programs, and so on).
Weather conditions	• Develop a set of regular activities that are always available regardless of weather (indoor cycling, aerobic dance, indoor swimming, calisthenics, stair climbing, rope skipping, mall walking, dancing, gymnasium games, and so on)
Travel	• Put a jump rope in your suitcase, and jump rope. • Walk the halls and climb the stairs in hotels. • Stay in places with swimming pools or exercise facilities. • Join the YMCA or YWCA (ask about reciprocal membership agreements). • Visit the local shopping mall and walk for half an hour or more. • Bring your MP3 player to listen to your favorite aerobic exercise music.
Family obligations	• Trade babysitting time with a friend, neighbor, or family member who also has small children. • Exercise with the kids—go for a walk together, play tag or other running games, get an aerobic dance or exercise tape for kids (there are several on the market), and exercise together. You can spend time together and still get your exercise. • Jump rope, do calisthenics, ride a stationary bicycle, or use other home gymnasium equipment while the kids are busy playing or are sleeping. • Try to exercise when the kids are not around (e.g., during school hours or their nap time).
Retirement years	• Look upon your retirement as an opportunity to become more active instead of less. Spend more time gardening, walking the dog, and playing with your grandchildren. Children with short legs and grandparents with slower gaits are often great walking partners. • Learn a new skill you've always been interested in, such as ballroom dancing, square dancing, or swimming. • Now that you have the time, make regular physical activity a part of every day. Go for a walk every morning or every evening before dinner. Treat yourself to an exercycle and ride every day while reading a book or magazine.

Adapted from U.S. Department of Health and Human Services, Centers for Disease Control and Prevention, 2011.

TABLE 4.2 **Suggestions for Overcoming Barriers to Healthy Dietary Choices**

Dislike vegetables	• Explore the wide range of different vegetables that are available and choose some you're willing to try. • Try mixed dishes that include vegetables, like stir-fries, vegetable soups, or pasta with marinara sauce. • When eating out, choose a vegetable (other than french fries) as a side dish.
Don't or can't drink milk	• You don't need to drink milk, but you do need the nutrients it provides. You can get these nutrients from yogurt, from fortified soy milk (soy beverage), or from low-fat cheese. • Milk or other dairy foods can also be incorporated into lots of foods and drinks including lattes, puddings, and soups.
Family resists trying new foods	• Exposure to a new item may take more than a few tries before the new food is accepted. • Be a good role model by showing your willingness to try new foods. • Encourage family members to pick out a new food to try.
Cost of fresh fruits and vegetables	• Buy fresh fruits and vegetables that are in season; they are easy to get, have more flavor, and are usually less expensive. • You can also try canned or frozen. For canned items, choose fruit canned in 100% fruit juice and vegetables with "low sodium" or "no salt added" on the label. • Check the local newspaper, online, and at the store for sales, coupons, and specials that will cut food costs.
Don't know what to eat	• Follow the *Dietary Guidelines* (see chapter 3 for details) including a focus on vegetables, fruits, whole grains, low- or no-fat dairy, seafood, legumes, and nuts. • Keep to a lower intake of sugar-sweetened food and beverages and refined grains. • Become knowledgeable on how to read the food labels.
Difficulty eating healthfully when dining out	• To help keep portion sizes in check, consider ordering a side dish or appetizer-size portion rather than a regular entrée. • Select water or other drink without added sugars. • Opt for a salad and ask for the dressing on the side so you can control the amount. • Select steamed, grilled, or broiled dishes rather than foods fried in oil or cooked in butter. • Avoid buffets and "all-you-can-eat" options and order an item from the menu instead.

Sources: USDA Center for Nutrition Policy and Promotion and Health Canada.

Preventing Relapse

Relapse prevention skills help you maintain your behavioral change efforts even when faced with situations that may increase the likelihood of a lapse or a poor health choice (2). Learning to avoid situations can help you avoid a complete relapse. For example, consider the time you plan to exercise. If you know that mornings are typically a rushed time for you, don't schedule a workout class at that time, as you may be more likely to skip the class. On the nutritional front, buffets, by their "all-you-can-eat" nature, encourage overconsumption. If possible, select other options when dining out or simply order an entrée from the menu, thus encouraging portion control in advance. By anticipating circumstances that could derail your exercise and nutrition goals, you can plan ahead to avoid those situations and help yourself stay on track.

Another way to prevent relapse is to develop a plan for high-risk situations (2). Life situations arise that may disrupt your progress toward health and fitness goals. Don't let this be discouraging. Instead, plan for it. Your exercise program is not an all-or-none endeavor. For example, when traveling for business, you may become stuck in the airport with a delayed flight. Rather than sit and fret about the delay (over which you have no control), take a brisk walk around the terminal. When traveling, consider staying in hotels that have fitness rooms. Although they are not ideal, typically you can find activities that will complement your program. If there is no fitness room, walk the halls or consider doing some calisthenics and stretching in your room. Ask the hotel staff about safe places to walk or jog in the neighborhood.

As with your exercise plan, your diet involves many small decisions made throughout the day, and planning ahead can help avoid lapses. A healthy diet includes focusing on a higher intake of some items (for example, vegetables, fruits, whole grains, low- or nonfat dairy, seafood, legumes, and nuts) while keeping to a lower intake of other items (for example, sugar-sweetened items, refined grains, saturated fats, and high-sodium items) (10). Rather than being discouraged by an overly stringent plan in which foods are placed into "good" versus "bad" categories, consider strategies for promoting a healthy pattern of eating. For example, for a tasty pasta dish, consider using whole-grain pasta rather than refined options along with a tomato-based sauce rather than a high-fat creamy sauce. Preplanning meals can be helpful at home as well as at work or school. Bringing a wholesome lunch or packing some nutritious snacks can help avoid reliance on fast food or vending machines during the day.

Unfortunately, plans and intentions to maintain a regular exercise program and make nutritious dietary choices can fail. Even then, use the situation to your advantage by taking the opportunity to explore what worked previously and what aspects led to a lapse (11). Researchers have actually found that lapses have the potential to strengthen one's resolve (6). Be willing to honestly consider what factors brought about the lapse, and use those insights to renew your focus on your health and fitness goals.

Dealing With Setbacks

Will you experience setbacks in your path to better health and fitness? Very likely. When sickness, travel, family responsibilities, work obligations, and other unavoidable situations arise, realize they are just short-term holdups, not permanent derailments. Have a return plan of action in place (2). When faced with a setback in your exercise program, you might have to reverse your timeline a bit. For example, after an illness, you should start back slowly rather than jumping right back to where you left off. Although you may feel frustrated at losing fitness, be encouraged that you are able to start again and build back up. Similarly, when you find that your dietary plan is off track, start once again with making healthy substitutions, and before you know it, you will be off and running toward a wholesome approach to your diet. Keep a positive mindset by realizing that a single missed workout or overconsumption at a holiday party is not the end of the world. With this approach to the inevitable setbacks that come along, you can keep moving toward your goals.

Self-Monitoring

Self-monitoring involves observing and recording your behaviors as well as your thoughts and feelings (1). Keeping tabs on your exercise and nutrition helps keep you on track. Just as regular car maintenance gives you worry-free driving, taking a few moments to check your body's progress ensures that you are still on course to meet your goals. One way to do this is to write down what you have accomplished each week along with your reflections on those activities.

Although logging your exercise accomplishments or your dietary choices can be done using paper and pencil (see figure 4.3 for a simple example of an exercise log), other options are available. Technology provides many interesting possibilities on monitoring behavior. For physical activity, consider a heart rate monitor, pedometer, or other commercial activity tracker. In addition to tracking physical activity, many smartphones have options to help monitor dietary intake. Whether recording on paper or using technology, monitoring your behaviors can help you check progress toward your goals. By tracking behavior as well as how you felt about the experience, you can reflect on your progress, including observation of barriers to achieving your goals.

No matter the method used, the key is to take time to reflect. Look for trends and patterns. Do you find that your approach to the weekend promotes or reduces your

FIGURE 4.3

Activity log.

Day	A-M-F-NM*	Time or distance	Comments (heart rate, rating of perceived exertion, health status, environmental conditions, etc.)
Sunday			
Monday			
Tuesday			
Wednesday			
Thursday			
Friday			
Saturday			
Weekly summary	A: # workouts = _____; # minutes =_____		
	M: # workouts = _____; # minutes =_____		
	F: # workouts = _____; # minutes =_____		
	NM: # workouts = _____; # minutes =_____		
Next week's goal			

*A = aerobic; M = muscular; F = flexibility; NM = neuromotor.

From ACSM, 2017, *ACSM's complete guide to fitness and health*, 2nd ed. (Champaign, IL: Human Kinetics). Adapted from B. Bushman and J.C. Young, 2005, p. 188.

activity? As seasons change, do you struggle to maintain a regular exercise routine? Does eating out affect your dietary choices or are you able to maintain a healthy approach to your food and beverage selections? What dietary substitutions have you made, and how have they influenced your overall diet? A reflective and mindful approach can help you to make any needed adjustments in order to continue moving toward your goals.

Writing a Contract

How strong is your intention to be active and make healthy dietary choices? What are you doing to bridge the gap between your intentions and taking action? Many of the techniques discussed throughout this chapter promote this link. You may also find developing a contract to be effective. Contract components may include a clearly stated goal (remember the SMARTS characteristics), benefits of reaching the goal, what steps will be taken to meet the goal, what activities promote meeting the goal, what barriers inhibit reaching the goal and how you will overcome those barriers, and short-term goal(s). See figure 4.4 for an example of an exercise contract (3).

Taking a Long-Term Approach

One final consideration regarding behavior change and motivation relates to the development of a long-term, or lifetime, approach. In spite of advertisements that promise fitness or extreme weight loss in a week, the reality is that changes take time and require an ongoing commitment. Modern society has conditioned everyone to value things that are instant and disposable. This "now" perspective conflicts with the long-term commitment needed for building a healthy life. This mismatch in values likely contributes to the high dropout rate observed among new exercisers and the difficulty people have sustaining new behaviors.

Immediate pleasure is not always the outcome of exercise participation. Rather, physical discomfort such as muscle aches may occur, especially in the early weeks after starting a new program or advancing your exercise level in a given area. Changes in diet can be a challenge, and benefits to health or changes in body weight are not immediately apparent. Acknowledge the challenges you may face in the short term and experience each moment for what it is. Balance the challenges and effort in the short term with the greater feeling of well-being that will result in the long term.

FIGURE 4.4

Sample behavior contract.

Goal: Walk 10,000 steps on each day for a full week as noted on my pedometer
Timeframe: 3 months from now
Benefits: Walking more throughout the day will promote my desire to be more active and reduce sedentary time. In addition, more activity will help me with my weight loss goals and will promote my overall health and fitness.

To reach my goal, I will:
- Wear my pedometer every day and keep track of my step count in my activity log
- Walk at least 15 minutes during my lunch hour and 15 minutes after dinner
- Take the stairs rather than the elevator
- Walk while talking on the phone to friends and family

Goal supporting activities:
- Keep an extra pair of walking shoes at work
- Find co-workers who are interested in walking with me
- Ask family members to join me for a walk after dinner
- Download some music I enjoy onto my phone so I can listen while I walk

Barriers and strategies to overcome barriers:
- When unable to walk outside due to the weather, I will walk on a treadmill or in the hallway of my building.
- When I have a work lunch that restricts my ability to walk over the lunch hour, I will include 10 minutes of walking before and after work.
- When I forget to wear my pedometer, I will continue with my typical activity and estimate number of steps from similar activity days.

Initial short-term goal: I will wear my pedometer each day for the upcoming week and record my number of steps. I will use this as a baseline to see how far I have to progress to reach 10,000 steps per day.

Signed: _____ Date: _____

Reevaluation dates (every two weeks):

Date: _____ Update to contract: _____

Date: _____ Update to contract: _____

Date: _____ Update to contract: _____

Adapted by permission from J. Buckworth, 2012, p. 432.

Deciding to take charge of your health and to improve your fitness is a powerful resolution. Understanding the basic components of fitness and what constitutes a healthy diet gives you the tools you need. With tools in hand, you must reflect on what is important to you. Putting your goals down on paper and examining your reasons for exercising and making nutritious dietary choices will give you a perspective that allows you to create an individualized approach. Effective planning considers goals, available resources, and social support. Finding ways to overcome barriers and recover from setbacks or temporary lapses is key to developing a lifelong approach to health. This is not a static process but an evolution that continues to be refined as you develop new and more challenging goals.

Part II

Exercise and Activity for Building a Better You

A complete exercise program includes activities that promote aerobic fitness, muscular fitness, flexibility, and neuromotor fitness. You will gain insight into the importance of each area and acquire the tools to create an individualized program that fits with your health status, fitness level, and personal goals. Chapters 5 to 8 contain specific activities that you can make part of your exercise program. No matter whether you are just starting out or are already a regular exerciser, these chapters guide you in taking the next steps in developing your complete exercise program.

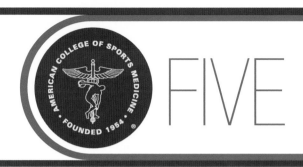

FIVE

Improving Your Aerobic Fitness

Consider how you can feel breathless when going up a flight of stairs quickly—your body is showing the need for oxygen. "Aerobic" means "with oxygen," and aerobic fitness, otherwise referred to as cardiorespiratory endurance, pertains to how well your body is able to take in oxygen and put that oxygen to use. Activities that involve large-muscle groups engaged in dynamic movement for prolonged periods of time are considered aerobic (2, 6). Your cardiovascular system (heart and blood vessels) and your respiratory system (lungs and air passages) work together during longer-duration activities to supply working muscles and organs with the oxygen they need. Examples of aerobic activities include walking, jogging, running, cycling, swimming, dancing, hiking, and team sports such as basketball and soccer.

Health and Fitness Benefits of Aerobic Activity

Regular and consistent aerobic activity improves your cardiorespiratory endurance. In other words, your heart, blood vessels, and lungs benefit from working harder than normal. Exercise improves your cardiorespiratory function by increasing the activity of these organ systems above what they experience at rest. Over time, your body adapts to these stresses and your fitness improves (2, 6).

Cardiorespiratory endurance is an important aspect of health for a number of reasons (2, 6, 8):

- Better cardiorespiratory endurance typically leads to higher levels of routine physical activity as you go about your day-to-day life. This in turn provides additional health benefits.

- Low levels of cardiorespiratory fitness are associated with higher risk of premature death from all causes, and specifically from cardiovascular disease. To look at this from a more positive perspective, increases in cardiorespiratory fitness are associated with a decreased risk of death from all causes.

- Aerobic fitness is an important foundation that allows you to engage in activities of daily living with greater ease.
- Increases in cardiorespiratory endurance allow you to more fully participate in recreational and sport activities.
- Aerobic activities that promote cardiorespiratory endurance also burn a relatively large number of calories and thus help to maintain appropriate body weight.

This is not an exhaustive list but does demonstrate the wide-ranging benefits of aerobic exercise for health as well as fitness.

Aerobic Fitness Assessments

Assessing aerobic fitness can provide helpful insights on your current status as well as on the progress you are making in your exercise program over time. Before engaging in any active measurement, be sure to complete the preparticipation screening steps (including follow-up with your health care provider if indicated) outlined in chapter 2. This process is intended to help verify your readiness for exercise testing and future physical activity. If you are already currently active and have no cardiovascular, metabolic, or renal disease, then you can consider any of the assessments described in the following section. If you have not been regularly active, or if you have noted any medical condition warranting lower exercise intensity or have any activity restrictions recommended by your health care provider, then select less intense assessments and

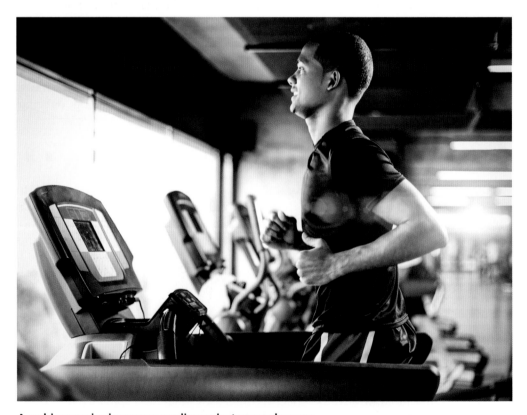

Aerobic exercise improves cardiorespiratory endurance.

consider consulting with your health care provider to ensure you are ready for exercise testing. Additional considerations are provided for each assessment described in the following sections.

Assessing Heart Rate

Perhaps the simplest fitness assessment reflecting aerobic fitness is heart rate, which is reported in beats per minute. Heart rate naturally increases during exercise. The higher the intensity, the faster your heart must beat to bring oxygen and nutrients to your working muscles. As you gain fitness, however, your heart rate will be lower at rest as well as in response to a given level of exercise. As a result of aerobic training, the heart becomes a better pump. Your heart can now do the same job while beating more slowly because it is able to push out more blood with each heartbeat. This is evidence of your body adapting to the exercise and improvement in your cardiorespiratory fitness.

You can determine your heart rate by finding a location on your body where an artery (a blood vessel carrying blood from the heart to the rest of the body) is close to the surface of the skin so you can feel your pulse, which is the slight surge in blood flow that occurs when the heart contracts. Common locations are the radial artery in the wrist and the carotid artery in the neck (see figure 5.1). Use the tips of your middle and index fingers to feel your pulse. If you use the carotid, be sure to keep the pressure light. Too much pressure at this location can alter your heart rate artificially.

Resting heart rate can be determined first thing in the morning or when you have been seated, relaxed, and inactive for a period of time. To measure resting heart rate you will need a timing device that displays time in seconds. Locate one of the arteries just described, and simply count the number of beats (pulses) you feel for 1 minute.

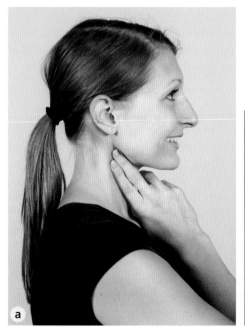
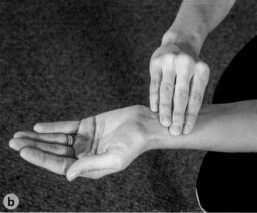

FIGURE 5.1   *(a)* Carotid and *(b)* radial artery pulse locations.

▪ Q&A

What is a typical resting heart rate for an adult?

For most adults, the number is between 60 and 100, but if your heart rate is lower than 60 or higher than 100 after multiple resting measurements, you should mention this to your health care provider.

Exercise heart rate is just as easy to measure as resting heart rate, but because heart rate steadily returns to a resting rate once you stop physical activity, finding your pulse and beginning your count immediately upon stopping is important. Take your pulse for 15 seconds and multiply the resulting number by 4. The answer is your exercise heart rate in beats per minute.

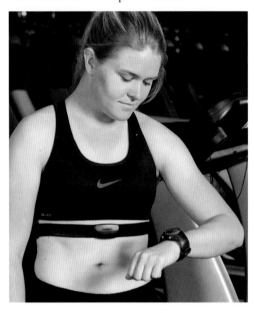

FIGURE 5.2   Heart rate monitor.

If manually taking your pulse is too difficult, consider making an investment in a heart rate monitor (an example is shown in figure 5.2). A heart rate monitor allows for a constant real-time readout of your heart rate by way of a transmitter (worn around the chest) that electronically communicates with a receiver that looks like a wristwatch. Heart rate is displayed on the receiver in beats per minute. The cost of heart rate monitors varies widely depending on their features (e.g., programmable heart rate zones, memory features to download to a computer after a workout, timekeeping functions). The simplest models that display only heart rate typically cost around $25. They are very durable and allow for easy checks of your heart rate during exercise.

Estimating Aerobic Fitness Level

Aerobic fitness is typically assessed by looking at maximal oxygen consumption, also called $\dot{V}O_{2max}$. $\dot{V}O_{2max}$ is a marker of your body's ability to take in and use oxygen. The higher this value is, the better your aerobic fitness is (2). Complex laboratory tests can most precisely determine your $\dot{V}O_{2max}$, but you can get a reasonable estimate from simple tests such as the Rockport One-Mile Walking Test or the 1.5-mile run test, both of which are described in this section. Other assessments are available for older people (e.g., 6-minute walk test) as well as younger individuals. For youth, a shorter-distance run test is often used (see One-Mile Run Test for Youth later in this chapter) (3).

Select one of these tests based on your current health status, as well as physical activity and perceived fitness level. The walking test is more appropriate if you are planning to begin an exercise program after a period of inactivity or currently engage in moderate levels of exercise. If you are healthy and more active, the run test is another option. Each test and the associated calculations produce an estimation of your aerobic capacity. Use that result and the numbers provided in table 5.1 to determine your fitness level by age and sex (2).

TABLE 5.1 Fitness Levels for Aerobic Capacity* in Males and Females

Males	Age				
	20 to 29	30 to 39	40 to 49	50 to 59	60 to 69
Superior	66.3 or higher	59.8 or higher	55.6 or higher	50.7 or higher	43.0 or higher
Excellent	57.1 to 66.2	51.6 to 59.7	46.7 to 55.5	41.2 to 50.6	36.1 to 42.9
Good	50.2 to 57.0	45.2 to 51.5	40.3 to 46.6	35.1 to 41.1	30.5 to 36.0
Fair	44.9 to 50.1	39.6 to 45.1	35.7 to 40.2	30.7 to 35.0	26.6 to 30.4
Poor	38.1 to 44.8	34.1 to 39.5	30.5 to 35.6	26.1 to 30.6	22.4 to 26.5
Very poor	38.0 or lower	34.0 or lower	30.4 or lower	26.0 or lower	22.3 or lower

Females	Age				
	20 to 29	30 to 39	40 to 49	50 to 59	60 to 69
Superior	56.0 or higher	45.8 or higher	41.7 or higher	35.9 or higher	29.4 or higher
Excellent	46.5 to 55.9	37.5 to 45.6	34.0 to 41.6	28.6 to 35.8	24.6 to 29.3
Good	40.6 to 46.4	32.2 to 37.4	28.7 to 39.9	25.2 to 28.5	21.2 to 24.5
Fair	34.6 to 40.5	28.2 to 32.1	24.9 to 28.6	21.8 to 25.1	18.9 to 21.1
Poor	28.6 to 34.5	24.1 to 28.1	21.3 to 24.8	19.1 to 21.7	16.5 to 18.8
Very poor	28.5 or lower	24.0 or lower	21.2 or lower	19.0 or lower	16.4 or lower

*Aerobic capacity or $\dot{V}O_{2max}$ expressed in mL·kg^{-1}·min^{-1}.

Adapted by permission from American College of Sports Medicine, 2018.

Rockport One-Mile Walking Test

The Rockport One-Mile Walking Test is a way to estimate $\dot{V}O_{2max}$ (2). To complete this test, you should have the ability to walk 1 mile continuously. Choose a day without windy weather for testing. Ideally, you should perform the One-Mile Walking Test using an outdoor or indoor running track so that you can be certain that the distance you walk is no more or less than 1 mile. A standard quarter-mile track would be ideal (four laps on the inside lane), but many tracks are metric. If you are on a 400-meter track, then you will need to complete four laps on the inside lane plus an additional 9.3 meters (equal to approximately 31 ft). If a track is not available, any measured course will work as long as the surface is smooth and the course is flat. Grab a comfortable pair of shoes and a stopwatch. Walk the course as rapidly as you can without jogging or running, and record the time it takes for you to complete the mile. You also need to take your pulse as previously described immediately after you complete the mile walk.

Computing your results from the Rockport One-Mile Walking Test takes a bit of work, but the math is very simple when you plug results into one of the formulas shown here (numbers in bold are constant in the equations and thus are predetermined):

Males

139.150

Minus (**0.1692** × ____ weight in kilograms)

Minus (**0.3877** × ____ age in years)

Minus (**3.2649** × ____ time in minutes)

Minus (**0.1565** × ____ heart rate in beats per minute)

= ____ Aerobic capacity

Females

132.835

Minus (**0.1692** × ____ weight in kilograms)

Minus (**0.3877** × ____ age in years)

Minus (**3.2649** × ____ time in minutes)

Minus (**0.1565** × ____ heart rate in beats per minute)

= ____ Aerobic capacity

To obtain your weight in kilograms, multiply your weight in pounds by 0.454. For the time factor, you might wonder how to account for the number of seconds. For example, suppose you completed the one-mile walk in 14 minutes and 25 seconds. The 25 seconds needs to be expressed as a fraction (decimal number) of a minute. To do that, simply divide the number by 60 (because there are 60 seconds in a minute). In this case, 25 seconds would be about 0.42 of a minute, so you would use the number 14.42 in your calculation of aerobic capacity.

The answer you calculate is your aerobic capacity and refers to the amount of oxygen your body can use each minute—more specifically, the number of milliliters of oxygen your body uses per unit of body weight every minute ($mL \cdot kg^{-1} \cdot min^{-1}$). The more oxygen your body can use, the better your aerobic fitness level is. Once you have determined your aerobic capacity, find your fitness classification level in table 5.1.

1.5-Mile Run Test

Just as the Rockport One-Mile Walking Test is a way to estimate aerobic capacity, so too is the 1.5-mile (2.4 km) run (2). Because of the higher intensity and longer distance of this test, it is not appropriate for beginners, anyone with symptoms of or known heart disease, or anyone with risk factors or other health concerns as determined by a health screening or a health care provider.

To perform this test, choose a day without windy weather and use an outdoor or indoor running track. If you are on a quarter-mile track, this will involve six laps in the inside lane. If you are using a 400-meter track, it will involve six laps plus an additional 14 meters (46 ft) to complete the full distance of 1.5 miles. Wear a comfortable pair of running shoes and have a stopwatch handy. Because this test requires you to run as fast as you can for 1.5 miles, you should walk a lap or two to warm up. At the track, run as rapidly as you can for 1.5 miles, timing yourself to the nearest second. For this test, there is no need to record your heart rate. This test is challenging, so be sure to walk a lap or two to cool down after completion, and rehydrate as needed afterward.

The math used to interpret your results is much simpler than that for the Rockport One-Mile Walking Test. Use the following formula to estimate your aerobic capacity:

Aerobic capacity = (483 ÷ _____ time in minutes) + 3.5

As with the One-Mile Walking Test, this calculated value is an estimate of your aerobic capacity, or $\dot{V}O_{2max}$. Because the number itself may not have much meaning, be sure to consult table 5.1 to check on your status compared to others of your age and sex (2). The higher the value, the better.

6-Minute Walk Test

Although some older adults may be comfortable completing the one-mile walk or 1.5-mile run test, another option is a 6-minute walk test (7). The 6-minute walk test could also be considered if you have been very inactive and are currently deconditioned. The test requires you to determine the distance you can walk in 6 minutes around a 50-yard (45.7 m) rectangular area (see figure 5.3 for the setup showing the number of yards walked). Focusing on a time rather than a particular distance covered allows individuals of all abilities to assess their fitness. Normal ranges for older adults are found in table 5.2. If your score is over the range listed, consider yourself above average; if your score falls short of the range, consider yourself below average (7).

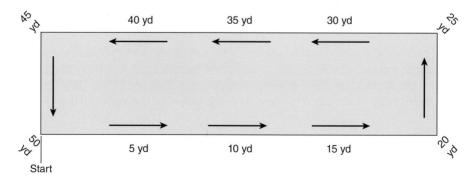

FIGURE 5.3   Setup for 6-minute walk.

Adapted by permission from R.E. Rikli and C.J. Jones, 2013, p. 76.

TABLE 5.2 **Normal Ranges for 6-Minute Walk Test for Older Adults in Yards**

	Age						
	60 to 64	**65 to 69**	**70 to 74**	**75 to 79**	**80 to 84**	**85 to 89**	**90 to 94**
Males	610 to 735	560 to 700	545 to 680	470 to 640	445 to 605	380 to 570	305 to 500
Females	545 to 660	500 to 635	480 to 615	435 to 585	385 to 540	340 to 510	275 to 440

Adapted by permission from R.E. Rikli and C.J. Jones, 2013 pp. 89, 90.

One-Mile Run Test for Youth

FitnessGram is an assessment for children that emphasizes personal fitness for health rather than comparisons among children (3). With this philosophy in mind, healthy ranges are given rather than fitness rankings. Youth are considered in the "healthy fitness zone" or "needs improvement" zone. For boys and girls between the ages of 10 and 17, a one-mile run test is used (if a child cannot run this entire distance, encourage walking at a fast pace). For the one-mile run test, the calculation to estimate aerobic capacity ($\dot{V}O_{2max}$) takes into account body mass index (BMI) as well as the time to complete the one-mile run (5).

Boys

> **108.94**
>
> Minus (**8.41** × _____ mile time in minutes)
>
> Plus (**0.34** × _____ mile time in minutes × _____ mile time in minutes)
>
> Plus (**0.21** × _____ age in years)
>
> Minus (**0.84** × _____ BMI)
>
> = _____ Estimated $\dot{V}O_{2max}$

Girls

> **108.94**
>
> Minus (**8.41** × _____ mile time in minutes)
>
> Plus (**0.34** × _____ mile time in minutes × _____ mile time in minutes)
>
> Minus (**0.84** × _____ BMI)
>
> = _____ Estimated $\dot{V}O_{2max}$

Note that this estimation can be used only for run times of 13 minutes or less. If the child requires more than 13 minutes to complete the one-mile run, then simply enter "13" into the formula for the mile time. To determine BMI, see figure 18.1. See table 5.3 for the healthy fitness zone for boys and girls between the ages of 10 and 17 (4).

TABLE 5.3 **FitnessGram Standards for Aerobic Capacity Based on the One-Mile Run for Youth***

Age	Boys	Girls
10	40.2 or higher	40.2 or higher
11	40.2 or higher	40.2 or higher
12	40.3 or higher	40.1 or higher
13	41.1 or higher	39.7 or higher
14	42.5 or higher	39.4 or higher
15	43.6 or higher	39.1 or higher
16	44.1 or higher	38.9 or higher
17	44.2 or higher	38.8 or higher

*The values listed represent the healthy fitness zone and indicate that the child has a sufficient fitness level to provide important health benefits. Being below the value listed indicates a need for improvement.

Adapted by permission from The Cooper Institute, 2017, pp. 86, 87.

Aerobic Workout Components

An aerobic workout should follow a consistent pattern to optimize safety as well as enjoyment (2). You should begin with a warm-up, which is followed by the main part of the workout, called the endurance conditioning phase. The workout is then wrapped up with a cool-down. See figure 5.4 for an overview of an aerobic exercise session.

Warm-Up

A warm-up that consists of a minimum of 5 to 10 minutes of low- to moderate-level activity is essential (2). The intent of the warm-up is to increase the temperature of the muscles, thus preparing the body for the demands of the endurance conditioning phase, or main focus, of the workout. A warm-up prepares your heart, lungs, and

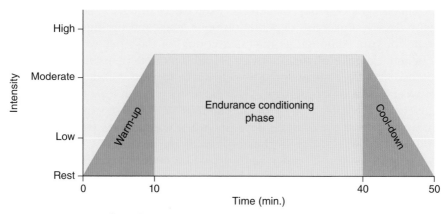

FIGURE 5.4 Overview of aerobic exercise session.

Adapted from B. Bushman and J.C. Young, 2005, p. 35.

muscles for the endurance conditioning phase of your aerobic training session (2) and may reduce the risk of injury (6). Think of the warm-up as an on-ramp to a freeway. The on-ramp gives you time to bring your vehicle up to the speed of traffic to avoid an accident. The faster the traffic is, the longer the on-ramp should be. In the same way, your warm-up should be longer if the intensity of the conditioning phase is high.

Warm-up activities may include some light calisthenics or lower-level activities similar to what you will be including in the conditioning phase. For example, if your program includes brisk walking for the conditioning phase, then the warm-up could include slower-paced walking. If the conditioning phase includes a more intense activity such as running, then jogging would be appropriate in the warm-up. The point is to gradually increase the intensity from resting levels to the intensity you plan for the conditioning phase.

Endurance Conditioning Phase

To continue with the freeway analogy, the endurance conditioning phase is the freeway itself—the main focus of your journey. The conditioning phase for aerobic activity is guided by the FITT-VP principle, which stands for frequency, intensity, time, type, volume, and progression (2). Frequency refers to the number of days per week you set aside time for exercise. Intensity reflects how hard you are working when exercising. Time simply refers to the duration you are active, on a daily or weekly basis. Type, or exercise mode, focuses on activities that involve large-muscle groups to improve cardiorespiratory fitness. Volume reflects the total amount of exercise and may be expressed in the number of calories burned. Progression refers to the manner in which the program is advanced over time as your fitness level improves.

Although FITT-VP nicely summarizes the conditioning phase, you will also want to add an "E"—the E stands for enjoyment. All the recommendations and information in the world mean little if you do not stick with your exercise program. Understanding the benefits of an exercise program (as outlined in chapter 1) may keep you active, but considering the time commitment you are making, you should also be sure you are having some fun. Suggestions for keeping exercise enjoyable are found later in this chapter. First, consider the nuts and bolts of an aerobic exercise program.

Frequency

The recommended frequency of aerobic exercise is three to five days per week. How many days you exercise depends on your goals and the intensity that is most appropriate for you. Although as few as a couple of days per week of activity can provide benefits, regular physical activity provides more benefits and has a lower risk of musculoskeletal injury than sporadic activity (2, 6). You will need as few as three days per week if you are engaging in vigorous activity, but at least five days per week is recommended if you plan on moderate-intensity activity. For example, if you enjoy running (a vigorous activity), three days per week will provide you with health and fitness benefits. However, if you plan on a walking program (a moderate-intensity activity), then at least five days per week would be better. If you enjoy mixing types and intensities of activity, then a weekly combination of three to five days of moderate and vigorous activity is recommended (2, 8). For example, you may walk a couple days per week and jog on another couple days. This would be considered two days per week of moderate activity (i.e., walking) and two days per week of vigorous activity (i.e., jogging), allowing you to meet the recommended amount of physical activity.

Intensity

As the intensity of activity increases, so do the potential health benefits. To promote health and fitness benefits, your exercise must place some stress on your cardiorespiratory system. In other words, you should notice an increase in your heart rate and breathing. When speaking of intensity, fitness professionals generally use the terms moderate and vigorous (2, 8). To help visualize this, consider moderate-intensity activity to be equivalent to brisk walking and vigorous-intensity activity to be equivalent to jogging or running (8).

A variety of simple methods are available to help you quantify the intensity of your exercise bout. One method is to monitor your relative level of effort. Although this is subjective (i.e., you determine how easy or hard you are exercising), a numerical scale can help guide you to appropriate levels of activity. The U.S. Department of Health and Human Services' *Physical Activity Guidelines for Americans* suggests a scale of 0 to 10. Sitting at rest is 0, and your highest effort level possible is 10 (8). Moderate-intensity activity is a 5 or 6 on this effort scale. Vigorous-intensity activity is at a level of 7 or 8. This method allows you to individualize your exercise based on your current level of cardiorespiratory fitness (8). For an example of applying this scale, see figure 5.5.

Another method, called the talk test, can also be used to establish exercise intensity (2). If you are working at an intensity that increases breathing rate but still allows you to speak without gasping for breath between words, you are likely exercising at a moderate intensity. The goal would be to exercise to the point at which speech would start to become more difficult. The *Physical Activity Guidelines for Americans* suggests that moderate-intensity activity allows you to talk but not to sing, whereas more vigorous activity results in an inability to say more than a few words without pausing for a breath (8).

Heart rate monitoring can also be helpful for determining your intensity level, although it is a bit more technical than the subjective measures of effort level and the talk test. Maximal heart rate can be estimated by subtracting your age in years from 220 (2). Thus for a 40-year-old, estimated maximal heart rate would be 180 beats per minute (i.e., 220 − 40 = 180). You will not be exercising at maximal heart rate, but rather at a percentage of that value; the percentage will depend on your target level of intensity (2). Multiply your estimated maximal heart rate by the activity factor from table 5.4 to determine your target heart rate.

_____ estimated maximal heart rate × _____ activity factor

= target exercise heart rate in beats per minute

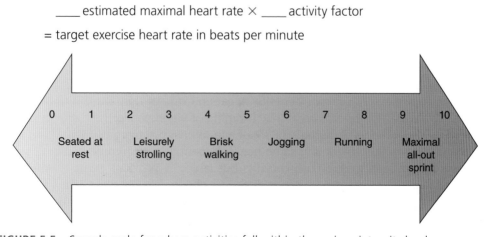

FIGURE 5.5   Sample scale for where activities fall within the various intensity levels.

TABLE 5.4   **Heart Rate Intensity Guidelines**

Intensity level	Percentage of maximal heart rate	Activity factor*
Very light	~55%	0.55
Light	~60%	0.60
Moderate	~70%	0.70
Vigorous	~85%	0.85

*Multiply activity factor by maximal heart rate to determine target heart rate.

Adapted by permission from American College of Sports Medicine, 2018.

Note that your heart rate can also be influenced by environmental conditions (e.g., hot, humid environments) as well as medications (e.g., beta-blockers used for migraines and heart disease can lower heart rate). The calculated value should be used in conjunction with relative perception of effort or the talk test (2). You can adjust your workload up or down depending on your perception of effort on a given day.

Recognize, too, that you can vary your intensity during the conditioning phase. Athletes often use interval training, which includes some time at higher intensity followed by lower-intensity exercise. This provides a unique stress on the body that translates into improved aerobic fitness. This principle can be used for general exercise programs as well (2). For example, if you are just beginning to exercise, you could include a few minutes at a faster walking pace within your conditioning phase. Alternating between lower and higher intensity provides variety as well as a stimulus to improve your aerobic capacity, no matter your current level of fitness.

Time

The duration of each of your exercise sessions is determined by the amount of time you are able to commit as well as your current fitness status. If you are a beginner, don't worry about some arbitrary time goal; rather, find an activity that you can do continuously for 10 minutes. Increase the duration of the exercise session as it becomes easier to complete. Add a couple of minutes per session until you reach about 30 minutes of aerobic exercise per day. Depending on your initial fitness level, this may take weeks or even a month or more. The key is to keep going and make progress.

If you have already been doing some exercise (or have now built up to 30 minutes of continuous activity) and feel comfortable with moderate-intensity activity for this length of time, decide whether you want to maintain your current intensity and go for a bit longer, or if you want to begin to increase the intensity. Time and intensity are like a teeter-totter. When you increase intensity, you generally decrease the length of the session. If you decrease intensity, you will need to increase the time you spend exercising to achieve full health benefits. A general rule of thumb from the *Physical Activity Guidelines for Americans* is that 1 minute of vigorous-intensity activity can be counted as the same as 2 minutes of moderate-intensity activity (8). For example, a 15-minute run would provide the same health benefit as a 30-minute walk.

Labels are difficult to apply universally, but table 5.5 provides some terminology related to activity status that was introduced in chapter 2. For the purposes of this book, beginners are those who currently have limited activity. As you can see in the table, beginners are focusing on very light to light activity and build up to 100 to 150 minutes per week of light to moderate activity. The intermediate level of activity reflects

TABLE 5.5   **Activity Status and Aerobic Training Focus**

Activity status	Aerobic training focus
Beginner (inactive with no or minimal physical activity and thus relatively deconditioned)	*No prior activity:* Focus is on very light to light activity for 20 to 30 min over the course of the day. Accumulating time in 10-min bouts is an option. Overall, your target is 60 to 100 min per week. *Some prior activity* (i.e., once you have met the target level of 60-100 min per week): Focus is on light- to moderate-level activity for 30 to 45 min per day. Accumulating time in 10-min bouts is an option. Overall, your target is 100 to 150 min per week.
Intermediate (somewhat active but overall only moderately conditioned)	*Some activity* (fair to average fitness): Focus is on moderate activity for 30 to 60 min per day. Overall, your target is 150 to 250 min per week.
Established (regularly engaging in moderate to vigorous exercise)	*Regular exerciser* (moderate to vigorous): Focus is on moderate- to vigorous-intensity activity for 30 to 90 min per day. Overall, your target is 150 to 300 min per week (duration depends on intensity).

people who are somewhat active and are moderately conditioned. The focus at this stage is increasing moderate-intensity aerobic activity to 150 to 250 minutes per week. Typically, people at this level are of fair to average fitness levels. Established exercisers are those who have been engaged in regular exercise for at least six months. Fitness levels vary according to genetic potential as well as personal fitness goals. Typically, established exercisers have average to excellent aerobic fitness.

The *Physical Activity Guidelines for Americans* recommends working toward a minimum of 150 minutes per week of moderate-intensity activity, or 75 minutes per week of vigorous-intensity activity (8). If you are already physically active at this level, then consider increasing your activity to gain additional health and fitness benefits. For you, a new target of 300 minutes per week of moderate-intensity activity, or 150 minutes per week of vigorous-intensity activity, would be a potential goal (8).

■ Q&A ■

How can interval training be designed to provide variety in an exercise program?

Interval training occurs when exercise intensity varies during an exercise session. This type of training provides many options, as you can change the number, duration, and intensity of various phases of the exercise session (2). For example, you could engage in moderate exercise at a level 5 (on the 10-point exertion scale) for 2 minutes followed by 3 minutes of vigorous exercise at a level 7 (on the 10-point exertion scale) and repeat that sequence four times for a total of 20 minutes for the exercise session. To provide variety, you can change the time spent or the intensity of each of the different intervals. For example, 2 minutes at level 6 followed by 2 minutes at level 8 could be repeated five times for a total of 20 minutes for the exercise session. The options are almost limitless and can be individualized based on your current health and fitness status (2).

Type or Mode

Aerobic activities are grouped into four categories along with recommendations on who would most appropriately engage in the given activity (see table 5.6) (2). Exercises in group A are recommended for everyone because they are relatively simple activities that can be started at a low level of effort. Group B activities are more vigorous and thus are most appropriate if you already have a good fitness base (i.e., you have been exercising regularly and have determined your fitness level to be at least in the fair to average range). Group C activities are those that have a definite skill component and thus may require some learning before being used as a fitness tool. Group D activities are recreational and, because intensity varies depending on the situation, are best reserved for people who are regularly active and have a good fitness base. Do not consider these groupings progressive (e.g., that group C activities are better than group B activities), but rather as a way to classify various aerobic exercises.

Volume

The concept of volume reflects a summary or overall amount of activity. One way to provide a summary of your aerobic exercise is to determine the calories you use when engaging in your aerobic activities each week. When considering the activity recommendations in the *Physical Activity Guidelines for Americans,* a reasonable target is at least 1,000 calories per week (2). Calculating calories burned can be helpful when you are interested in losing weight, but it is also a great way to pull together the four parts of your aerobic exercise prescription—frequency, intensity, time, and type of activity—into one number. Whether you do the same activity each day or change it up, you still can take a look at your weekly total to ensure that you are on track with just a few calculations.

TABLE 5.6   Aerobic Exercise Groupings

Exercise group	Group characteristics	Recommended participants	Examples
A	Endurance activities that can be done with minimal skill and with minimal fitness	Everyone	Walking, easy bicycling, slow dancing
B	Endurance activities that are more vigorous but can be done with minimal skill	Because of the higher intensity, adults who are regularly active and have at least an average level of fitness would be best suited.	Jogging, running, spinning, elliptical exercise, fast dancing
C	Endurance activities that require a certain level of skill to perform	Assuming that a skill level has been achieved, people should have at least an average level of fitness to be suited for these activities.	Swimming, cross-country skiing, skating
D	Recreational sports	Because of the changing exertion level due to competition or terrain, people should have at least an average level of fitness.	Basketball, tennis, soccer, downhill skiing, hiking

Adapted by permission from American College of Sports Medicine, 2018.

To keep things simple, researchers have created a unit of measure called a metabolic equivalent, or MET. A MET is equal to the oxygen cost at rest (i.e., 1 MET = resting level = 3.5 milliliters of oxygen per kilogram body weight per minute). Multiples of a MET are then applied to various activities. For example, walking at 3.5 miles per hour (5.6 km/h) is equal to 4 METs. In other words, you are working four times harder when walking at 3.5 miles per hour than you are when seated in a resting position. Metabolic equivalent values have been determined for a wide variety of activities (see table 5.7 for some examples of basic activities) (1).

Once you know the MET value for a given exercise, you can estimate how many calories you burned per minute by inserting that value into the following formula (numbers in bold are constants—in other words, they do not change):

____ MET value of activity × **3.5** × ____ body weight in kg ÷ **200**

= ____ calories burned per minute

Insert the MET value for the activity and then your body weight (to convert from pounds to kilograms, multiply your weight in pounds by 0.454 to determine your weight in kilograms). For an example on how this can be used, see Checking Volume of Aerobic Exercise.

TABLE 5.7   **MET Values for Selected Activities***

Activity	MET value
Bicycling outdoors, <10.0 mph (16 km/h), leisure riding	4.0
Bicycling outdoors, 10.0 to 11.9 mph (16 to 19.2 km/h)	6.8
Bicycling outdoors, 12.0 to 13.9 mph (19.2 to 22.4 km/h)	8.0
Bicycling outdoors, 14.0 to 15.9 mph (22.5 to 25.6 km/h)	10.0
Biking, stationary, 30 to 50 W, very light to light effort	3.5
Biking, stationary, 90 to 100 W, moderate to vigorous effort	6.8
Biking, stationary, 101 to 160 W, vigorous effort	8.8
Biking, stationary, 161 to 200 W, vigorous effort	11.0
Running, 5 mph (8 km/h)	8.3
Running, 6 mph (9.7 km/h)	9.8
Running, 7 mph (11.3 km/h)	11.0
Running, 8 mph (12.9 km/h)	11.8
Swimming laps, freestyle, light to moderate effort	5.8
Swimming laps, sidestroke	7.0
Swimming laps, backstroke	9.5
Swimming laps, breaststroke	10.3
Swimming laps, butterfly	13.8
Walking, 2.0 mph (3.2 km/h)	2.8
Walking, 2.5 mph (4 km/h)	3.0
Walking, 3.5 mph (5.6 km/h)	4.3
Walking, 4.5 mph (7.2 km/h)	7.0

*For a comprehensive list of activities and MET values, see http://prevention.sph.sc.edu/tools/compendium.htm.
Source: B.E. Ainsworth, W.L. Haskell, S.D. Herrmann, et al.

Progression

Progression is how an exercise program is advanced over time. Many factors must be considered, including current health and fitness status, training responses, and goals (2). The key is gradual progression rather than making abrupt or significant changes in one of the FITT components. If you are just starting, to optimize safety and avoid injury, the recommendation is "start low and go slow" (2). Table 5.5 reflects this concept of slowly increasing the volume of exercise. Rather than increasing frequency, intensity, and duration all at once, you want to gradually introduce changes. For example, initially, you may simply increase the time spent in activity. As you adjust to this level of activity, you may then want to cut back the time a bit and increase the intensity slightly. Reflect on the overall volume of exercise to help make sure your progression is gradual. As you make adjustments to your program, give yourself time at a particular volume of activity to ensure you are able to maintain this new level before trying to move forward.

Cool-Down

The cool-down should consist of a minimum of 5 to 10 minutes of low- to moderate-level activity (2). The cool-down provides an opportunity for body systems to gradually return to preexercise levels. A cool-down is recommended to allow the heart to slow down in a controlled manner, thus avoiding negative changes in heart rhythm. In addition, if you stop your activity too abruptly, blood that was circulating to the working muscles can pool in your legs, resulting in a drop in blood pressure. A cool-down also helps to gradually decrease body temperature, which naturally increased

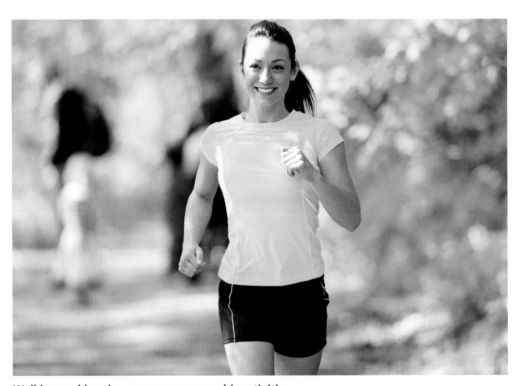

Walking and jogging are common aerobic activities.

Checking Volume of Aerobic Exercise

To compare two programs—one focused on walking and the other on jogging—take a look at the MET values to help you examine how intensity influences the number of calories burned.

Walking program: walking 3.5 miles per hour (5.6 km/h) for 50 minutes

Jogging program: running at 5 miles per hour (8 km/h) for 25 minutes

For this example, the calculations are done for a 150-pound (68.1 kg) person. The MET values for each activity are found in table 5.7.

Walking at 3.5 miles per hour (5.6 km/h) is equal to 4.3 METs, so using the formula provided previously, a 50-minute workout burns about 255 calories (determined by multiplying 5.1 calories per minute by the workout duration of 50 minutes), as follows:

$$(4.3 \text{ METs} \times 3.5 \times 68.1 \text{ kg}) \div 200 = 5.1 \text{ calories per minute}$$

Running at 5 miles per hour (8 km/h) is equal to 8.3 METs, so using the formula provided previously, a 25-minute workout would burn 248 calories (determined by multiplying 9.9 calories per minute by the workout duration of 25 minutes), as follows:

$$(8.3 \text{ METs} \times 3.5 \times 68.1 \text{ kg}) \div 200 = 9.9 \text{ calories per minute}$$

The two workouts burn approximately the same number of calories. Thus even though the activities are very different, the overall volume (which accounts for the type, duration, and intensity) is similar.

during the endurance phase. Activities included in a cool-down are similar to those in the warm-up, but the intensity needs to gradually diminish toward resting levels (2).

A proper cool-down is driven by both practical issues (e.g., avoiding fainting from a drop in blood pressure) and safety issues (e.g., avoiding negative changes in heart rhythm). The cool-down is like a freeway off-ramp. When shifting from freeway speeds to those appropriate on city streets, time is needed for an adjustment. In a similar way, the cool-down allows the body to adjust back toward normal resting levels. The higher the intensity of your conditioning phase, the longer your cool-down should be.

Your Aerobic Program

If you are just getting started with your exercise program, be sure to complete the preparticipation screening process found in chapter 2 (2). This screening can help you determine whether you should visit your health care provider before starting an exercise program. Of course, regardless of the outcome, consulting with your personal health care provider is always appropriate. In addition, you need to consider your current fitness level and begin at a point suitable to your current status. Over time, with regular activity, you will progress and improve.

Your personal exercise prescription takes into account the frequency, intensity, time, and type of activity. Take walking, for example, which is the most commonly reported exercise and is a great activity for the start of an exercise program (walking is a group A activity as shown in table 5.6). Figure 5.6 shows an example of a progressive walking and jogging program. You can determine where to enter into the exercise progression based on your current level of fitness.

FIGURE 5.6

Sample walking and jogging program.

Stage	Time point	Warm-up	Workout*	Cool-down
Beginner	Initial week	Slow, easy walking pace for a couple of minutes	Walk at a pace that involves a light level of exertion (level 3 or 4) for 10 min at least twice a day for a total of 20 min each day (three days per week). Your weekly total should be 60 min.	Slow, easy walking pace for a couple of minutes
	Progression	Slow, easy walking pace for 5 min	Each week add 10 min to your weekly total until you reach 100 min of activity (e.g., 20 min five days per week). Stay at this duration and increase your intensity over the next couple of weeks from light (level 3 or 4) to moderate (level 5 or 6). Once you are comfortable with this time and intensity for a couple of weeks, continue to add 10 to 15 min per week until you reach 150 min.	Slow, easy walking pace for 5 min
	Final week	Easy walking pace for 5 to 10 min	Walk at a pace that involves a moderate level of exertion (level 5 or 6) for 30 to 60 min (three to five days per week). Your weekly total should be 150 min.	Easy walking pace for 5 to 10 min
Intermediate	Initial week	Easy walking pace for 5 to 10 min	Walk at a pace that feels moderate (level 5 or 6) for 30 to 60 min (three to five days per week). Your weekly total should be 150 min.	Easy walking pace for 5 to 10 min
	Progression	Easy walking pace for 5 to 10 min	Continue to increase exercise duration by 10 to 15 min per week to approach 200 to 250 min of moderate activity accumulated on a weekly basis. Another option is to introduce a slightly more vigorous activity, such as jogging, realizing that the time needed will be less (typically 2 min of moderate activity equals 1 min of vigorous activity).	Easy walking pace for 5 to 10 min
	Final week	Easy walking pace for 5 to 10 min	Walk at a pace that feels moderate (level 5 or 6) for 30 to 60 min (three to five days per week). Your weekly total should be 200 to 250 min (moderate intensity). Or: Combine moderate and vigorous walking on alternate days.	Easy walking pace for 5 to 10 min
Established	Continue, maintain	Easy walking pace for 5 to 10 min	Walk at a pace that feels moderate (level 5 or 6). Your weekly total should be 200 to 300 min (moderate intensity). Or: Jog (level 7 or 8). Your weekly total should be 100 to 150 min (vigorous intensity). Or: Combine moderate and vigorous walking on alternate days.	Easy walking pace for 5 to 10 min

*Level of exertion is on a scale of 0 to 10 (sitting at rest is 0, and your highest effort level is 10).

Once you feel comfortable with 30 minutes of continuous moderate-intensity activity, you may be interested in other activity options. Swimming, a group C activity, is another excellent aerobic activity if you have basic swimming skills or are willing to gain those skills. Follow the time and intensity progression described in figure 5.6, substituting swimming (using different strokes for variety) for walking and jogging.

Figure 5.7 provides a sample program for someone with a membership at a health club. Activities at the club, when done at a low intensity, would fall into group A, but as the person's fitness level improves, the intensity increase will likely result in a shift to group B exercise.

FIGURE 5.7

Sample cross-training program at a health club.

Stage	Time point	Warm-up	Workout*	Cool-down
Beginner	Initial week	Slow, easy walking pace for a couple of minutes	Pick one activity each day at a light level of exertion (level 3 or 4) for 10 min at least twice a day for a total of 20 min each day (three days per week). Select from walking on the treadmill or stationary biking. Your weekly total should be 60 min.	Slow, easy walking pace for a couple of minutes
	Progression	Slow, easy walking pace for 5 min	Each week add 10 min to your weekly total until you reach 100 min of activity (e.g., 20 min five days per week). Potential activities include treadmill walking, stationary biking, and using a stair climber. Stay at this duration and increase your intensity over the next couple of weeks from light (level 3 or 4) to moderate (level 5 or 6). Once you are comfortable with this time and intensity for a couple of weeks, continue to add 10 to 15 min per week until you reach 150 min.	Slow, easy walking pace for 5 min
	Final week	Easy walking pace for 5 to 10 min	Exercise at an intensity that involves a moderate level of exertion (level 5 or 6) for 30 to 60 min (three to five days per week). Activities may include treadmill walking; stationary biking; or using a stair climber, elliptical trainer, rowing machine, or Nordic ski machine. Your weekly total should be 150 min.	Easy walking pace for 5 to 10 min
Intermediate	Initial week	Easy walking pace for 5 to 10 min	Exercise at a level that feels moderate (level 5 or 6) for 30 to 60 min (three to five days per week) using a treadmill, stationary bike, stair climber, elliptical trainer, or Nordic ski machine. Your weekly total should be 150 min.	Easy walking pace for 5 to 10 min

> *continued*

Figure 5.7 *> continued*

Stage	Time point	Warm-up	Workout*	Cool-down
	Progression	Easy walking pace for 5 to 10 min	Continue to increase exercise duration by 10 to 15 min per week to approach 200 to 250 min of moderate activity accumulated on a weekly basis. Another option is to introduce slightly more vigorous activity a couple of days per week, such as jogging on the treadmill, taking a spinning class, or joining a step aerobics class, realizing that the time needed will be less (typically, 2 min of moderate activity equals 1 min of vigorous activity).	Easy walking pace for 5 to 10 min
	Final week	Easy walking pace for 5 to 10 min	Exercise at a level that feels moderate (level 5 or 6) for 30 to 60 min (three to five days per week). Your weekly total should be 200 to 250 min (moderate intensity). Or: Combine moderate and vigorous walking on alternate days.	Easy walking pace for 5 to 10 min
Established	Continue-maintain	Easy walking pace for 5 to 10 min	Exercise at an intensity that feels moderate (level 5 or 6). Your weekly total should be 200 to 300 min (moderate intensity). Or: Exercise at a higher intensity (level 7 or 8). Your weekly total should be 100 to 150 min (vigorous intensity). Or: Combine moderate and vigorous walking on alternate days.	Easy walking pace for 5 to 10 min

*Level of exertion is on a scale of 0 to 10 (sitting at rest is 0, and your highest effort level is 10).

The examples in figures 5.6 and 5.7 show a progression from beginner to established exerciser. Depending on your current status, you may be at the start of the table as a beginner or already in the established, or maintenance, phase. If you are just beginning to exercise, progress slowly and base your advancement on how your body is responding to the exercise. If you are in the established, or maintenance, phase, keep tracking your activity. Also, stay focused on the FITT-VP factors as discussed previously, and if you are becoming bored with your current activity program, consider other modes of exercise or joining an exercise group.

As you move along in your exercise journey, increase the duration (time) first; once you are comfortable with the activity at the longer session length, then consider increasing the intensity. To avoid injury, do not increase the session duration and intensity at the same time. Although placing a stress on the body is necessary for improvement, excessive overload can result in injury as well as frustration. To keep steady forward progress, refer to table 5.5 for general guidance.

In addition, as you examine the sample programs, once again consider the FITT-VP factors as discussed earlier and how each relates to your fitness goals. Don't forget about enjoyment. As you create your plan of action, consider the types of activities that you enjoy and that also are accessible to you. Joining a health club can be a great way to increase your access to a variety of activities (equipment as well as group classes). If you don't want to join a health club, you can easily find aerobic activities at no cost. Walking and running trails are becoming more common in cities; many malls open their doors early to allow walkers to use the corridors before the stores open; and your local library has many aerobic exercise videos that you can use in the privacy of your own home. To get started, you need to pick a day and take the first step—literally as well as figuratively.

Cardiorespiratory (or aerobic) fitness is important for promoting health and, in particular, is associated with a reduced risk of cardiovascular disease. An aerobic exercise session includes a warm-up, a conditioning phase, and a cool-down. The warm-up and cool-down are links between the resting state and the exercise portion of your workout. The main focus, the endurance conditioning phase, is guided by the FITT-VP principle: frequency, intensity, time, type, volume, and progression. General recommendations are as follows: three to five days per week (frequency), moderate to vigorous level of exertion (intensity), 20 to 30 minutes or more per session (time), large-muscle group activity (type of activity), total of 1,000 calories burned per week (volume), and gradual increases over time (progression). In addition, tracking aerobic fitness assessments periodically is a helpful way to determine current status and the effectiveness of your aerobic exercise program.

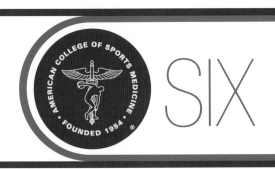

Enhancing Your Muscular Fitness

Muscular fitness is a global term that includes muscular strength, endurance, and power. Muscular strength refers to the ability to lift a heavy weight one time, muscular endurance is the ability to lift a lighter load several times, and muscular power refers to ability to exert maximum effort in a very short period of time. Muscle-strengthening activities that involve all the major muscle groups are recognized as an essential component of an overall fitness program for both adults and youth (1, 6).

Just as aerobic fitness is improved by stressing the heart and lungs, muscular fitness requires a stress, or resistance, to be placed on the muscles. Resistance training (also called strength training) involves the use of a variety of activities that include free weights (barbells and dumbbells), weight machines, elastic tubing, medicine balls, stability balls, and body weight. Resistance training does not refer to one specific mode of conditioning but rather to an organized process of exercising with various types of resistance to enhance muscular fitness.

When correctly performed and sensibly progressed over time, resistance training can be a safe, effective, and enjoyable method of exercise for people of a wide range of ages, fitness levels, and health conditions (1, 20). While resistance training has been a part of sport programs for many years, public health recommendations now aim to increase participation in muscle-strengthening activities for all youth and adults (28, 33). With instruction on developing proper exercise technique and guidance on sensibly progressing the exercise program, resistance training can offer observable health and fitness value.

Health and Fitness Benefits of Resistance Training

To maintain your physical capacity, you must make a lifestyle choice to include resistance training on a regular basis. Unfortunately, physical capacity and muscle strength decrease dramatically with age in adults who do not engage in resistance training (3,

Resistance Training Terminology

Following are definitions of some common terms used in the design of a resistance training workout:

Atrophy—A reduction in muscle fiber size.

Concentric—A type of muscle action that occurs when the muscle shortens.

Eccentric—A type of muscle action that occurs when the muscle lengthens.

Hypertrophy—An enlargement in muscle fiber size.

Muscular endurance—The ability to repeat or maintain muscle contraction.

Muscular strength—The ability to exert maximal force in a single effort.

Repetition—One complete movement of an exercise.

Repetition maximum (RM)—The maximum amount of weight that can be lifted for a predetermined number of repetitions with proper exercise technique.

Set—A group of repetitions performed without stopping.

Spotter—A training partner or fitness professional who can provide assistance in case of a failed repetition.

30). Resistance training results in stronger muscles and therefore an increased capacity for force production, which is not achievable with solely aerobic-based training. Because muscles function as the engine of your body, they must be used regularly to avoid disuse atrophy (i.e., a reduction in muscle size) and age-related declines in physical performance.

You don't need to be a competitive athlete to benefit from resistance training; it is equally important from a health and fitness perspective. The benefits of resistance training include favorable changes in body composition, metabolic health, and quality of life. Resistance training activities can increase lean muscle mass, reduce body fat, fortify bone, lower blood pressure, improve blood lipid and cholesterol levels, and enhance your body's ability to use glucose (2, 12). These benefits can optimize your day-to-day functioning while limiting the development of chronic diseases such as diabetes, heart disease, and osteoporosis (30, 32). Of paramount importance, regular participation in a resistance training program can help adults preserve their muscle health to maintain independent physical functioning with advancing age (23, 27).

Skeletal muscle represents about 40 percent of one's total body weight and influences a variety of physiological processes and disease risk factors (26). The increase in muscle tissue that results from resistance exercise is accompanied by an increase in resting metabolic rate; the decrease in muscle tissue that results from a sedentary lifestyle is accompanied by a decrease in resting metabolic rate. Muscle mass declines about 5 percent each decade after age 30, and this loss can reach 10 percent per decade after age 50 (15). This gradual decrease in muscle mass and metabolism is associated with the gradual increase in body fat that typically occurs with age. Calories that were previously used by muscle tissue (now smaller as a result of disuse) are stored as fat. On the other hand, resistance training raises resting metabolic rate and results in more calories burned on a daily basis. In theory, if you resistance train and gain 2 pounds (~1 kg) of muscle mass, your resting metabolic rate should increase by about 20 calories per day (29). Thus, performing resistance training throughout your life can help you recharge your metabolism, facilitate physical function, and maintain your health (30).

In addition to the effect of muscle on metabolism, another benefit of regular resistance training is an increase in bone mineral density that may reduce the risk of osteoporosis (8, 9, 11). On top of the direct effect of strength-building (and weight-bearing) exercises on bone, the act of muscles pulling on bones during resistance exercises may also be a potent stimulus for new bone formation in certain people. This potential benefit is of particular importance to women who are at increased risk of functional limitations as a result of age-related losses of bone mass.

Strong muscles serve as shock absorbers and balancing agents that help dissipate the repetitive landing forces from weight-bearing activities for active people and also reduce the risk of falling in older adults (3, 31). As such, a resistance training program that requires agility and balance may be the most effective way to enhance movement control and avoid injury (1, 10). Moreover, strength-building activities are particularly important for decreasing physical discomfort associated with low back pain, which is a growing health care concern (31).

Regular participation in resistance training activities that are consistent with your needs, goals, and abilities can improve muscle function, enhance quality of life, and lower the risk of premature all-cause mortality (18, 25). The health and fitness benefits are clear. You can also realize benefits linked to personal appearance. Firm, toned muscles are possible with regular resistance training. Whether you are seeking to improve in recreational or sport activities or just to look and feel better, resistance training should be part of your fitness program.

Assessments for Muscular Fitness

There is not one test of muscular fitness that is best. Rather, different tests can be used to safely and effectively assess muscular strength or muscular endurance in various age groups. This section describes several assessments that can be used.

Assessing Muscular Strength

A common assessment of muscular strength is called the one-repetition maximum (1RM), in which the goal is to lift as much weight as possible on a strength exercise with proper

■ Q&A

What is the typical impact of aging on muscle and metabolism?

As a person ages, decreases in muscle along with a lower resting metabolic rate result in less than optimal changes in body composition. For example, consider a 160-pound (72.6 kg) male with 15 percent body fat at age 30. He therefore has 24 pounds (10.9 kg) of fat weight and 136 pounds (61.7 kg) of lean weight, which consists of muscle, bone, blood, skin, organs, and connective tissue. If he weighs the same (160 pounds) at age 50, his body composition will have changed by about 20 pounds (9 kg)—10 pounds (4.5 kg) less lean weight and 10 pounds (4.5 kg) more fat—and he will now be 21 percent body fat. Of course, this increase in percentage of body fat and decrease in lean weight would have a negative impact on his appearance, health, and fitness.

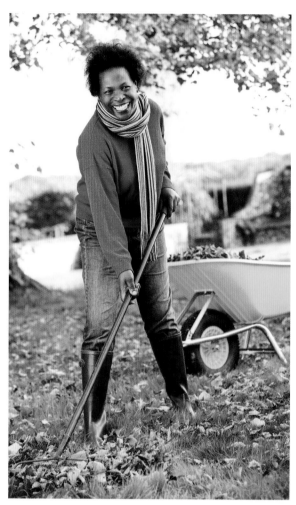

Muscular fitness is a part of recreational and daily activities.

technique for one repetition only. This test is time-consuming and should be performed under the supervision of a qualified fitness professional. Also, familiarization and practice sessions are critical to ensure that the test is safe and accurate (20).

Another option is to estimate your 1RM by lifting a submaximal weight multiple times. While different exercises can be used for this assessment, the use of multijoint exercises such as the leg press and chest press is common. With a few calculations you can estimate your 1RM and compare your performance to that of others of your age and sex.

First, multiply the number of repetitions you can perform on a given exercise by 2.5. Try to select a weight you can lift about 10 to 15 times with proper form (note that if you can lift the weight more than 20 times, the results will be more accurate if you rest and then repeat the test with a heavier weight). Subtract that number from 100 to determine the percentage of your theoretical 1RM. Then, divide that number by 100 to produce a decimal value. Finally, divide the weight you lifted by that decimal value to estimate your 1RM on that exercise.

For example, if a 35-year-old female can lift 60 pounds (27 kg) on the chest press exercise 10 times, then she can use the following steps to estimate her 1RM:

> 10 repetitions × 2.5 = 25
> 100 − 25 = 75
> 75 ÷ 100 = 0.75
> 60 pounds ÷ 0.75 = 80 pounds = estimated 1RM

To compare her performance with others of her same age and sex, the 1RM is divided by body weight. In the previous example, if the individual's body weight is 145 pounds (66 kg), then she can complete the calculation (80 / 145 = 0.55) and use the result (0.55) to assess her performance with table 6.1 (and to assess lower body strength with table 6.2). Note that the ratio of weight lifted to body weight is the same whether you use pounds or kilograms. For a 35-year-old female, her upper body strength is in the "fair" category. With regular resistance training she will see her strength improve as she tracks her progress. A weight she could lift only 10 times will be lifted more often before fatiguing, or she will be able to lift a heavier weight for those same 10 repetitions.

TABLE 6.1   **Interpretation of Upper Body Strength for Males and Females***

	Age					
Males	**20 or younger**	**20 to 29**	**30 to 39**	**40 to 49**	**50 to 59**	**60+**
Superior	1.76 or higher	1.63 or higher	1.35 or higher	1.20 or higher	1.05 or higher	0.94 or higher
Excellent	1.34 to 1.75	1.32 to 1.62	1.12 to 1.34	1.00 to 1.19	0.90 to 1.04	0.82 to 0.93
Good	1.19 to 1.33	1.14 to 1.31	0.98 to 1.11	0.88 to 0.99	0.79 to 0.89	0.72 to 0.81
Fair	1.06 to 1.18	0.99 to 1.13	0.88 to 0.97	0.80 to 0.87	0.71 to 0.78	0.66 to 0.71
Poor	0.89 to 1.05	0.88 to 0.98	0.78 to 0.87	0.72 to 0.79	0.63 to 0.70	0.57 to 0.65
Very poor	0.88 or lower	0.87 or lower	0.77 or lower	0.71 or lower	0.62 or lower	0.56 or lower
	Age					
Females	**20 or younger**	**20 to 29**	**30 to 39**	**40 to 49**	**50 to 59**	**60+**
Superior	0.88 or higher	1.01 or higher	0.82 or higher	0.77 or higher	0.68 or higher	0.72 or higher
Excellent	0.77 to 0.87	0.80 to 1.00	0.70 to 0.81	0.62 to 0.76	0.55 to 0.67	0.54 to 0.71
Good	0.65 to 0.76	0.70 to 0.79	0.60 to 0.69	0.54 to 0.61	0.48 to 0.54	0.47 to 0.53
Fair	0.58 to 0.64	0.59 to 0.69	0.53 to 0.59	0.50 to 0.53	0.44 to 0.47	0.43 to 0.46
Poor	0.53 to 0.57	0.51 to 0.58	0.47 to 0.52	0.43 to 0.49	0.39 to 0.43	0.38 to 0.42
Very poor	0.52 or lower	0.50 or lower	0.46 or lower	0.42 or lower	0.38 or lower	0.37 or lower

*Bench press weight ratio = weight lifted divided by body weight.

Data provided by The Cooper Institute. Physical Fitness Assessments and Norms for Adults and Law Enforcement (2013). Used with permission.

TABLE 6.2   **Interpretation of Lower Body Strength for Males and Females***

Males	Age				
	20 to 29	30 to 39	40 to 49	50 to 59	60+
Well above average	2.27 or higher	2.07 or higher	1.92 or higher	1.80 or higher	1.73 or higher
Above average	2.05 to 2.26	1.85 to 2.06	1.74 to 1.91	1.64 to 1.79	1.56 to 1.72
Average	1.91 to 2.04	1.71 to 1.84	1.62 to 1.73	1.52 to 1.63	1.43 to 1.55
Below average	1.74 to 1.90	1.59 to 1.70	1.51 to 1.61	1.39 to 1.51	1.30 to 1.42
Well below average	1.73 or lower	1.58 or lower	1.50 or lower	1.38 or lower	1.29 or lower

Females	Age				
	20 to 29	30 to 39	40 to 49	50 to 59	60+
Well above average	1.82 or higher	1.61 or higher	1.48 or higher	1.37 or higher	1.32 or higher
Above average	1.58 to 1.81	1.39 to 1.60	1.29 to 1.47	1.17 to 1.36	1.13 to 1.31
Average	1.44 to 1.57	1.27 to 1.38	1.18 to 1.28	1.05 to 1.16	0.99 to 1.12
Below average	1.27 to 1.43	1.15 to 1.26	1.08 to 1.17	0.95 to 1.04	0.88 to 0.98
Well below average	1.26 or lower	1.14 or lower	1.07 or lower	0.94 or lower	0.87 or lower

*Leg press weight ratio = weight lifted divided by body weight.

Data provided by The Cooper Institute, 1994. Used with permission. Study population for the data set was predominantly white and college educated. A Universal DVR machine was used to measure the 1RM.

Assessing Muscular Endurance

As with muscular strength, various assessments can provide insight into one's muscular endurance status. This section describes the push-up test as well as some age-specific assessments for children and older adults.

Push-Up Test for Adults

The push-up test is commonly used to measure muscular endurance, which is the ability of a muscle or muscle group to exert force repeatedly over time. Many activities of daily life such as carrying groceries and household chores require repeated or sustained muscular actions. Like muscular strength, muscular endurance can be different in upper body and lower body muscles.

The goal of the push-up test is to perform as many push-ups as possible with proper form. Note that there are two different ways to perform this test for adults, one for males and one for females. For males the toes are the rear pivot point (see figure 6.1), but for females the knees are in contact with the ground (see figure 6.2). For both males and females, proper form includes keeping the back straight while pushing up to a straight-arm position and then lowering the body until the chin touches the floor. It is important to perform the push-up test as shown so you can accurately assess your performance using table 6.3.

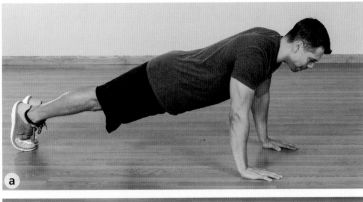

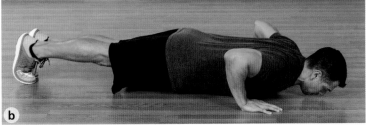

FIGURE 6.1   Push-up for males.

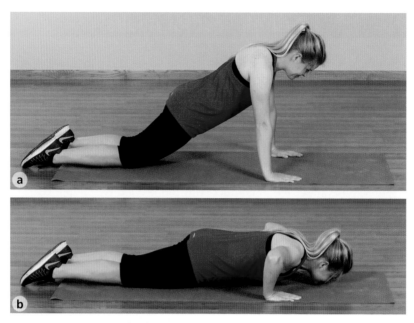

FIGURE 6.2   Push-up for females.

TABLE 6.3   **Push-Up Test Norms for Adults**

Males	Age				
	20 to 29	**30 to 39**	**40 to 49**	**50 to 59**	**60 to 69**
Excellent	36 or more	30 or more	25 or more	21 or more	18 or more
Very good	29 to 35	22 to 29	17 to 24	13 to 20	11 to 17
Good	22 to 28	17 to 21	13 to 16	10 to 12	8 to 10
Fair	17 to 21	12 to 16	10 to 12	7 to 9	5 to 7
Needs improvement	16 or fewer	11 or fewer	9 or fewer	6 or fewer	4 or fewer
Females	**Age**				
	20 to 29	**30 to 39**	**40 to 49**	**50 to 59**	**60 to 69**
Excellent	30 or more	27 or more	24 or more	21 or more	17 or more
Very good	21 to 29	20 to 26	15 to 23	11 to 20	12 to 16
Good	15 to 20	13 to 19	11 to 14	7 to 10	5 to 11
Fair	10 to 14	8 to 12	5 to 10	2 to 6	2 to 4
Needs improvement	9 or fewer	7 or fewer	4 or fewer	1 or none	1 or none

Curl-Up and Push-Up Tests for Youth

FitnessGram includes healthy fitness zone ranges for curl-ups and push-ups (4, 5). For the curl-up test, the two pieces of tape used to help guide the extent of the curl-up are placed 3 inches (7.6 cm) apart for 5- to 9-year-olds and 4.5 inches (11.4 cm) apart for 10- to 19-year-olds. Heels must stay in contact with the mat, and no pauses or rest periods are allowed (see figure 6.3 for an example of a youth performing a curl-up). Movement should be controlled (about one curl every 3 seconds or a total of 20 per minute). If the heels come up, if the fingers do not touch the far tape, or if the child is unable to maintain a continuous cadence, the test is over and the final count should be recorded (a total of 75 curl-ups is considered maximal). Healthy ranges are shown in table 6.4.

For the push-up test, the hands are placed slightly wider than the shoulders and the legs are out straight (see figure 6.4). The back should remain in a straight line from head to toes throughout the test. The body is lowered until the elbows are at a 90-degree angle and the upper arms are parallel with the floor. Then, arms should be straightened fully to return to the starting position. The test is continued as long as these form requirements are met and the movement is continuous (no rest stops are allowed). Record the maximal number completed. Boys and girls follow the same protocol. Healthy ranges are found in table 6.4.

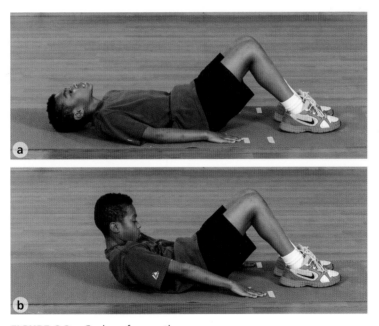

FIGURE 6.3   Curl-up for youth.

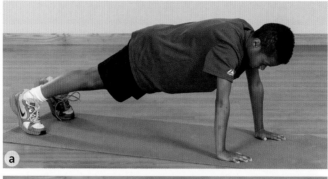

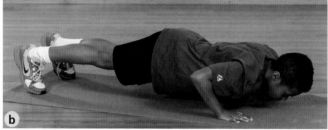

FIGURE 6.4   Push-up for youth.

TABLE 6.4   FitnessGram Standards for Healthy Fitness Zone* for Curl-Ups and Push-Ups for Youth

	Curl-up		Push-up	
Age	Boys	Girls	Boys	Girls
5	2 or more	2 or more	3 or more	3 or more
6	2 or more	2 or more	3 or more	3 or more
7	4 or more	4 or more	4 or more	4 or more
8	6 or more	6 or more	5 or more	5 or more
9	9 or more	9 or more	6 or more	6 or more
10	12 or more	12 or more	7 or more	7 or more
11	15 or more	15 or more	8 or more	7 or more
12	18 or more	18 or more	10 or more	7 or more
13	21 or more	18 or more	12 or more	7 or more
14	24 or more	18 or more	14 or more	7 or more
15	24 or more	18 or more	16 or more	7 or more
16	24 or more	18 or more	18 or more	7 or more
17	24 or more	18 or more	18 or more	7 or more
17+	24 or more	18 or more	18 or more	7 or more

*The values listed represent the healthy fitness zone and indicate that the child has a sufficient fitness level to provide important health benefits. Being below the value listed indicates a need for improvement.

Adapted by permission from The Cooper Institute, 2017, pp. 86, 87.

Chair Stand Test for Older Adults

The chair stand test is used to assess lower body strength in older adults, which is important in daily activities such as climbing stairs; walking; and getting out of a chair, bathtub, or car. For the chair stand test, fold your arms across your chest and count the number of times that you can stand from a seated position in 30 seconds (see figure 6.5) (24). Normal ranges are shown in table 6.5; if your score is over the range listed, consider yourself above average and if your score falls short of the range listed, consider yourself below average.

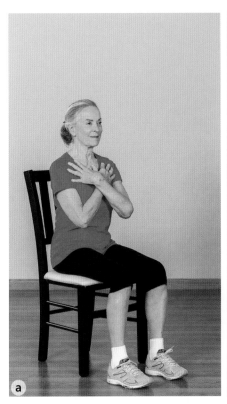 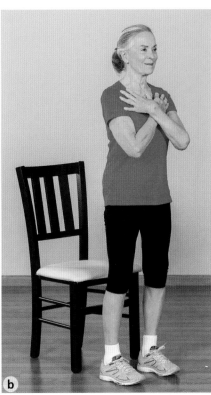

FIGURE 6.5   Chair stand for older adults.

Arm Curl Test for Older Adults

An arm curl test is used to assess upper body strength in older adults, which is important for daily activities such as carrying groceries or small children. The arm curl assessment, as shown in figure 6.6, is used to determine upper body muscular fitness. This test involves counting the number of dumbbell curls you can complete in 30 seconds. Men should use an 8-pound (3.6 kg) dumbbell, and women should use a 5-pound (2.3 kg) dumbbell. Normal ranges are shown in table 6.5; if your score is over the range listed, consider yourself above average and if your score falls short of the range listed, consider yourself below average.

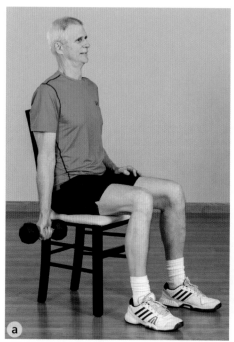 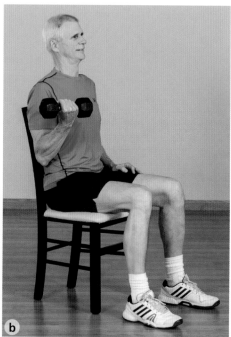

FIGURE 6.6   Arm curl for older adults.

TABLE 6.5   **Normal Ranges for Fitness Test Scores for Older Adults**

Males	Age						
	60–64	65–69	70–74	75–79	80–84	85–89	90–94
Chair stand test (number of stands)	14–19	12–18	12–17	11–17	10–15	8–14	7–12
Arm curl test (number of repetitions)	16–22	15–21	14–21	13–19	13–19	11–17	10–14
Females	**Age**						
	60–64	65–69	70–74	75–79	80–84	85–89	90–94
Chair stand test (number of stands)	12–17	11–16	10–15	10–15	9–14	8–13	4–11
Arm curl test (number of repetitions)	13–19	12–18	12–17	11–17	10–16	10–15	8–13

Adapted by permission from R.E. Rikli and C.J. Jones, 2013, pp. 89, 90.

Muscular fitness assessments that are consistent with each individual's training experience and fitness goals can provide useful information. In addition to comparing performance to that of others of the same age and sex, periodic assessments can help to gauge the effectiveness of your resistance training program. For safety purposes, individuals with health concerns should seek consultation from a health care provider before performing any fitness test.

Fundamental Principles of Resistance Training

Improvements in muscular fitness occur only if the resistance training program is based on sound training principles and is prudently progressed over time (7, 21). Although factors such as your initial level of fitness, genetics, nutrition, and motivation will influence the rate and magnitude of adaptation that occurs, you can maximize the effectiveness of your resistance training by addressing three fundamental principles: progressive overload, regularity, and specificity.

Progressive Overload

The progressive overload principle states that to enhance muscular fitness, you must exercise at a level beyond the point to which your muscles are accustomed. This goes back to the idea of having to stress the muscle to get a positive response. Doing the same workout month after month will not maximize benefits. The principle of progression refers to consistently boosting the training stimulus or load at a rate that is compatible with the training-induced adaptations that are occurring (21). Following the principle of progressive overload requires that you provide your muscles with a new stimulus when they have adapted to the current overload. You can do this in a variety of ways:

- *Increase the number of repetitions.* Typically, 8 to 12 repetitions is recommended for muscular fitness (for middle-age and older adults starting exercise, 10 to 15 repetitions is recommended). People focusing on strength development may select fewer repetitions, whereas those focusing on muscular endurance may include up to 15 to 20 repetitions (1).

- *Increase the number of sets for a given muscle group.* You could do additional sets of the same exercise, or you could add another exercise that targets the same muscle group. For example, the chest muscles could be trained with two sets of the chest press or one set of the chest press and one set of the dumbbell fly.

- *Increase the resistance.* The increase in weight needed will vary depending on the exercise but is often prescribed according to the increments available (e.g., next-weight dumbbell, increasing by one plate on a weight machine).

When providing an overload, select one of these options at a time. Although you want to provide a new stress on the muscle, you do not want to overtax the muscle or supporting structures to the point of injury.

Although every training session does not have to be more intense than the last session, the principle of progressive overload states that the training program needs to be increased gradually over time to realize gains. For example, if you have been able to easily complete a given workout for a couple of exercise sessions, it may be time to make changes to provide an overload once again in order to keep the resistance training program fresh, challenging, and effective. If you are able to perform a given exercise for one or two repetitions over your target number for two training sessions in a row, this indicates that you are ready to increase the resistance while returning to the original target repetition range.

Regularity

The principle of regularity states that exercise must be performed several times per week on a habitual basis to enhance physical fitness. Although training once per week may maintain training-induced gains, more frequent workouts are needed to optimize gains in health and fitness (1). In short, the adage "use it or lose it" is true because you will lose strength gains if you do not progress your program over time and perform resistance training on a regular basis (21). Although consecutive days of heavy strength training for the same muscle groups are not recommended, regularly training each major muscle group two to three times per week, with at least 48 hours separating training sessions for the same muscle group, is recommended to enhance muscular fitness.

Specificity

The principle of specificity refers to the distinct adaptations that take place as a result of the training program. In essence, every muscle or muscle group must be trained to make gains in muscular fitness (see figure 6.7 for the location of the major muscle groups in the body). Exercises such as the squat and leg press can be used to enhance lower body strength, but these exercises will not affect upper body strength. What's more, the adaptations that take place in a given muscle or muscle group will be as simple or as complex as the stress placed on them. For example, because tennis requires multijoint and multidirectional movements, it seems prudent for tennis players to perform resistance exercises that mimic the movements of the sport. For tennis players who need strong leg muscles to move across the court, lunges are unbeatable exercises to improve lower body performance. Lunges performed in different directions actually simulate steps used in game situations.

The specificity principle can also be applied to the design of resistance training programs for adults who want to enhance their abilities to perform activities of daily life such as stair climbing and household chores, which also require multijoint and multidirectional movements. For example, climbing stairs may be difficult as a result of poor lower body strength. By sensibly progressing from single-joint exercises such as leg extensions to multijoint exercises such as leg presses and dumbbell step-ups, you can improve your stair-climbing ability. These multijoint exercises specifically strengthen the quadriceps and gluteals, which are used in stair climbing.

Resistance Training Workout Components

The general format of an aerobic training session (as described in chapter 5) can be applied to resistance training as well. Before beginning a session, you should perform a warm-up to prepare your muscles for the conditioning phase of the workout. The conditioning phase is the main focus, and you should follow it with a cool-down.

Warm-Up

The warm-up for resistance training should include 5 to 10 minutes of low- to moderate-intensity aerobic activities and muscular endurance activities (lower resistance with a

Resistance Training Guidelines for Healthy Adults

Following are a few guidelines for resistance training if you are a healthy adult (1):

- Select a weight that allows you to perform 8 to 12 repetitions per set (10 to 15 repetitions for middle-age and older adults who are starting exercise).
- Train each major muscle group for a total of two to four sets (beginners can benefit from one set, which may reduce soreness and enhance adherence).
- Perform each set to the point of muscle fatigue but not failure.
- Rest for 2 to 3 minutes between sets to improve muscular fitness.
- Perform 8 to 10 exercises with proper technique.
- Resistance train two to three days per week on alternate days (48 hours is recommended between sessions to allow the muscles to recover).
- Continually progress the training program to optimize long-term adaptations.

higher number of repetitions, such as 10 to 15 repetitions). These activities will increase your body temperature and prepare your body for the demands of the resistance training workout (1).

Muscle Conditioning Phase

Despite various claims about what constitutes the best resistance training program, it does not appear that one optimal combination of sets, repetitions, and exercises promotes long-term adaptations in muscular fitness in everyone. Rather, you can alter many program variables to achieve desirable outcomes provided that you follow the fundamental training principles as discussed in this chapter. The program variables to consider are choice of exercise, order of exercise, training weight (which determines the number of repetitions), number of sets, repetition velocity, and rest periods between sets and exercises (see Resistance Training Guidelines for Healthy Adults).

Exercise Choice

A limitless number of exercises can be used to enhance muscular fitness. Exercises can generally be classified as single joint (i.e., body part specific) or multijoint (i.e., structural). The dumbbell biceps curl and leg extension are examples of single-joint exercises that isolate a specific body part (biceps and quadriceps, respectively), whereas the chest press and squat are multijoint exercises that involve two or more joints. Although it is important to incorporate multijoint exercises into a resistance training program, be sure to select exercises that are appropriate for your exercise technique experience and training goals. When learning any new exercise, start with a light weight to master the technique of the exercise before increasing the weight. To maximize gains and minimize the risk of injury, all resistance training exercise should be performed with proper exercise technique in a controlled manner.

Your choice of exercise should also promote muscle balance across joints and between opposing muscle groups (e.g., quadriceps and hamstrings). Of particular importance is the inclusion of exercises for the abdominal and low back musculature. It is not uncommon for beginners to focus on strengthening the chest and biceps and not spend adequate time strengthening the abdominal muscles and lower back.

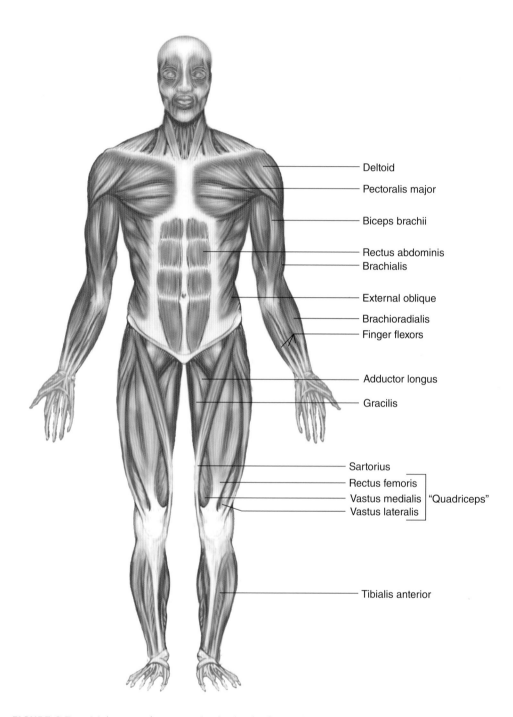

Deltoid

Pectoralis major

Biceps brachii

Rectus abdominis
Brachialis

External oblique

Brachioradialis
Finger flexors

Adductor longus

Gracilis

Sartorius
Rectus femoris
Vastus medialis   "Quadriceps"
Vastus lateralis

Tibialis anterior

FIGURE 6.7a Major muscle groups in the body: front view.

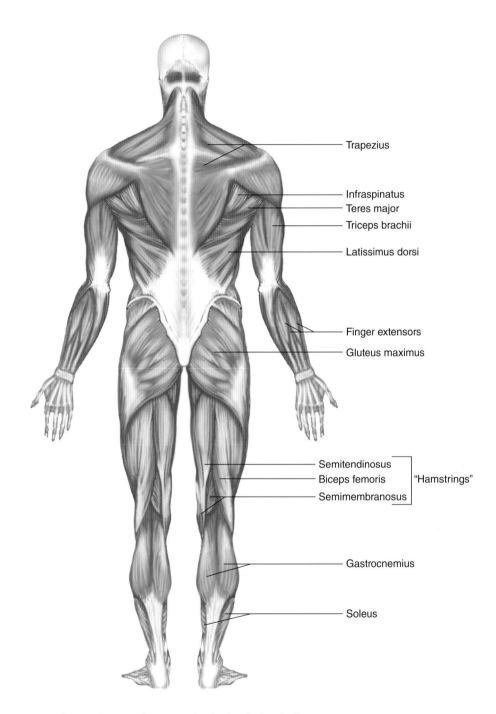

FIGURE 6.7b Major muscle groups in the body: back view.

Strengthening the midsection, or trunk area, may not only enhance body control during performance of free weight exercises such as the squat, but may also reduce the risk of injury (10). The resistance training program suggestions in this chapter promote muscle balance by including the appropriate muscle groups (see table 6.6 and figure 6.8).

Exercise Order

There are many ways to arrange the sequence of exercises in a resistance training session. Traditionally, large-muscle group exercises are performed before smaller-muscle group exercises, and multijoint exercises are performed before single-joint exercises.

TABLE 6.6   Resistance Training Workout Muscle Guide

Body area	Exercise
Hips and legs (gluteals, quadriceps, hamstrings)	Machine leg press (p. 128)
	Dumbbell squat (p. 129)
	Dumbbell step-up (p. 129)
	Ankle weight hip flexion and extension (p. 130)
	Band leg lunge (p. 131)
Legs (quadriceps)	Machine leg extension (p. 131)
	Ankle weight knee extension (p. 132)
Legs (hamstrings)	Machine leg curl (p. 132)
	Ankle weight knee flexion (p. 133)
Chest (pectoralis)	Machine chest press (p. 133)
	Dumbbell chest press (p. 134)
	Band seated chest press (p. 134)
	Modified push-up (p. 135)
	Push-up (p. 107-108)
Back (latissimus dorsi)	Machine lat pulldown (p. 135)
	Machine seated row (p. 136)
	Dumbbell one-arm row (p. 136)
	Band seated row (p. 137)
Shoulders (deltoid)	Machine overhead press (p. 137)
	Dumbbell lateral raise (p. 138)
	Dumbbell or band upright row (p. 138-139)
Arms (biceps)	Machine biceps curl (p. 139)
	Dumbbell or band biceps curl (p. 140)
Arms (triceps)	Machine triceps press (p. 141)
	Dumbbell lying triceps extension (p. 141)
	Band triceps extension (p. 142)
Low back (erector spinae)	Machine back extension (p. 142)
	Prone plank (p. 143)
	Kneeling hip extension (p. 143)
Abdominal muscles	Machine abdominal curl (p. 144)
	Curl-up (p. 144)
	Diagonal curl-up (p. 145)

Following this exercise order allows you to use heavier weights on the multijoint exercises because fatigue will be less of a factor.

Perform more challenging exercises earlier in the workout when your neuromuscular system is less fatigued. In general, it seems reasonable to follow the priority system of training in which exercises that will most likely contribute to enhanced muscular fitness are performed early in the training session. The sample resistance training programs presented in this chapter include exercises that reflect this sequence (see table 6.6 and figure 6.8).

Number of Repetitions

One of the most important variables in the design of a resistance training program is the amount of weight used for an exercise (7). Gains in muscular fitness are influenced

FIGURE 6.8

Sample resistance training programs.

Stage*	Exercises**	Number of sets	Number of repetitions	Number of days per week***
Beginner	*Moving through this level typically takes about two to three months, although you should remain at this level until you feel comfortable enough to advance.*			
	Do a total of six exercises. Select one exercise from each of the following body areas: hips and legs, chest, back, shoulders, low back, and abdominal muscles.	1 to 2	8 to 12 (10 to 15 for older adults)	2 to 3
Intermediate to established	*Moving through the intermediate to the established level typically takes 3 to 12 months depending on your level of consistency.*			
	Do a total of 10 exercises. Select one exercise from each of the following body areas: hips and legs, quadriceps, hamstrings, chest, back, shoulders, biceps, triceps, low back, and abdominal muscles.	2	8 to 12 (10 to 15 for middle-age and older adults starting exercise)	2 to 3
More advanced (complete all 15 exercises)	Do a total of 10 exercises. Select two exercises from each of these larger-muscle group areas: hips and legs, quadriceps, hamstrings, chest, and back.	2 to 3	8 to 12	2 to 3
	Do a total of five exercises. Select one exercise from each of these smaller-muscle group and trunk areas: shoulders, biceps, triceps, low back, and abdominal muscles.	2	8 to 12	2 to 3

*The time spent at each stage will depend on your muscular fitness level. Transition slowly between the stages (e.g., over time a beginner can add additional exercises or increase the number of sets to move toward the intermediate level of resistance training).

**Different exercises can be performed on different days.

***Schedule your training days so that at least 48 hours separates training sessions that target the same muscle group.

by the amount of weight lifted, which is inversely related to the number of repetitions you can perform. As the weight increases, the number of repetitions you can perform decreases. Although you should never sacrifice proper form, the training weight should be challenging enough to result in at least a modest degree of muscle fatigue during the last few repetitions of a set. If this does not occur, you will not achieve the desired gains from your resistance training program.

Because heavy weights are not required to increase the muscular strength of beginners, weights corresponding to about 60 to 80 percent of the 1RM for 8 to 12 repetitions are recommended for adults (10 to 15 repetitions for middle-age and older adults with limited resistance training experience) (1). Although weights that can be lifted more than 15 times are effective for increasing local muscular endurance, light weights rarely result in meaningful gains in muscular strength. If you are a beginner, the best approach is to first establish a target repetition range (e.g., 8 to 12), and then by trial and error determine the maximum load you can handle for the prescribed number of repetitions. If multiple sets of an exercise are performed, the first set may be performed for 12 repetitions before fatigue occurs whereas the last set may be performed for about 8 repetitions.

Although it may take two to three workouts to find your desired training weight on all exercises, keep in mind that the magnitude of your effort will determine the outcome of your strength training program. For example, training within an 8RM to 12RM zone means that you should be able to perform no more than 12 repetitions with a given weight using proper exercise technique. Simply performing an exercise for 8, 9, 10, 11, or 12 repetitions does not necessarily mean you are training within the 8RM to 12RM zone. You should be stopping because of the onset of muscle fatigue, not just because you have reached a predetermined number. However, regardless of the number of repetitions, it is important to maintain proper technique on every repetition to optimize adaptations and reduce the risk of injury.

Number of Sets

The number of sets performed in a workout is directly related to the overall training volume, which reflects the amount of time the muscles are being exercised. For beginners, even one set can provide benefits. Healthy adults should perform two to four sets for each muscle group to achieve muscular fitness goals (1). Although single-set protocols can enhance your muscular strength if you are a beginner, multiple-set pro-

---

■ Q&A

When should the weight lifted be increased?

Consider how many repetitions are currently possible. For example, initially it may be possible to lift a 20-pound (9 kg) barbell only eight times. As training continues and muscular fitness improves, this repetition number increases from 8 to 12 before fatigue (i.e., repetitions number 11 and 12 are a bit of a struggle to complete). Increasing the repetitions is one way to overload the muscle. When you are able to easily complete 12 repetitions in two consecutive training sessions, this is evidence that the muscles have adapted to the overload and now it is time to progress to a higher weight to provide greater resistance. The repetition number will drop back and the process of increasing number of repetitions from 8 to 12 will start over again.

tocols have proven more effective in the long term, with evidence of a dose response for the number of sets per exercise (14, 19). That is, greater gains in muscular fitness can be expected with additional sets per exercise (up to a point). What's more, you do not need to perform every exercise for the same number of sets. As a general recommendation, perform more sets of large-muscle group exercises than of smaller-muscle group exercises.

You can use different combinations of sets and exercises to vary the training stimulus, which is vital for long-term gains. For example, if you complete one set of two different exercises for the same muscle group (e.g., leg press and leg extension), the quadriceps on the front of the thigh will have performed two sets. From a practical standpoint, your health status, fitness goals, and time demands should determine the number of sets you perform per muscle group.

Repetition Velocity

Strength-building exercises should be performed at a controlled, or moderate, velocity during the lifting and lowering phases. Movement control can be defined as the ability to stop any lifting or lowering action at will without momentum carrying the movement to completion. Uncontrolled, jerky movements not only are ineffective but also may result in injury. Intentionally slow velocities with a relatively light weight (e.g., a 5-second lifting phase and a 5-second lowering phase) may be useful to enhance muscular endurance, but this type of training is not recommended to optimize gains in muscular strength (20). Although different movement speeds have proven effective, if you are a beginner, you should perform each repetition at a moderate speed, with about 2 seconds for the lifting phase and 3 seconds for the lowering phase. A longer lowering phase places more emphasis on the eccentric muscle action, which is important for muscle growth and strength development (20).

Rest Periods Between Sets and Exercises

The length of the rest period between sets and exercises is an important but often overlooked training variable. In general, the length of the rest period influences energy recovery and training adaptation. For example, if your primary goal is muscular strength, heavier weights and longer rest periods of 2 to 3 minutes are needed, whereas if your goal is muscular endurance, lighter weights, higher repetitions, and shorter rest periods of 30 to 60 seconds are required (20). Obviously, the heavier the weight is, the longer the rest period should be if the training goal is to maximize strength gains.

Cool-Down

The cool-down brings the body systems back to resting levels. Just as the warm-up led into the conditioning phase, the cool-down helps to transition the body from the higher demands of the conditioning phase to the lower levels of physiological demand seen at rest. Shifting to moderate-intensity and then low-intensity aerobic and muscular endurance activity will lower your heart rate and blood pressure gradually and safely (1). See Safety First for additional ways to maximize safety when training.

Types of Resistance Training

Provided that you adhere to the fundamental principles of training, you can use almost any type of resistance training to enhance muscular fitness. Some equipment is relatively

Safety First

Your resistance training program should be based on your health status, fitness training experience, and goals. As discussed in chapter 2, you should assess your health status before participating in strength-building activities. In some cases, specialized exercise programs are needed for those with preexisting medical conditions such as high blood pressure, heart disease, or diabetes. Thus, if you have a medical concern or issue, you should consult with your health care provider before resistance training.

Recognizing that resistance training to improve general fitness is different from training to enhance sport performance will further promote the development of and adherence to safe, effective, and enjoyable programs. If you have little experience with resistance training, you are strongly encouraged to seek instruction from a qualified fitness professional, because most injuries are the result of improper exercise technique or excessive loading (13, 17). Qualified fitness professionals can provide instruction on proper warm-up procedures, offer advice on specific methods of progression, and monitor the magnitude of your effort, which in turn can have a positive impact on training adaptations (16, 22).

Knowing proper breathing techniques will help you avoid the Valsalva maneuver, which can occur if you hold your breath while lifting. Not exhaling can increase pressure in the chest cavity, which can increase blood pressure to harmful levels. To avoid this effect, continue to breathe normally by inhaling before you start the lift, exhaling during the lifting–exertion phase (as you lift against gravity), and then inhaling again as you return to the starting position. Using this technique will allow you to lift weight correctly and safely.

Following are general safety recommendations for designing and performing a resistance training program:

- *Maintain a regular breathing pattern when lifting and lowering weights.* Do not hold your breath; rather, inhale before you start the lift, exhale during the lift, and inhale as you return to the starting position.

- *Make sure the exercise environment is well lit, clean, and free of clutter.* Tripping or falling over resistance training equipment can be avoided by following this guideline.

- *Learn proper exercise technique from a qualified fitness professional.* If you have little

easy to use; other equipment requires balance, coordination, and high levels of skill. A decision to use a certain type of resistance training should be based on your health status, fitness goals, training experience, and access to professional fitness instruction if needed. Common types of resistance training involve the use of weight machines; free weights; body weight exercises; and a broadly defined category that involves the use of balls, bands, and elastic tubing (table 6.7 summarizes the advantages and disadvantages of various types of resistance training). These types of resistance training typically include dynamic movements that involve a lifting (concentric) and lowering (eccentric) phase through a predetermined range of motion.

Weight machines train all the major muscle groups and can be found in most fitness centers. They are relatively easy to use because the exercise motion is controlled by the machine. For this reason, weight machines are a good option if you have not done resistance training before, are relatively new to this type of training, or are out of shape or deconditioned. Also, weight machines are ideal for isolating muscle groups. As a result, they often do not mimic sport activities or activities of daily life as well as some free weight exercises do. For general health and convenience, however, they

experience with resistance training, have someone with appropriate qualifications show you how to do resistance training exercises and assist you with making any needed adjustments.

- *Perform warm-up and cool-down activities.* Taking time for warming up and cooling down helps your body to transition safely into and out of your workout.

- *Move carefully around the strength training area.* Resistance training by its nature is equipment intensive. Dumbbells, barbells, and weight plates are all potential tripping hazards.

- *Do not use broken or malfunctioning equipment.* Check for frayed belts or cables before using any resistance training machine. Fittings should be tight, and all belts and cables should be in good condition.

- *Use collars on all plate-loaded barbells and dumbbells.* Collars are devices placed on the ends of barbells and dumbbells to hold the individual weight plates in position. Without these fasteners in place, the weight plates could shift or even fall off, causing injury.

- *Be aware of proper spotting procedures when using free weights.* A spotter is a person who is in a position to assist you when you are using free weights. Because free weights are not supported by cables or any other devices, a spotter's role is to help guide or lift a weight if you have difficulty with the resistance.

- *Avoid jerky, uncontrolled movements while resistance training.* Maintaining controlled movements maximizes the benefits of your workout and also helps you avoid injury.

- *Periodically check all training equipment.* Checking equipment for cleanliness as well as any signs of wear and tear (e.g., frayed cables or belts) and making needed corrections will help keep your resistance training sessions safe and enjoyable.

- *Regularly clean equipment pads that come in contact with the skin.* Pads become soiled with sweat; maintaining a routine of wiping off contacted surfaces promotes good hygiene.

TABLE 6.7   Comparison of Various Types of Resistance Training

Type	Cost	Portability	Ease of use	Muscle isolation	Functionality	Exercise variety	Space requirement
Weight machines	High	Limited	Excellent	Excellent	Limited	Limited	High
Free weights	Low	Variable	Variable	Variable	Excellent	Excellent	Variable
Body weight	None	Excellent	Variable	Variable	Excellent	Excellent	Low
Balls and cords or bands*	Very low	Excellent	Variable	Variable	Excellent	Excellent	Low

*Medicine balls, stability balls, and elastic cords or bands.

What would be a good circuit of exercises at a fitness center?

Depending on available equipment, you will want to select exercises that target the major muscle groups. The following is an example of a program for an established exerciser with 10 body areas targeted:

- *Hips and legs:* Machine leg press or dumbbell squat
- *Quadriceps:* Machine leg extension
- *Hamstrings:* Machine leg curl
- *Chest:* Machine or dumbbell chest press
- *Back:* Machine lat pull-down or machine seated row
- *Shoulders:* Machine overhead press or dumbbell lateral raise
- *Biceps:* Machine biceps curl or dumbbell biceps curl
- *Triceps:* Machine triceps press or dumbbell lying triceps extension
- *Low back:* Machine back extension
- *Abdominal muscles:* Machine abdominal curl

provide an effective method of resistance training. Although weight machines fit the typical male or female, smaller body size may require a seat pad or back pad to adjust body position to create a better fit.

Free weights, such as barbells and dumbbells, are inexpensive and can be used for a wide variety of exercises that require greater balance and coordination. Although it may take longer to master proper exercise technique using free weights compared to weight machines, proper fit is not an issue because one size fits all. Free weights also offer a greater variety of exercises than weight machines because they can be moved in many directions. Another benefit of free weights is that they require the use of additional stabilizing and assisting muscles to hold the correct body position to perform an exercise correctly. As such, free weight training can occur in different planes of motion and is ideal for enhancing performance during activities of daily life. This is particularly true regarding the use of dumbbells because they train each side of the body independently. However, unlike weight machines, several free weight exercises, such as the bench press, require the aid of a spotter who can assist the lifter in case of a failed repetition. Spotters should be able to handle the weight lifted and should know when to intervene.

Body weight exercises such as push-ups, pull-ups, and curl-ups are among the oldest modes of strength training. Obviously, a major advantage of body weight training is that equipment is not needed and a variety of exercises can be performed. On the other hand, a limitation of body weight training is the difficulty in adjusting the body weight to the strength level of the person. Exercise machines that allow you to perform body weight exercises such as pull-ups and dips using a predetermined percentage of your body weight are available. Even if you do not have the strength to lift your entire body weight, these machines provide assistance, allowing participants of all abilities to incorporate body weight exercises into their strength training programs and feel good about their accomplishments.

Stability balls, medicine balls, and elastic tubing are inexpensive, safe, and effective alternatives to weight machines and free weights. Stability balls are lightweight, inflatable balls (about 45 to 75 centimeters in diameter) that add the elements of balance and coordination to any exercise. Medicine balls come in a variety of shapes and sizes (about 2 pounds to over 20 pounds, or 1 kilogram to over 9 kilograms) and stress muscles as you hold, catch, and throw them. Training with elastic rubber cords, or bands, involves generating force to stretch the cord and then returning the cord in a controlled manner to its unstretched state. The more the cord is stretched, the greater the force needed to move through the range of motion. Different colors of cords reflect different amounts of resistance.

■ Q&A

Can muscular fitness be improved without access to a fitness center?

Although membership at a fitness center has many advantages, you can also improve your muscular fitness at home. Resistance bands and ankle weights are relatively inexpensive purchases. In addition to exercises that use body weight, these can target the major muscle groups. For example, a beginner program with six exercises might look like this:

- *Hips and legs:* Ankle weight hip flexion and extension or band leg lunge
- *Chest:* Band seated chest press or modified push-up
- *Back:* Band seated row
- *Shoulders:* Band upright row
- *Low back:* Prone plank or kneeling hip extension
- *Abdominal muscles:* Curl-up

Your Resistance Training Program

Your resistance training program needs to take into account your current muscular fitness level. Beginner, intermediate, and more advanced sample programs are outlined in figure 6.8 (for a workout guide that groups exercises into the appropriate body areas, see table 6.6). If you have no resistance training experience or have not trained for several months or years, you should begin resistance training by following a general program in which weights are light to moderate and the focus is on learning proper exercise technique. Also, it is always a good idea for beginners to receive instruction on proper exercise technique and training guidelines from a qualified fitness professional.

Avoid the common mistake of doing too much too soon. Give your body a chance to adapt gradually to the physical stress of resistance training while making fitness gains. Use the initial weeks to increase your body's ability to tolerate the stress of resistance training gradually to minimize muscle soreness. The aim is to develop healthy habits early on so that resistance training becomes an enjoyable, meaningful, and long-lasting experience. Regardless of how much weight others can lift, go slowly during the first few weeks as you build a foundation for more advanced training programs in the future.

As indicated in the sample programs in figure 6.8, if you are a beginner, you should perform one or two sets of six exercises with a moderate weight. Of course, regardless of your level of experience, you should use lighter loads when you are learning a new exercise or attempting to correct any flaws in your exercise technique. Also, keep in mind that you do not have to perform every exercise for the same number of sets. This preparatory period is designed to gradually enhance your physical abilities as you start the process of resistance training. If you have a very low level of fitness, you may need a longer period of time before you can participate in a resistance training program designed to maximize gains in muscular fitness. A major goal of this training phase is to learn correct form and technique for a variety of upper body, lower body, and midsection exercises while practicing proper training procedures. Table 6.6 outlines resistance training exercises that use weight machines, free weights (dumbbells), and your own body weight.

Once you are comfortable with the level of exercise at the beginner level, you are ready to move to the intermediate level. Typically, this takes around two to three months, although this time may be shorter or longer depending on your initial fitness level. The intermediate level begins once you have progressed through the beginner level, or you can start at this level if you are already engaging in some resistance training. The intermediate activities are broader in scope than the beginner activities and also increase the overall volume (increasing the number of exercises and sets). Depending on the consistency of your training, you may spend three months to a year or more at the intermediate level.

After 6 to 12 months of consistent training, you may appropriately be classified as "established." At this point you can continue with the intermediate-level exercise format but increase the weight, or resistance, over time (recall the concept of progressive overload). Figure 6.8 includes a "more advanced" category for those looking to increase their focus beyond health-related levels of resistance training. More advanced resistance training can provide additional muscular fitness benefits and includes exercises for different body parts on separate days of the week (thus increasing the overall training volume and the time you spend training).

By varying the program variables such as the choice of exercise and number of sets, you will start to achieve specific goals in health and fitness. Although every workout does not need to be more intense than the previous one, varying your program helps to prevent boredom and training plateaus that eventually lead to a lack of adherence and dropout. As you perform additional sets, keep in mind that your effort determines your training outcomes. Thus, feelings related to exercise exertion should be an expected and welcome part of the training process. A major goal is to gain confidence in your ability to perform strength-building exercises while maximizing training adaptations.

After the first few months of resistance training, improvements in muscular fitness occur at a slower rate. People who started resistance training with great enthusiasm sometimes become disappointed when gains in muscle strength are less dramatic during the third month of training. You need to understand that a workout that was effective during the first few months may not be effective in the long term. Once your body adapts to the training program, no additional gains will take place unless the training program is altered. In short, to make continual gains in muscular fitness and achieve specific health and fitness goals, you need to work harder and engage in a more challenging training program. This is particularly important if you want to maximize gains in muscular fitness (21).

Because of the demands of training, you need to allow time for adequate recovery between workouts for a given muscle group. For example, more advanced lifters may perform a whole-body workout only twice per week or a greater number of sessions per week using a split routine in which only certain muscle groups are selected on a given day. For example, a lifter may train the lower body on Monday and Thursday and the upper body on Tuesday and Friday. In any case, all lifters should appreciate the importance of adequate recovery between demanding resistance training workouts.

For continued gains in muscular fitness, you must sensibly alter your resistance training program over time so your body is continually challenged to adapt to the new demands (21). To clarify, every workout does not need to be harder than the previous workout; rather, a systematic progression of the exercise program is needed for long-term gains in muscular fitness. Even though beginners will improve at a faster rate than more experienced lifters, manipulating the program variables every couple of weeks will limit training plateaus and reduce the likelihood that you become bored with your training program and lose your enthusiasm for resistance training.

Although improving at the same rate over the long term is not possible, you have to place greater demands on the musculoskeletal system gradually if you want to

Resistance Training That Works for You

A total-body resistance training workout is an effective way to improve muscular fitness and physical performance. Although resistance training programs that split the body into selected muscle groups are popular, a total-body workout performed two to three days per week on nonconsecutive days is appropriate for most people. Such a program gives you time to learn proper exercise technique and develop a fitness base for more advanced training. The idea is to start with a general resistance training program and gradually make it more specific as your strength and confidence improve.

Because the ultimate goal is the adoption of muscular fitness exercises as a lifestyle choice, your resistance training program should be consistent with your current fitness status and personal goals. In addition, you need to consider the time you have available for training, the equipment you can access, and your strength training experience. Consider the following questions before beginning a resistance training program:

- Do you have health concerns that may limit your participation in a resistance training program?
- Do you currently participate in an exercise program?
- How much resistance training experience do you have?
- What type of resistance training equipment is available at home or at your gym?
- How much time do you have for resistance training during the week?
- What are your specific training goals?
- Would individualized instruction from a qualified fitness profession be beneficial?

Once you have answered these questions, you are ready to design a safe, effective, and enjoyable resistance training program that is consistent with your goals. This chapter provides guidance whether you are just starting or are already doing resistance training and are looking for ways to continue to improve. To make continual gains in health and fitness, you must continue, progress, and modify your program.

Using a workout card to monitor your training progress can be very helpful. On the card, record the exercises, weight lifted, and number of repetitions and sets. It is also a good idea to exercise with a training partner or fitness instructor who can serve as a spotter on selected exercises and provide assistance when needed.

make steady gains in muscular fitness. In addition to increasing the amount of weight you lift, you can also progress your training program in other ways. You can perform additional repetitions with the current weight, add more sets to your program, and incorporate different exercises or types of equipment into the program to provide progressive overload. The key to long-term training success is to make gradual changes in the program to keep it effective, challenging, and fun.

Resistance training is an essential component of adult fitness programs and can offer observable health and fitness gains when properly performed and sensibly progressed over time. The importance of the training-induced changes from resistance training should not be underestimated because they can have a meaningful impact on your physical function and quality of life (20, 30). Although many exercise options are available, resistance training programs based on sound training principles and consistent with your needs, goals, and abilities are most likely to result in favorable adaptations. In general, perform resistance training two to three days per week (with 48 hours between sessions), do two to four sets of 8 to 12 repetitions of each exercise (10 to 15 repetitions for middle-age and older adults starting exercise), and target each of the major muscle groups.

Resistance Training Exercises

Descriptions and photos for each of the exercises in the sample programs are included here (see table 6.6 for a guide showing you which exercises work specific body areas). In general, the photos depict the two ends of the range of motion for each exercise. Be sure to control your movement to reap the full benefits from each exercise.

Machine Leg Press

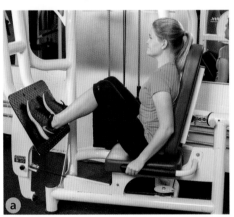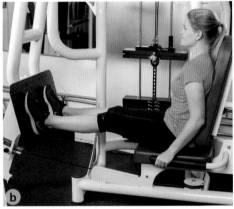

Adjust the machine so your knees are bent about 90 degrees, with feet flat on the foot pads *(a)*. Your knees and feet should be in line with your hips. Exhale and push your feet and legs forward by pushing through your heels until your knees are nearly straight *(b)*. Do not lock your knees.

Dumbbell Squat

Choose your desired or appropriate dumbbell weights. Spread your feet about shoulder-width apart; your knees and feet should be in line with your hips (a). Bend slightly at the hips and then bend your knees until your thighs are parallel to the floor (b). Your knees should not go beyond your toes. Pause briefly; then return to the starting position. Keep your chest up throughout the movement to avoid excessive forward lean.

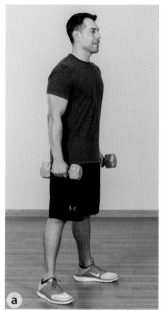
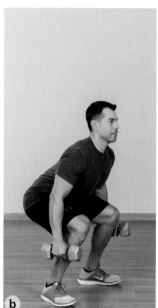

Dumbbell Step-Up

Choose your desired or appropriate dumbbell weights. Stand with a dumbbell in each hand facing a step (or bench). Place one foot on the step (a) and then step up with the other foot while keeping torso upright (b). Step back down and return to the starting position. Repeat with opposite leg. Begin with body weight only to learn proper form.

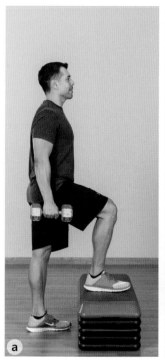
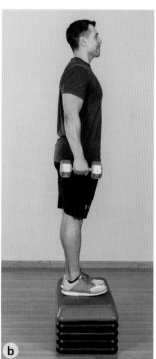

Ankle Weight Hip Flexion

Ankle weights are needed for this exercise. Stand tall with one hand on the back of a chair for balance *(a)*. Without leaning forward, lift one knee toward your chest in a marching motion *(b)*, pause briefly, and then return your knee to the starting position and repeat on the opposite side.

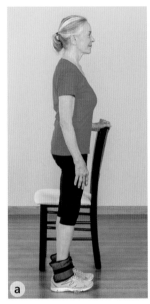
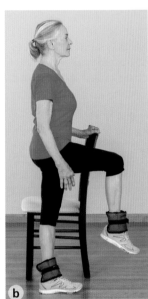

Ankle Weight Hip Extension

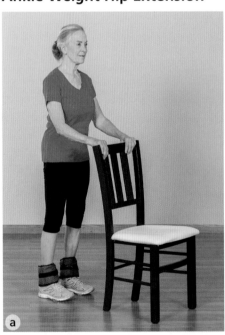
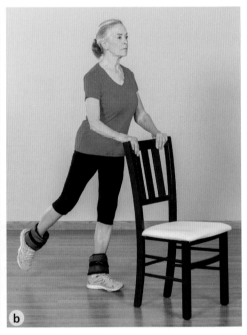

Ankle weights are needed for this exercise. Stand about 12 inches (30.5 cm) from a chair with your feet slightly apart. Bend forward slightly and hold on to the back of the chair for balance *(a)*. Lift one leg backward without moving your upper body forward or bending your knee *(b)*. Pause briefly; then return to the starting position and repeat on the opposite side.

Band Leg Lunge

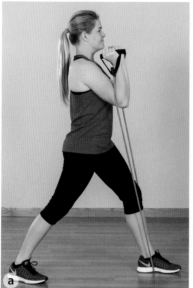 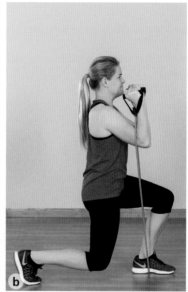

Start in a stride position with one foot in the middle of the band and the other foot extended behind your body. Pull the band tight by bending your elbows to allow your hands to be at shoulder height *(a)*. Lower your body toward the floor while keeping your shoulders over your hips and your front knee over the ankle of your front foot *(b)*. Return to the starting position and perform the desired number of repetitions. Repeat on the opposite side.

Machine Leg Extension

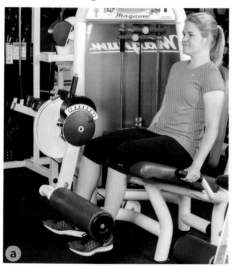 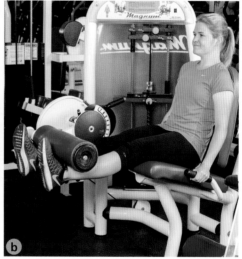

Adjust the machine so your knee joints are in line with the machine's axis of rotation and the leg pads are just above your ankles *(a)*. Straighten both knees until they are fully extended *(b)*, pause briefly, and then return to the starting position and repeat.

Ankle Weight Knee Extension

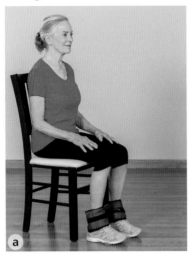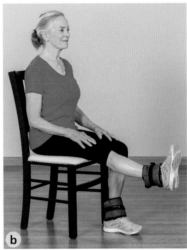

Ankle weights are needed for this exercise. Sit tall in a chair with your feet flat on the floor (a). Lift one leg by straightening your knee until the leg is parallel to the floor (b). Pause briefly; then return your leg to the starting position and repeat on the opposite side.

Machine Leg Curl

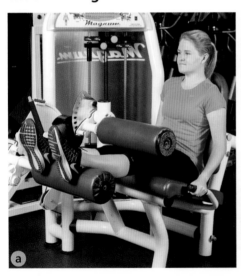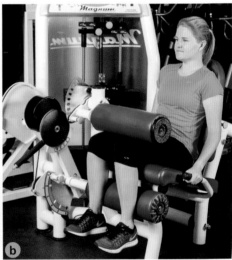

Adjust the machine so your knees are in line with the machine's axis of rotation and the roller pads are under your ankles (a). Grasp both handles. Pull the roller pad toward your hips until both knees are bent at least 90 degrees (b). Pause briefly; then return to the starting position and repeat.

Ankle Weight Knee Flexion

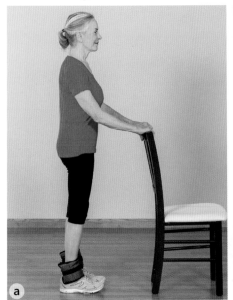
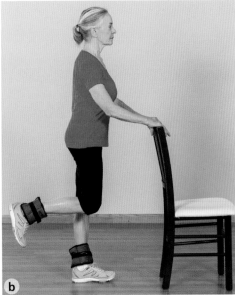

Ankle weights are needed for this exercise. While wearing ankle weights, stand tall behind a chair and grasp the chair back *(a)*. Bend one knee and raise your foot toward your buttocks without moving your thigh *(b)*. Pause briefly; then return to the starting position. Repeat on the other side.

Machine Chest Press

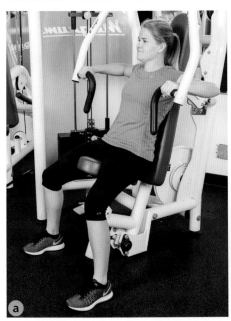
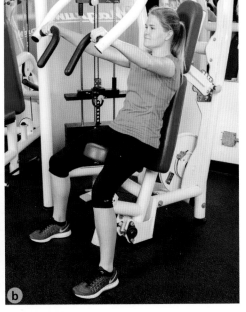

Adjust the seat so that the handles are aligned at midchest level. Sit with your back against the seat pads and grasp the bar handles with an overhand grip *(a)*. Push the handles forward until your elbows are straight and fully extended but not locked *(b)*. Pause briefly; then return the handles to the starting position and repeat.

Dumbbell Chest Press

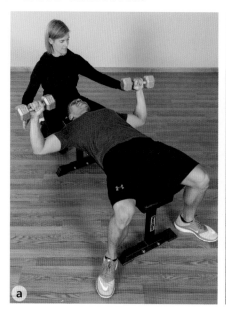 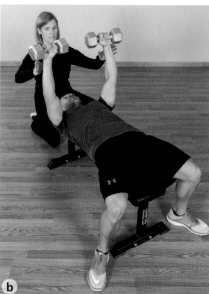

Choose your desired or appropriate dumbbell weight. Lie on a bench with your knees bent and your feet flat on the floor. Your head, shoulders, back, and buttocks must maintain contact with the bench during the exercise. Hold the dumbbells at the side of your chest with your thumbs wrapped around the handles and your elbows bent about 90 degrees (a). Press the dumbbells upward over your chest until your arms are straight (b). Return to the starting position and repeat. A spotter should be nearby to assist you if needed.

Band Seated Chest Press

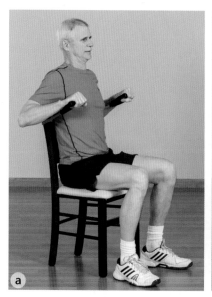 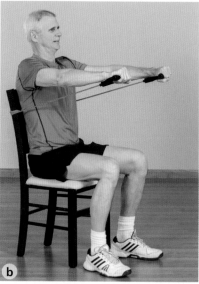

Choose a band color or thickness. Sit in a chair and wrap the band around the back of the chair. Hold the ends of the band at chest level with your elbows bent (a). The band tension should be tight. Press both arms straight out in front of your body (b). Pause briefly; then return to the starting position and repeat.

Modified Push-Up

Stand 2 to 3 feet (61-91 cm) from a wall and place your palms on the wall at shoulder height *(a)*. Your palms should be placed slightly wider than your shoulders. Keeping your back straight, bend your elbows until your nose almost touches the wall *(b)*. Pause briefly; then press away from the wall and return to the starting position. Moving your feet farther away from the wall increases the difficulty of this exercise. As you gain more strength in your upper body, prog-

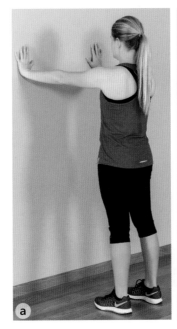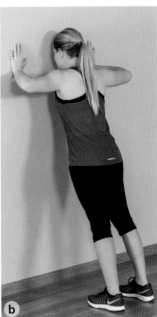

ress to bent-knee push-ups on the floor (see figure 6.2) and finally to full push-ups (see figure 6.1).

Machine Lat Pull-Down

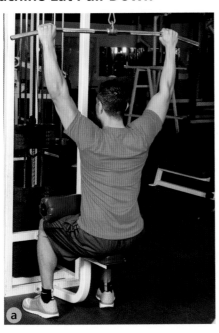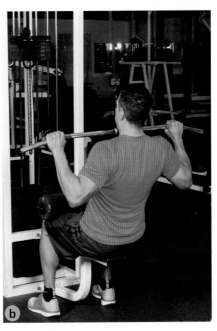

Adjust the seat height and extend your arms overhead to grasp the bar *(a)*. Your palms should face forward with your hands slightly wider than shoulder width. Lean back slightly, and pull the bar downward to the top of your chest *(b)*. Tuck your chin to allow the bar to freely pass in front of your face. Focus on pulling your elbows in toward your body. Return to the starting position and repeat.

Machine Seated Row

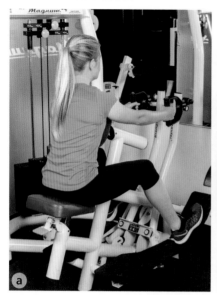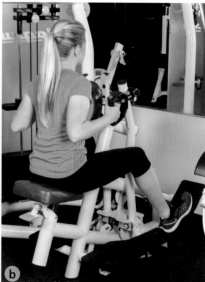

Move the seat so your shoulders are level with the machine handles and your chest is against the chest pad. Grasp the handles and sit tall with your chest up *(a)*. Pull the handles backward while moving your shoulder blades together *(b)*. Return to the starting position and repeat.

Dumbbell One-Arm Row

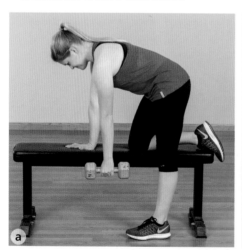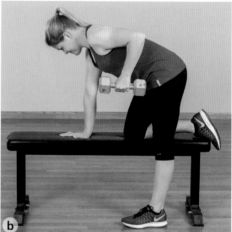

Choose your appropriate or desired dumbbell weight. Stand near the left side of the bench and place your right knee and the palm of your right hand on the bench, keeping your right arm straight and your torso almost horizontal. Hold the dumbbell in your left hand with your palm toward the bench *(a)*. Pull the dumbbell toward the side of your chest by bending at the elbow and the shoulder *(b)*. Return to the starting position and perform the desired number of repetitions. Repeat on the opposite side.

Band Seated Row

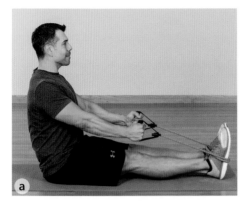
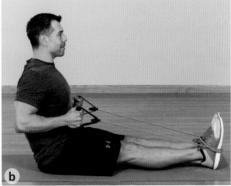

Choose a band color or thickness. Sit on the floor and wrap the band securely around both feet. The middle of the band should be placed at the center of your feet. Point your toes slightly forward to prevent the band from slipping. Fully straighten your elbows with your palms facing each other *(a)*. The band tension should be tight in both your hands. Pull the band toward the sides of your body while keeping your back straight *(b)*. Pause briefly; then return to the starting position and repeat.

Machine Overhead Press

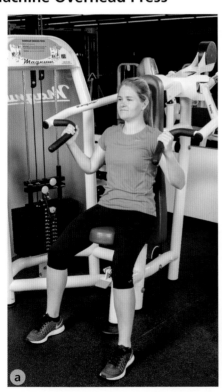
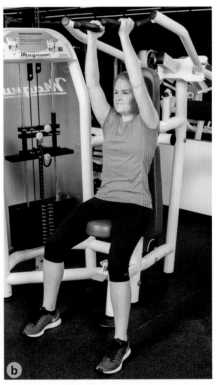

Adjust the seat height so the handles are aligned with or slightly above your shoulders. Grasp the handles and sit up straight with your head, shoulders, and back against the pad and your feet flat on the floor *(a)*. Push the weight up over your head until your arms are fully extended but not locked *(b)*. Pause briefly and return to the starting position.

Dumbbell Lateral Raise

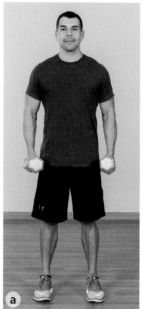
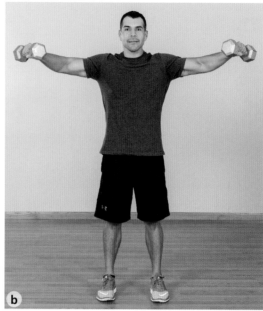

Choose your appropriate or desired dumbbell weight. Stand with your feet shoulder-width apart. Hold a dumbbell at the side of your body with your palms facing in and your elbows slightly bent (a). Raise both arms out to the sides until they are horizontal (b). Pause briefly; then return to the starting position and repeat.

Dumbbell Upright Row

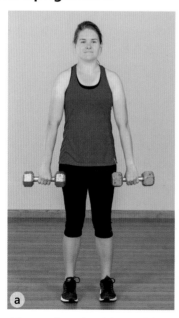
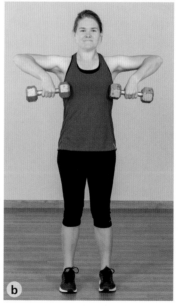

Stand tall with your feet shoulder-width apart. Hold a dumbbell in each hand with your palms facing your thighs and your elbows pointing outward (a). Bend at the elbows and lift both dumbbells to shoulder level (b). Keep your elbows pointed outward during the upward movement. Pause briefly; then lower the weights to the starting position and repeat.

Band Upright Row

Choose your appropriate or desired band. Stand with both feet placed about shoulder-width apart on top of the band. Grasp one end of the band in each hand and stand erect *(a)*. Your palms should be facing your thighs, and the band tension should be tight. Bend at the elbows and pull the band to shoulder level *(b)*. Keep your elbows pointed outward during the upward movement. Pause briefly; then lower your arms to the starting position and repeat.

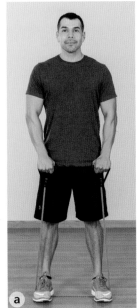
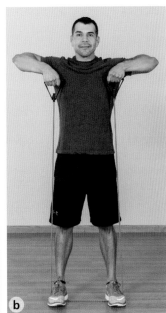

Machine Biceps Curl

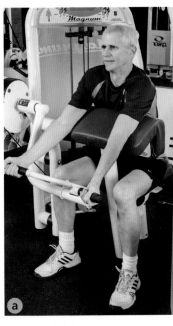
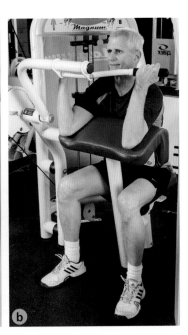

Adjust the seat height so your upper arms are resting flat against the arm pad and your elbow is aligned with the machine's axis of rotation. Grasp the handles firmly and position your body so your chest is up and your shoulders are back *(a)*. Curl your hands toward your shoulders until your elbows are fully flexed *(b)*. Return to the starting position and repeat.

Dumbbell Biceps Curl

Choose your appropriate or desired dumbbell weights. Stand tall with your feet shoulder-width apart. Hold the dumbbells with your palms facing forward and your elbows at the sides of your body (a). Raise both dumbbells by bending your elbows until they are fully flexed (b). Keep your elbows at your sides during the entire movement. Lower the dumbbells to the starting position and repeat. This exercise can also be performed in a seated position with alternating arms.

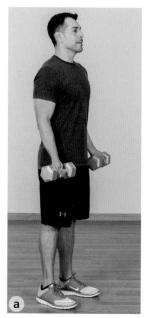
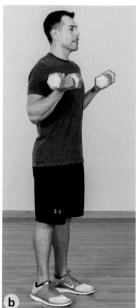

Band Biceps Curl

Choose a band thickness or color. Stand with both feet placed about shoulder-width apart on top of the band. Grasp one end of the band in each hand and stand erect (a). Your palms should be facing forward, and the band tension should be tight. Bend your elbows until they are fully flexed (b). Keep your elbows at your sides during the entire lift. Lower your arms to the starting position and repeat. This exercise can also be performed in a seated position with alternating arms.

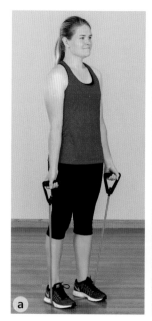
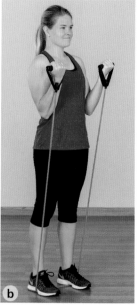

Machine Triceps Press

Stand tall with hands placed approximately shoulder-width apart on the bar. Grasp the bar and position your body so your chest is up and shoulders are back *(a)*. Move the bar from the starting position until your elbows are fully extended but not locked *(b)*. Return to the starting position and repeat.

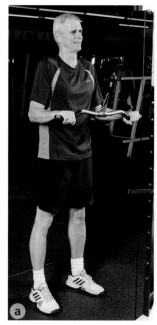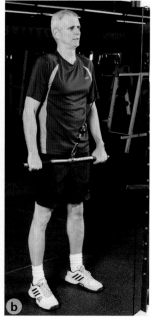

Dumbbell Lying Triceps Extension

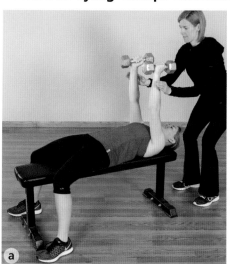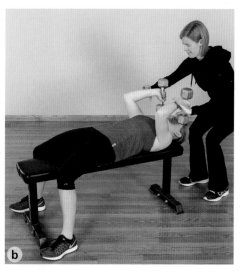

Choose an appropriate or desired dumbbell weight. Lie on a bench with your knees bent and your feet flat on the floor. Your head, shoulders, back, and buttocks must maintain contact with the bench during this exercise. Hold a dumbbell in each hand with your thumb wrapped around the dumbbell and both arms fully extended above your shoulders *(a)*. Bend your elbows and slowly lower the dumbbells toward (but not touching) the side of your head *(b)*. Return to the starting position and repeat. A spotter should be nearby to assist you if needed.

Band Triceps Extension

Choose a band thickness or color. Stand straight with your feet about shoulder-width apart. Hold one end of the band in your left hand placed near your low back and the other end in your right hand placed behind your neck *(a)*. Move your arm up so the right elbow straightens overhead without moving your left arm *(b)*. Pause briefly; then slowly return your right hand to the starting position and perform the desired number of repetitions. Repeat on the opposite side.

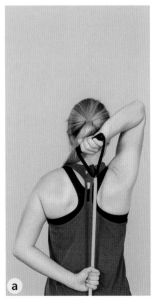
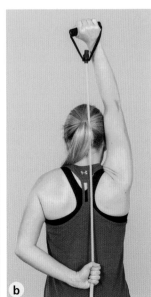

Machine Back Extension

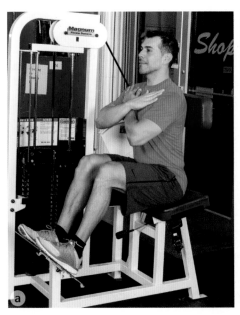
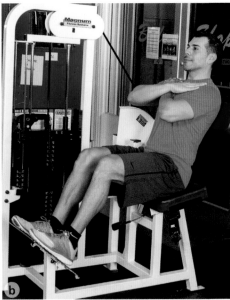

Adjust the seat so your navel is aligned with the machine's axis of rotation. Sit with your back against the pad, your feet on the foot pad, and your arms folded across your chest *(a)*. Slowly lean backward (extending the torso) with the back in contact with the pad *(b)*. Pause briefly; then return to the starting position and repeat.

Prone Plank

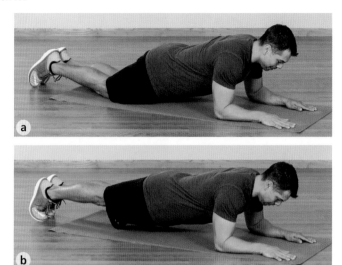

Lie facedown on the floor with your feet behind your body. Support your weight on your knees and forearms *(a)*. Keep your back flat and your head in line with your torso. Breathe normally as you hold the position for the desired number of seconds. To increase difficulty, lift your knees and support your weight on your toes and forearms *(b)*.

Kneeling Hip Extension

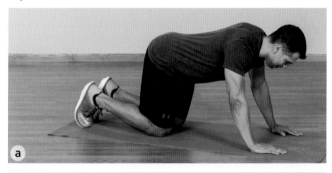

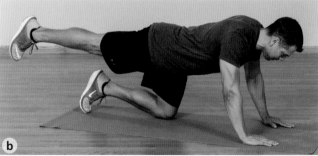

Kneel down in the crawl position with your arms directly below your shoulders *(a)*. Extend your right leg backward until it is parallel to the floor while keeping your shoulders and hips level *(b)*. Pause briefly; then return to the starting position and repeat on the opposite side.

Machine Abdominal Curl

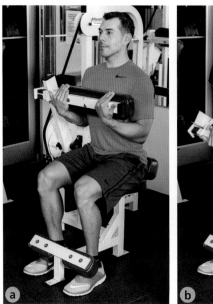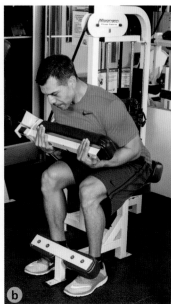

Adjust the seat so your navel is aligned with the machine's axis of rotation *(a)*. Curl your torso forward while fully flexing your trunk *(b)*. Pause briefly; then return to the starting position and repeat.

Curl-Up

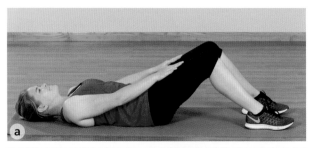

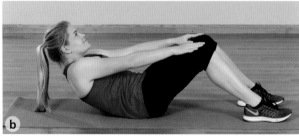

Lie on your back with your knees bent and your feet flat on the floor *(a)*. Place your hands on your thighs. Curl your shoulders and upper back off the floor while sliding your hands up your thighs toward your kneecaps *(b)*. Your low back should remain in contact with the floor. Pause briefly; then return to the starting position and repeat.

Diagonal Curl-Up

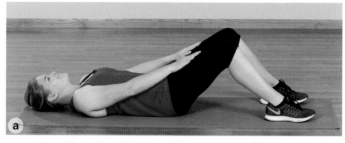

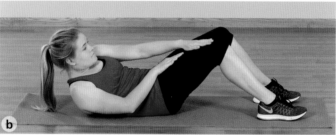

Lie on your back with your knees bent and your feet flat on the floor *(a)*. Place your hands on your thighs. Curl your shoulders and upper back off the floor while sliding your left hand toward your right kneecap *(b)*. Your low back should remain in contact with the floor. Pause briefly; then return to the starting position and repeat on the opposite side.

Regular participation in strength-building exercises that enhance muscular fitness can offer observable health and fitness value. Muscles and bones get stronger and activities of daily life become easier to perform. A well-designed resistance training program should target all the major muscle groups and should be sensibly progressed over time to optimize adaptations and maintain interest.

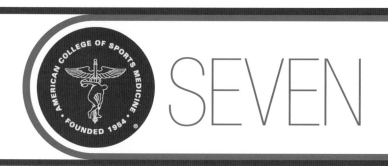

SEVEN

Increasing Your Flexibility

Flexibility may not have the same health benefits as aerobic or muscular fitness, but it is an important part of your overall physical fitness. Many activities require flexibility (e.g., golfing, swimming, dancing), and daily activities are also affected by flexibility (e.g., reaching, bending, twisting) (2, 3). Flexibility varies between individuals and is affected by joint types, differing muscle lengths, ligaments, tendons, muscles, skin, and age (17). Understanding flexibility and its role in exercise programming is essential for a well-balanced exercise regimen.

Flexibility Factors

Flexibility is the ability of a joint and surrounding muscle to move through a full or optimal range of motion (6). Improving range of motion at a joint eliminates awkward and inefficient movements, allowing you to move more fluidly. You can appreciate this throughout your day-to-day activities and in any recreation or sports you may do. Maintaining or improving your range of motion through flexibility exercises helps you move more efficiently (3, 4, 7). For example, if you improve range of motion in your hips and hamstring muscle groups, which are located at the back of your thighs, you can ease the task of reaching down to pick up a grocery bag or bending over to tie your shoes, as well as increase your stride when jogging or running.

Several factors influence flexibility, including age, sex, joint structure, and physical activity level (4, 17). Females tend to have a slightly greater range of motion at most joints than males do. This is usually explained by differences in joint structure and is often observed in joints in the upper body (e.g., shoulders, elbows, wrists, neck), with the exception of the trunk, in which males tend to have a greater range of motion than females (9). Flexibility typically decreases with age, resulting in many significant changes in the neck, shoulder, and trunk region (9, 19). You can minimize these changes by adhering to a regular stretching program. Specific activities you can incorporate into your stretching routine are outlined in this chapter.

■ Q&A

How can routine activities affect flexibility?

Routine daily activities including desk work can cause slumped-forward shoulders (internally rotated humerus) as well as lower back pain. To combat this, it is important to include dynamic and static stretches of the chest, shoulders, neck, and hips.

Health and Fitness Benefits of Flexibility

Compared to less active people, active people have greater flexibility in the joints they use (14). For example, people who walk more tend to have greater flexibility in their hips and spine than people who walk less. And limited motion of a specific joint can lead to a loss in flexibility. If you spend several hours per day driving or sitting at a computer, you may find that your shoulders round forward as a result of decreased range of motion at your shoulder joints. A focus on stretching and body position can help you avoid such losses in flexibility and allow you to keep a strong upright posture.

In addition, improvements in flexibility may enhance performance in certain skills that require greater flexibility (e.g., dancing, golf) (8). However, unless you have poor flexibility at a specific joint, increasing flexibility beyond a normal range of motion does not benefit performance or decrease the risk of injury. Contrary to popular belief, there is not sufficient evidence to support the contention that preexercise stretching prevents all injuries (although there may be potential benefits related to acute injuries in repetitive activities like running [5]), or that pre- and postexercise stretching prevents muscle soreness (5, 13). However, you may experience relaxation or stress relief from participating in flexibility-focused exercises.

Assessments for Range of Motion

Several tests can be administered for flexibility assessment if one has access to some rather simple pieces of equipment such as these:

- Masking tape
- Chair
- Measuring stick (yardstick or meter stick)
- Ruler

Flexibility testing is similar to stretching exercises in that a brief warm-up should be administered before attempting the assessment. On average, 5 minutes of brisk cardiovascular activity like a brisk walk, moderate cycling, or marching in place is typically enough to increase the heart rate and provide pliability to the muscle structures.

■ Q&A

Does stretching prevent or reduce muscle soreness?

Researchers have not proven that stretching before or after an exercise session adds benefits or protection against muscle soreness (11). Stretching has not been found to attenuate the structural mechanisms that contribute to soreness, including microtears to the muscle fibers, accumulation of calcium ions, cellular inflammation, or swelling.

This chapter describes a small subset of tests that are available to assess flexibility. Each joint and body segment is unique. Two assessments covered in this chapter are the sit-and-reach and the back-scratch test. These tests provide a snapshot of flexibility in the trunk and hips as well as the upper arm and shoulder.

Sit-and-Reach Assessments

The sit-and-reach is one of the most common tests of flexibility and reflects hamstring flexibility (muscles on the back of the thigh) and possible low back flexibility as well (3). There are various versions of the assessment for adults, older adults, and children.

Sit-and-Reach Test for Adults

The setup for the adult sit-and-reach test requires a yardstick and masking tape. The following steps outline the setup and measurement (10):

- A yardstick is placed on the floor and tape is placed across it at a right angle to the 15-inch (38 cm) mark. Sit with the yardstick between your legs, with legs extended at right angles to the taped line on the floor. Heels of the feet (with shoes removed) should touch the edge of the taped line and be about 10 to 12 inches (25-30 cm) apart (see figure 7.1a).
- Slowly reach forward with both hands as far as possible, holding this position approximately 2 seconds (see figure 7.1b). Be sure that you keep the hands parallel and do not lead with one hand or bounce. Fingertips can be overlapped and should be in contact with the yardstick.
- The score is the most distant point (recorded in inches) reached with the fingertips. The best of two trials should be recorded. To assist with the best attempt, you should exhale and drop your head between your arms when reaching. Make sure that your knees stay extended. Do not bend the knees as you reach forward, but also, do not press the knees down. Breathe normally during the test; you should not hold your breath at any time.
- You can track your score over time, realizing that a higher score indicates improving flexibility.

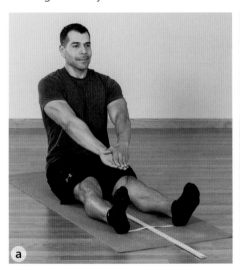 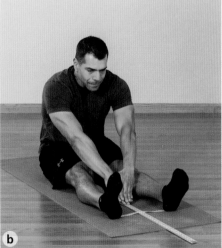

FIGURE 7.1   Sit-and-reach for adults.

Chair Sit-and-Reach Test for Older Adults

The sit-and-reach test for older adults can be done while sitting in a chair rather than on the floor (16). In addition to a sturdy chair, you will also need a ruler. Note that if you have pain when flexing, have severe osteoporosis, or have had recent knee or hip replacement, this assessment should not be attempted. The following steps outline the setup and results:

- Start in a sitting position on a chair placed securely against a wall. Move forward until you are sitting on the front edge of the chair. The crease between the top of the leg and the buttocks should be even with the edge of the chair seat.
- Keep your right leg bent and foot flat on the floor; the left leg is extended straight in front of the hip, with heel on floor and foot flexed (at approximately 90 degrees) (see figure 7.2a). With the left leg as straight as possible (but not hyperextended), slowly bend forward at the hip joint, reaching as far toward or past your toes on your left foot as possible (see figure 7.2b). Your hands should be one on top of the other with the tips of the middle fingers even. Continue breathing normally; do not hold your breath. Exhale as you reach forward and avoid bouncing or forcing the movement. Hold your reach for 2 seconds. Practice the movement twice.
- Now switch the position of your feet and keep your left leg bent and foot flat on the floor with the right leg extended straight in front of you. Repeat the test in this position.
- Whichever position results in the farthest reach is used for scoring purposes. Repeat the test two more times in this position. Using a ruler, record the number of inches short of reaching the toes (minus score) or beyond the toes (plus score). The tip of your toes at the end of your shoe represents a zero score.

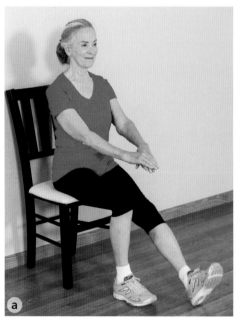 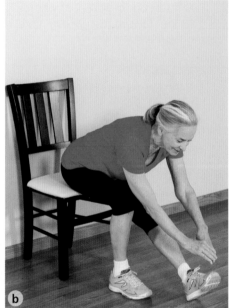

FIGURE 7.2 Chair sit-and-reach for older adults.

- Use table 7.1 to interpret the results of your sit-and-reach test. Normal ranges are shown; if your score is over the range listed, consider yourself above average and if your score falls short of the range listed, consider yourself below average.

TABLE 7.1   Normal Ranges for Chair Sit-and-Reach for Older Adults in Inches

	Age						
	60 to 64	65 to 69	70 to 74	75 to 79	80 to 84	85 to 89	90 to 94
Males	−2.5 to +4.0	−3.0 to +3.0	−3.0 to +3.0	−4.0 to +2.0	−5.5 to +1.5	−5.5 to +0.5	−6.5 to −0.5

	Age						
	60 to 64	65 to 69	70 to 74	75 to 79	80 to 84	85 to 89	90 to 94
Females	−0.5 to +5.0	−0.5 to +4.5	−1.0 to +4.0	−1.5 to +3.5	−2.0 to +3.0	−2.5 to +2.5	−4.5 to +1.0

Adapted by permission from R.E. Rikli and C.J. Jones, 2013, pp. 89, 90.

Sit-and-Reach Test for Youth

This version of the sit-and-reach test focuses mainly on hamstring flexibility. The sit-and-reach test used in the FitnessGram for youth requires a 12-inch-high (30.5 cm) box and a yardstick (18). The following steps outline the setup and results:

- The yardstick is placed on the box with the zero end of the yardstick facing the child and the 9-inch (22.9 cm) mark at the nearest edge of the box. One foot is placed against the box and the other is flat on the floor next to the knee of the straight leg (see figure 7.3).
- The child reaches forward with back straight and head up. After measuring one side, have the child reverse the position of the legs and repeat.
- Record the number of inches for both the right and left sides to the nearest half inch (1.3 cm).
- Rather than determining a range, the test establishes a standard score to be met (or not). For boys ages 5 to 17, this is 8 inches (20.3 cm). For girls the standard increases with age: For 5- to 10-year olds, the standard is 9 inches (22.9 cm), for 11- to 14-year olds it is 10 inches (25.4 cm), and for 15- to 17-year olds it is 12 inches (30.5 cm).

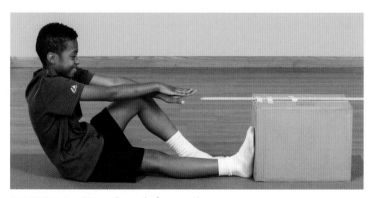

FIGURE 7.3   Sit-and-reach for youth.

Shoulder Flexibility Assessments

Shoulder flexibility can affect a person's capability to perform activities of daily living such as brushing one's hair or reaching for a seat belt. The most common test for shoulder flexibility is the back-scratch test. Note that this test should not be attempted by anyone with neck or shoulder injuries or problems such as pinched nerves or frozen shoulder.

Back-Scratch Test for Adults

The only equipment you will need is a ruler. The following steps outline the setup and results (15):

- In a standing position, place your preferred hand behind the same-side shoulder, palm toward back and fingers extended, reaching down the middle of the back as far as possible (elbow pointed up).
- Then place your other hand behind the back, palm out, reaching up as far as possible in an attempt to touch or overlap the extended middle fingers of both hands (see figure 7.4). Do not attempt to grab your fingers and pull.
- Practice for two trials before measuring.
- The distance of overlap or distance between the tips of the middle fingers is measured to the nearest 1/4 inch. A minus score (–) is given to represent a distance short of touching; a plus score (+) represents the amount of an overlap.
- You can track your score over time. If hands can touch (or overlap), shoulder flexibility is a strong point, but if hands are short of reaching, shoulder flexibility is an area in which to seek improvement.

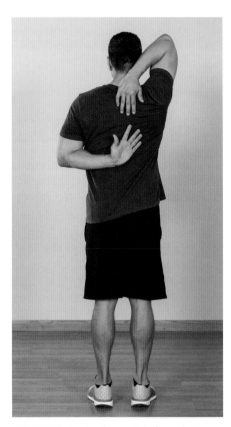

FIGURE 7.4 Back-scratch for adults.

Back-Scratch Test for Older Adults

This test requires only a ruler. The following steps outline the setup and results (16):

- In a standing position, place your right hand behind your right shoulder, palm toward back and fingers extended, reaching down the middle of the back as far as possible (elbow pointed up).
- Then place your left hand behind the back, palm out, reaching up as far as possible in an attempt to touch or overlap the extended middle fingers of your right hand (see figure 7.5).
- Practice for two trials and then repeat with your hands in the opposite position: left hand behind your left shoulder, reaching down toward your right hand that is placed behind your back.
- Whichever hand placement results in the closest reach should be used for scoring. Repeat the assessment twice with your hands in this position. Be sure to breathe normally and avoid bouncing or abrupt movements.
- The distance of overlap or distance between the tips of the middle fingers is measured to the nearest 1/2 inch. A minus score (−) is given to represent a distance short of touching (record the distance separating the middle fingers of each hand); a plus score (+) represents the amount of an overlap.
- Check your score in table 7.2. Normal ranges are shown; if your score is over the range listed, consider yourself above average and if your score falls short of the range listed, consider yourself below average.

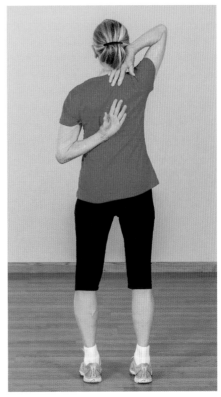

FIGURE 7.5   Back-scratch for older adults.

TABLE 7.2   **Normal Ranges for Back-Scratch Test for Older Adults in Inches**

	Age						
	60 to 64	65 to 69	70 to 74	75 to 79	80 to 84	85 to 89	90 to 94
Males	−6.5 to 0.0	−7.5 to −1.0	−8.0 to −1.0	−9.0 to −2.0	−9.5 to −2.0	−9.5 to −3.0	−10.5 to −4.0
Females	−3.0 to +1.5	−3.5 to +1.5	−4.0 to +1.5	−5.0 to +0.5	−5.5 to +0.0	−7.0 to −1.0	−8.0 to −1.0

Adapted by permission from R.E. Rikli and C.J. Jones, 2013, pp. 89, 90.

Shoulder Stretch Test for Youth

No equipment is needed for this assessment. The objective is to touch the fingertips of opposite hands by reaching over the shoulder and under the elbow (18). The following steps outline the setup and results:

- Reach with the right hand, palm toward the back, over the right shoulder and down the back while at the same time placing the left hand, palm facing out, behind the back, and reach up toward the fingers of the right hand (see figure 7.6). Do the fingers touch?
- Then repeat with hands in the opposite position. Again, do the fingers touch?
- The scoring for this assessment is a simple "yes" or "no" response. The scoring is considered for both the right and left positions.

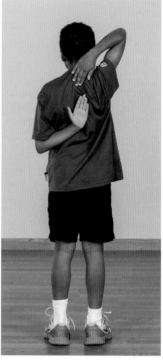

FIGURE 7.6   Shoulder stretch for youth.

Flexibility Program Components

Flexibility, like resistance training, is specific to the muscle groups and joints that are stretched. Thus, it is important to target all the major muscle groups (see figure 6.7, *a* and *b*, for the locations of the major muscle groups in the body).

A flexibility routine should be completed after a thorough warm-up of at least 5 minutes or after a cardiorespiratory or resistance training session. Increasing the temperature of the muscle increases its ability to stretch (1). Warm muscles have a greater elastic response than cold muscles do (3). The FITT-VP principle can be applied to your flexibility program, including the frequency, intensity, time, type, volume, and pattern of stretching activities.

Frequency

To improve flexibility, perform flexibility exercises at least two to three days per week for a minimum of 10 minutes (3). Note that this is considered a minimum; stretching on a daily basis as part of a warm-up or cool-down is effective in improving range of motion.

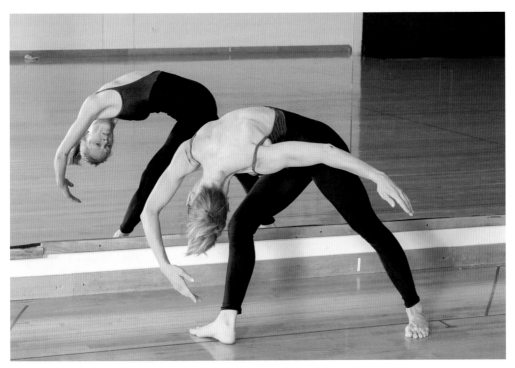

Flexibility does not have to reach this level to provide benefits.

Intensity

The question of how far to stretch (i.e., the intensity of the stretch) is a common one. Typically, stretching exercises are done to the point of mild tightness without discomfort within the range of motion of the joint(s) (3). If a given stretch creates discomfort, release slightly—a stretch should not be painful. Over time, you may be able to move the joint farther as your flexibility improves, but the stretch should never cause pain. If it does, back off slightly.

Time

You should hold a single flexibility exercise for 10 to 30 seconds (3, 5). In general, longer hold times have not been found to provide additional benefits for improving joint range of motion (3). However, older adults may benefit from holding the stretch for 30 to 60 seconds (3).

Type

Two of the most common methods of stretching to improve flexibility are static and dynamic. Both methods involve moving a joint or joints to the end of the range of motion. With static stretching, the position is held, whereas dynamic stretching involves continuous movement of the joint(s). Static stretching is more commonly used after an activity because some activities requiring strength, power, or endurance may be

■ **Q&A** ▬▬▬▬▬▬▬▬▬▬▬▬▬▬▬▬▬▬▬▬▬▬▬▬▬▬▬▬▬▬▬

Should you perform static or dynamic stretches before or after a workout?

You may want to perform dynamic stretching before the workout, as these activities encourage large movements that raise the heart rate and increase blood flow to the muscles, tendons, and ligaments. Incorporating a dynamic warm-up has the potential to reduce injury as well as to prepare the body for the upcoming workout (12). But don't forget the static stretches following the workout. The musculoskeletal system is warm and ready for these lengthening exercises.

---

impaired by static stretching before the activity (3). Dynamic stretching can be done before activity, following a general warm-up of the muscles (20).

Static

Static stretching is undoubtedly the most common method used to improve flexibility. Static stretching consists of slowly moving a joint to the point at which you feel tension and then holding that stretch for 10 to 30 seconds (3). Remember, do not place your joints in any position that causes pain. As you hold the stretch, the tension should lessen as the muscle lengthens. Each static stretch should be repeated two to four times to accumulate 60 seconds per stretch.

Dynamic

Dynamic stretching involves moving parts of your body through a full range of motion while gradually increasing the reach and speed of the movement in a controlled manner. An example of this is arm circles; you begin with small, slow circles and gradually progress to larger and faster circles until you reach the full range of motion of the shoulder joint. Many people think dynamic stretching involves bouncing or jerking motions—it does not! The goal is to move the joint in a controlled manner within a normal range of motion in order to minimize the risk of injury (4). To avoid the muscle soreness that often results from novel movements, introduce dynamic stretches into your stretching program gradually, particularly if you are not accustomed to this type of stretching. Dynamic movements are typically repeated 5 to 12 times within a time frame that varies depending on the motion (approximately 30 to 60 seconds).

Volume and Pattern

In order to improve joint range of motion over time, a total of 60 seconds of flexibility exercise per joint is recommended (3). This is accomplished by repeating shorter-duration stretches, for example, repeating a 30-second stretch twice or repeating a 15-second stretch four times. Typically a body-wide stretching routine can be completed in less than 10 minutes per session (3).

Your Flexibility Program

Stretching can be done any time a muscle is warmed up and should be included before sports or activities requiring a high degree of flexibility. Stretching can be included

Flexibility Stretches to Avoid

Many stretches that have been accepted in the past have been found to cause unnecessary strain on the joints and muscles. Although not everyone engaging in these activities will incur injury, it is sensible to avoid certain stretches and focus on those included at the end of this chapter. Table 7.3 lists a few stretches to avoid and suggested alternatives.

Also note that in some situations, stretching a muscle may not be appropriate. For example, if a muscle or joint has been injured, stretching exercises would typically be postponed unless prescribed as part of a treatment plan by a health care provider.

TABLE 7.3 Stretches to Avoid and Suggested Alternatives

Stretch to avoid		Reason to avoid	Alternative stretch
Standing toe touch		May strain the lower back	Seated hamstring stretch (page 168)
Hurdler stretch		May put strain on the bent knee	Prone quadriceps stretch (page 169)
Overrounding of the back		May stress the neck and low back	Pillar–overhead reach (with slight torso rotation to involve trunk muscles) (page 163)
Hyperextension of the back		Ineffective at stretching the abdominal muscles and may put stress on the back	
Full neck circle		Hyperextends the neck	Forward and lateral flexion (page 169)

before or after the conditioning phase of general fitness activities. Although not conclusive, some research suggests that static stretching could interfere with sports that require muscular strength, power, or endurance (3). Thus, in the following sample programs, dynamic stretching follows the warm-up (before the conditioning phase of the workout), and static stretching is part of the cool-down.

Sample Stretching Program After a Warm-Up

After a thorough warm-up, dynamic stretches can be performed to improve the efficiency of the movements you will do during your conditioning period of cardiorespiratory or resistance training. Dynamic stretches should begin with small ranges of motion and progress to larger ranges of motion. You should repeat each movement 5 to 12 times or move continuously for 30 to 60 seconds. Figure 7.7 outlines a dynamic stretching program you can use after a warm-up.

Sample Stretching Program After a Conditioning Period

After a conditioning period, use static stretching to improve your flexibility. Figure 7.8 outlines a sample progressive static stretching program. When you begin a flexibility program, start with level 1 stretches, which are the most basic. Begin by holding static stretches for 10 seconds and slowly progress to holding the final position for up to 30 seconds, repeating each stretch two to four times. Once you are comfortable with level 1 stretches, progress to level 2 and then to level 3 stretches. The progression of certain stretching exercises (e.g., quadriceps) moves from a lying to seated to standing position. As you move through these levels, you will need more balance to perform the exercise.

If you are having trouble placing your body in the required positions, you can use a towel to provide some extension. For example, when doing the triceps stretch with

---

FIGURE 7.7

Sample dynamic stretching program.

Body part	Stretch*
Arms and shoulders	Arm circle Shoulder shrug
Hips and buttocks	Pendulum leg swing (front to back) Pendulum leg swing (side to side) Internal and external hip rotation Hip circles Side shuffle
Quadriceps	Butt kick
Hamstrings	High knees
Ankles	Dynamic foot range of motion
Full body	Soldier walk Wood chop Power skip

*The descriptions and photos of these stretches can be found at the end of the chapter, beginning on page 173.

FIGURE 7.8

Sample progressive static stretching program.

| Body part | Stretches by level of progression* | | |
	Level 1	Level 2	Level 3
Neck	Forward flexion Lateral flexion Levator scapulae stretch	Forward flexion Lateral flexion Levator scapulae stretch	Forward flexion Lateral flexion Levator scapulae stretch
Shoulders	Arms across chest	Arms across chest Wall hold	Arms across chest Wall hold
Upper back	Arm hug	Kneeling cat	Pillar–overhead reach
Low back	Supine rotational stretch	Supine rotational stretch	Supine rotational stretch
Chest	Chest stretch	Progressive chest stretch	Progressive chest stretch
Biceps	Biceps wall stretch	Biceps wall stretch	Biceps wall stretch
Triceps	Elbow behind the head	Elbow behind the head	Elbow behind the head
Hips and buttocks	Seated hip rotator stretch Butterfly stretch Kneeling hip flexor stretch	Supine hip rotator stretch Butterfly stretch Standing hip flexor stretch	Supine hip rotator stretch Butterfly stretch Standing hip flexor stretch
Hamstrings	Seated hamstring stretch	Standing hamstring stretch	Standing hamstring stretch
Quadriceps	Prone quadriceps stretch	Side-lying quadriceps stretch	Standing quadriceps stretch
Calves	Seated calf stretch	Standing calf step stretch (gastrocnemius) Standing calf stretch (soleus)	Standing calf step stretch (gastrocnemius) Standing calf stretch (soleus)

*The descriptions and photos of these stretches can be found at the end of the chapter.

the elbow behind the head later in this chapter, you could hold a towel in the hand of the arm you are stretching and provide assistance with the stretch by gently pulling on the towel with the other hand placed behind your back rather than on the elbow. When using a stretching aid, be careful not to jerk or pull your limb into an awkward or painful position.

Flexibility Stretches

The exercises to improve flexibility that have been listed throughout this chapter are provided here, organized by type—either static or dynamic. Each stretch includes a description and photos to help you perform it correctly.

STATIC STRETCHES

Static stretches, as discussed in detail previously in this chapter, are simple exercises that you can use to improve your flexibility. Remember to always warm up before stretching.

Neck

Forward flexion: Facing forward, move your head forward to tuck your chin into your chest; hold.

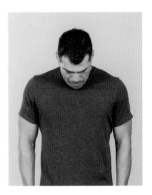

Lateral flexion: Facing forward, allow your head to tilt to the side so your ear moves toward your shoulder; hold. Repeat on the other side.

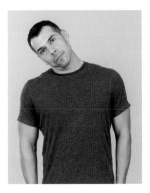

Levator scapulae stretch: Sit up straight on a chair. Put your hand up over your shoulder and bring your elbow back, pointing your elbow up to the ceiling. Use your left hand to pull your head forward and to the left; hold. Repeat on other side (6).

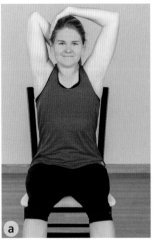
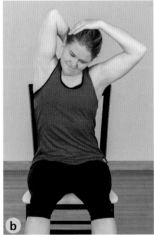

Shoulders

Arms across chest: Facing forward, straighten your right arm and draw it across your chest. Your arm should be as straight as possible, and you should feel gentle tension in your right shoulder. Grasp your right arm with your left hand and apply gentle pressure with your left hand to increase the tension in your right shoulder. Repeat on the other side.

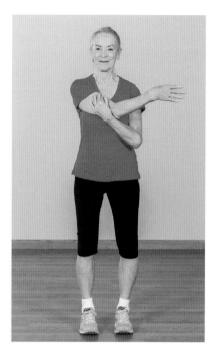

Wall hold: Stand with your right side facing a wall. Place your hand on the wall at shoulder height with elbow straight and thumb pointing down *(a)*. Turn your body away from the wall and maintain the rotation of your arm; hold *(b)*. Repeat on the other side.

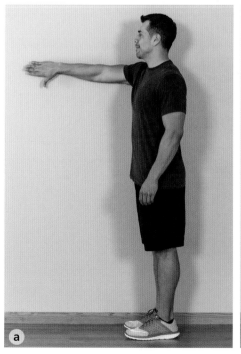

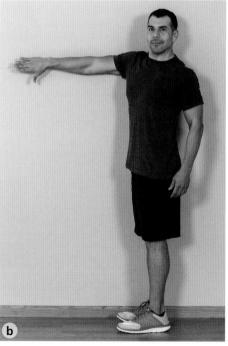

Upper Back

Arm hug: Cross your arms around your body with your elbows pointing forward. Let your upper body round, and squeeze your arms toward each other.

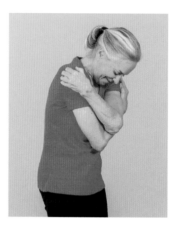

Kneeling cat: Adopt a crawl position on your hands and knees *(a)*. Draw in your abdominal muscles and contract your buttocks, and then round your spine throughout its entire length *(b)*.

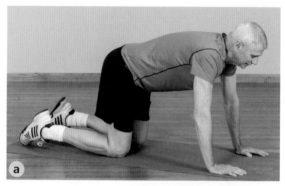

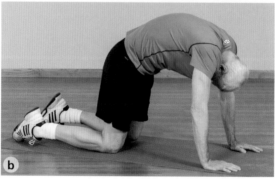

Pillar–overhead reach: Facing forward, stand upright and extend your arms above your head, keeping your shoulders in a neutral position (in line with your hips). Interlock your fingers and use your palms to press upward. You can also involve your trunk muscles (torso) by slightly rotating to one side of your body and back. Hold when you feel tension in your torso on the side opposite the reach; repeat on other side.

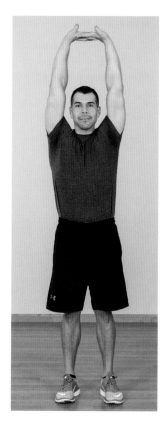

Low Back

Supine rotational stretch: Lie face up on the floor and bend your knees so that your feet are flat on the floor. Straighten your arms out from your sides across the floor to stabilize your upper body *(a)*. Slowly move both legs with your knees bent to the right side of your body while keeping your upper back against the floor and your abdomen oriented toward the ceiling *(b)*. Repeat by moving your legs to the left side.

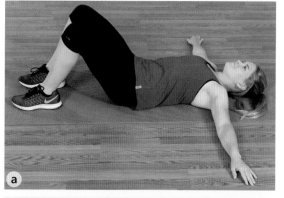

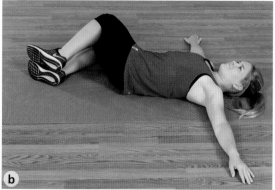

Chest

Chest stretch: In this stretch, your shoulders should be relaxed, not elevated. Straighten your arms toward your back, keeping them at or a little below shoulder height. A good cue for this stretch is "open arms wide."

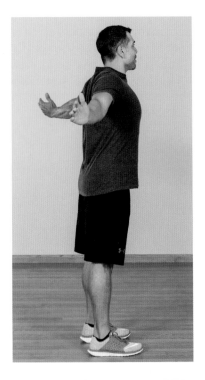

Progressive chest stretch: Place your arms against an open doorway and lean forward until you feel gentle tension across your chest. This exercise also stretches the biceps.

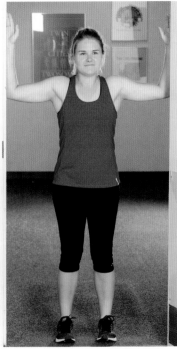

Biceps

Biceps wall stretch: Position your arm from your hand to your inner elbow against a wall and turn your body away from it, exhaling slowly. Repeat on the other side.

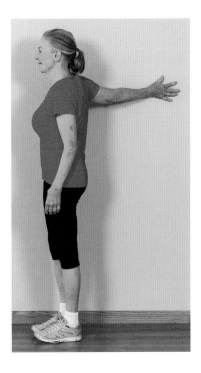

Triceps

Elbow behind the head: Facing forward, bring your right arm up, bend from your elbow, and drop your hand behind your head, trying to reach your left shoulder with your right hand. The left hand can be placed on the right elbow to assist with this stretch. Repeat on the other side.

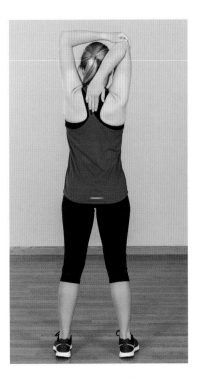

Hips and Buttocks

Seated hip rotator stretch: Sit upright on a sturdy chair that won't move. Cross your right ankle onto your bent left knee *(a)* and gently press down on your right knee until tension develops in the outer portion of your right thigh *(b)*. Repeat on the other side.

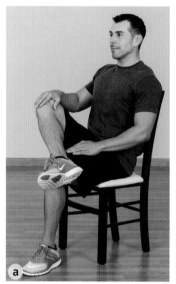 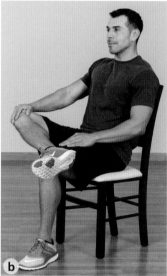

Supine hip rotator stretch: Lie faceup on floor with your knees bent so your feet are flat on the floor and cross your right ankle onto your bent left knee *(a)*. Lift your left foot off the floor and wrap your hands around your left leg and draw it into your body *(b)*. Focus on opening up your right knee until tension develops in the outer portion of your right thigh. Repeat on the other side.

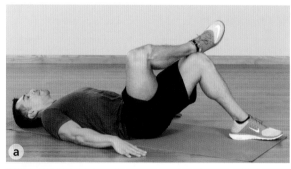

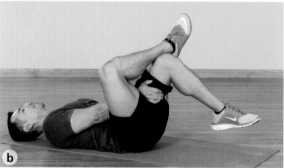

Butterfly stretch: Sit upright on the floor with the soles of your feet together. Draw your knees to the floor and lean forward from your hips and use your elbows to press your legs downward.

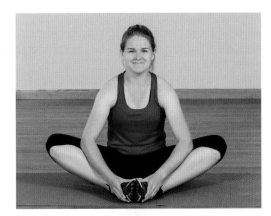

Kneeling hip flexor stretch: Kneel on both knees with your upper body lifted. Plant your left foot on the floor until you reach a 90-degree angle with both your front and back legs *(a)*. Shift your weight forward while keeping your upper body lifted *(b)*. Repeat on the other side.

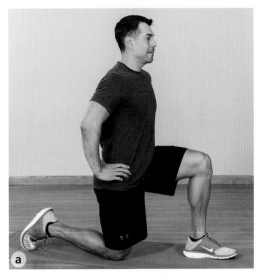

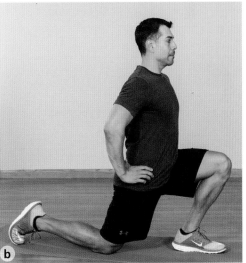

Standing hip flexor stretch: Stand erect and keep your hands on your hips. Step forward with your left foot into a lunge position *(a)*. Your left foot will be in front of your body and your right foot will be behind your body; your right heel may be elevated to facilitate this movement. Shift your hips forward and maintain this position, feeling tension develop in your hips, quadriceps, and buttocks *(b)*. Repeat on the other side.

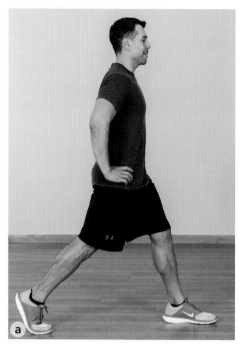 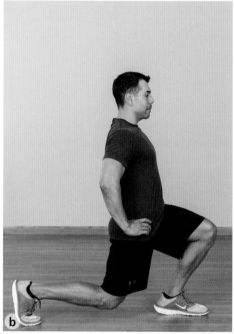

Hamstrings

Seated hamstring stretch: Sit upright on the floor with both legs straight and hands resting on your legs *(a)*. Slowly walk your hands forward toward your feet, keeping your chest lifted *(b)*.

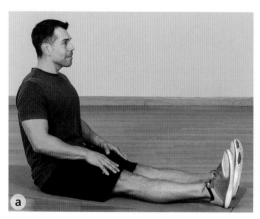 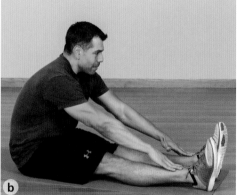

Standing hamstring stretch: Standing upright, bring your right foot slightly ahead of your left foot. Slowly draw your hips back while slightly bending your left knee and straightening your right knee *(a)*. Bring the toes of your right foot off the floor and toward your body *(b)*. Hold and then return to the starting position. Repeat with the other leg.

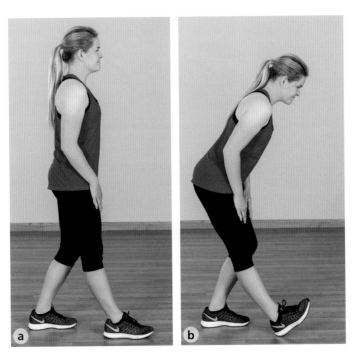

Quadriceps

Prone quadriceps stretch: Lie facedown on the floor with your legs straight. Draw your right heel back toward your buttocks using your left hand. Be sure to keep your knees together.

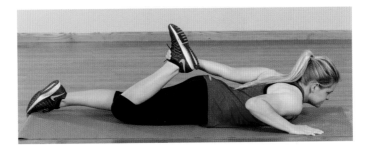

Side-lying quadriceps stretch: Lie on the floor on your right side. Bend your left knee, keeping your knees and hips in a straight line (keep your knees together and do not twist your leg to the side). Draw your left heel back toward your buttocks with your left arm. Repeat on the other side.

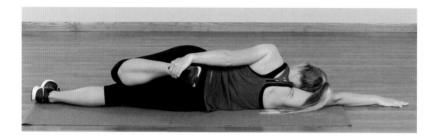

Standing quadriceps stretch: While in a standing position (you can hold on to a chair for support), bend your right knee toward your buttocks. Grasp your right ankle with your left hand. Be sure to keep your knees close together and your ankle behind your buttock; do not twist your leg outward. Gently pull your thigh back slightly. Repeat on the other side.

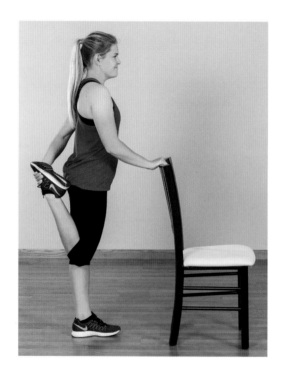

Calves

Seated calf stretch: Sit upright with both legs straightened out in front of you *(a)*. Draw your toes toward your upper body *(b)*.

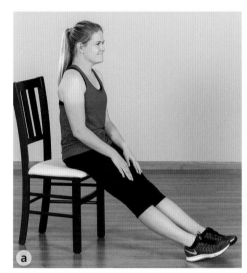 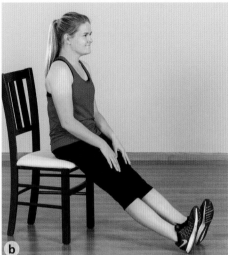

Standing calf step stretch: Stand with your legs extended on the edge of an immovable step and grasp a banister or handrail for support. Move your right foot so your heel back is off the edge of the step *(a)*. Slowly drop your right heel until tension develops in your right calf *(b)*. Repeat on the other side.

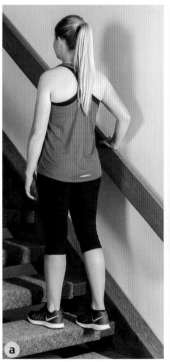 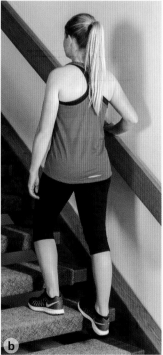

Standing calf stretch (gastrocnemius): Stand about 3 feet (0.9 m) from a wall and put your right foot behind you, ensuring that your toes are facing forward. Keep your heel on the ground and lean forward with your right knee straight. Rotating the toes in and out slightly will target the medial and lateral parts of this muscle separately. Repeat on other side.

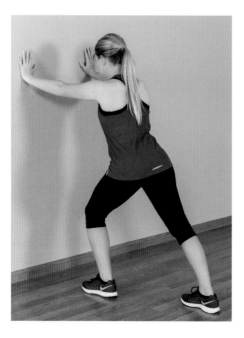

Standing calf stretch (soleus): Stand away from a wall and put your right foot behind you and be sure your toes are facing forward. Lean forward at the ankle while bending the right knee and keeping your heel on the ground. Because the knee is flexed, tension is taken off the gastrocnemius and placed on the soleus. Repeat on other side.

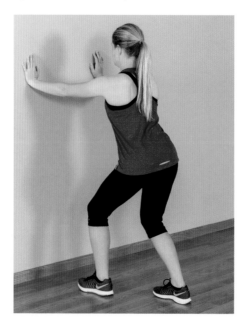

DYNAMIC STRETCHES

Dynamic stretches, as discussed in detail previously in this chapter, are more active than static stretches. Remember to always warm up before any stretching activity.

Arms and Shoulders

Arm circle: Stand with your feet shoulder-width apart and your knees slightly bent. Raise both arms to the side at shoulder height with your palms out. Make small circles with your arms extended, gradually increasing the size of the circles.

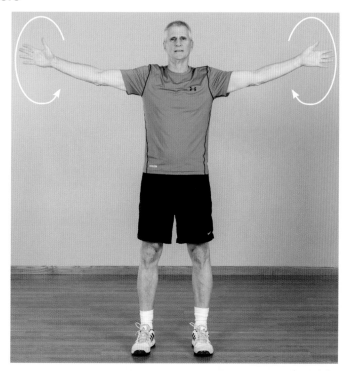

Shoulder shrug: Lift both shoulders toward your ears *(a)* and then lower them away from your ears *(b)*.

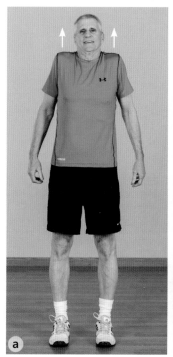
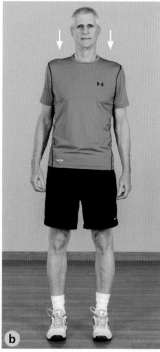

Hips and Buttocks

Pendulum leg swing (front to back): Place your right hand on the back of a chair for balance. Lift your left leg and swing it forward (in front of your body) *(a)* and back (behind your body) *(b)*. Begin with small swings and progress to larger swings. Switch to the opposite leg.

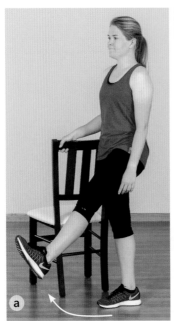
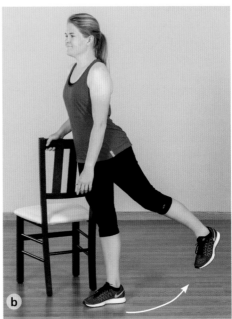

Pendulum leg swing (side to side): Place both hands on the back of a chair for balance. Swing your left leg out to the left *(a)*, and back across your body to the right *(b)*. Begin with small swings and progress to larger swings. Switch to the opposite leg.

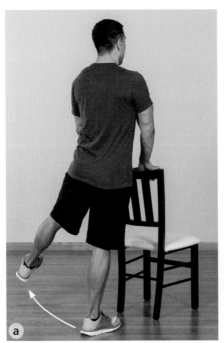
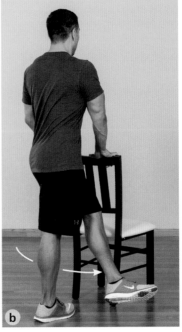

Internal hip rotation: Stand upright with your feet shoulder-width apart. Raise your left foot toward the side of your body and tap the outside of your left heel with your left hand. Allow your knee to rotate inward. Switch and tap the outside of your right heel with your right hand. Alternate tapping each foot. Progress to walking forward while alternating feet.

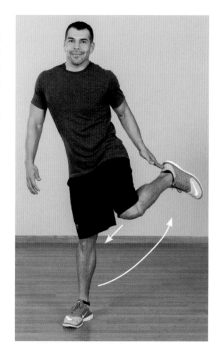

External hip rotation: Stand upright with your feet shoulder-width apart. Raise your left foot in front of your body and tap the inside of your left heel with your right hand. Allow your knee to point away from your body. Switch and tap the inside of your right heel with your left hand. Alternate tapping each foot. Progress to walking forward while alternating feet.

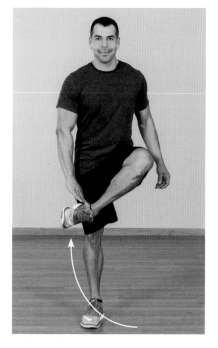

Hip circles: Place your hands on your hips and feet spread wider than your shoulders. Make circles with your hips in a clockwise direction for 6 to 10 repetitions. Then repeat in a counterclockwise direction.

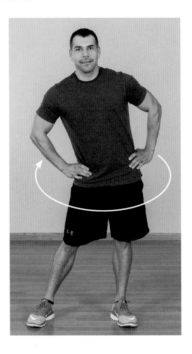

Side shuffle: Stand with your feet shoulder-width apart, your knees slightly bent, and your hands on your hips. Take one step to the left with your left foot *(a);* then bring your right foot in to meet your left foot *(b)*. Begin with small steps, progress to larger steps, and then progress to a shuffle. Switch to the opposite direction.

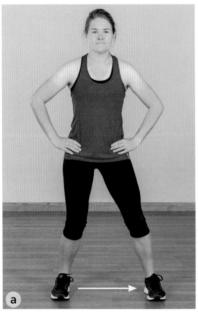
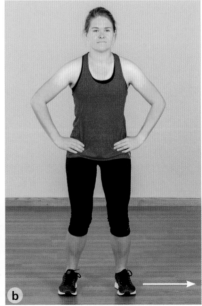

Quadriceps

Butt kick: Begin marching in place. Pull your heel in closer toward your buttock with each step. Progress to moving forward (walking or jogging) while kicking your buttocks.

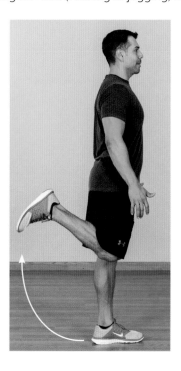

Hamstrings

High knees: Begin marching in place. Raise your knees higher and higher with each step. Progress to moving forward (walking or jogging) with high knees.

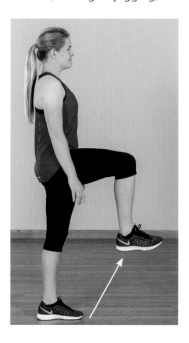

Ankles

Dynamic foot range of motion: Sit upright in a chair with both legs together and straightened in front of you. Point your toes away from your body and pull your toes toward your body *(a)*. Rotate your feet clockwise and counterclockwise *(b)*.

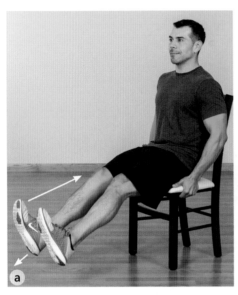 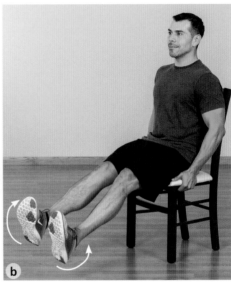

Combined Movements

Soldier walk: Simultaneously rotate your right arm forward and raise your left leg (straight). Reach your right hand toward your left lower leg and toes. Switch to the opposite side. Progress to alternating to the opposite side and then to walking while alternating sides.

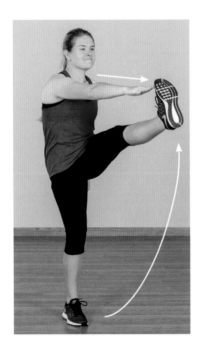

Wood chop: Stand with your feet wider than shoulder width. Reach both arms down toward the outside of your left foot while bending your knees slightly *(a)*. Move your arms diagonally across your body and end by reaching above your right shoulder *(b)*. Switch to the opposite side.

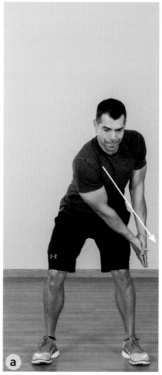
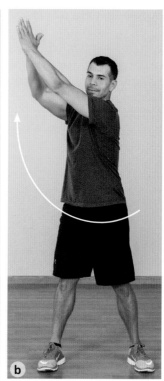

Power skip: Skip across the field using powerful explosive movements. Use big arm swings starting from the side of the body through the frontal plane and reaching for the sky. Use high knee lifts moving the opposite arm (i.e., as the left leg moves forward, the right arm reaches upward).

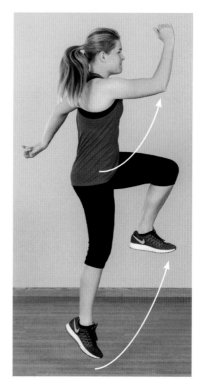

Stretching exercises are recommended as an essential component of any exercise training program due to the improvement in range of motion and physical functioning. Improving flexibility can be accomplished through various stretching techniques, for example static or dynamic methods. Stretching exercises can be incorporated into the warm-up to help prepare the body for more vigorous activity, or following the conditioning period of a workout to enhance flexibility. And while the research in flexibility training is still emerging, following the guidelines set forth in this chapter will help you to improve your flexibility in a safe and effective manner.

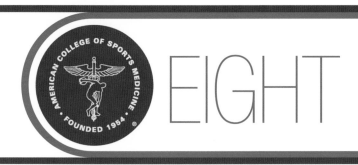

Sharpening Your Functional Fitness

The importance of training specific body systems to improve health, fitness, and function has been discussed in the previous chapters. When trained properly, the cardiorespiratory and muscular systems provide individuals with the strength and stamina needed to perform a variety of simple and complex activities ranging from sitting, standing, and stepping to skipping rope, walking down stairs, or even running a marathon. Historically, the emphasis of health and fitness programs has been on challenging the cardiorespiratory and muscular systems and improving aerobic capacity, muscular fitness, and flexibility. However, over the past few decades, the importance of training another essential body system known as the neuromuscular system has been established.

The neuromuscular system is a complex and interconnected network that links the brain, spinal cord, and extremity nerves with sensory receptors and muscles located throughout the body. The role of the neuromuscular system is to integrate sensory information and, based on this information, to coordinate the appropriate muscle actions needed to produce a desired movement. The relationship between the various components of the neuromuscular system is similar to that of a musical conductor and the musicians in an orchestra. The conductor (the brain and spinal centers) is charged with directing the musicians (the muscles) in order to perform a specific musical piece. The conductor communicates with the musicians and directs them on how and when to play their instruments so that the correct notes are played with sufficient clarity, pitch, precision, and tempo (sensory information). If conducted effectively, the musicians execute a highly complex and precisely orchestrated musical performance (the desired motor task). Like the conductor directing musicians, the neuromuscular system uses sensory cues to control the muscles' actions with sufficient precision, coordination, and speed.

The neuromuscular system coordinates every motor task completed throughout the day, and the amazing part is that the majority of these tasks are performed with little to no conscious effort. Even a simple task like getting dressed requires coordinated muscle activity. While getting dressed, did you consider engaging the muscles of your trunk, hips, and legs as you leaned forward to put on your shoes? Most likely you did not put a lot of thought into engaging all the muscles that were needed to carry out this activity. You simply considered the task that needed to be completed, and the right muscles were activated at precisely the right time. This is your neuromuscular system at work, and it has the extraordinary job of coordinating every muscle action for every movement you perform throughout the day.

The neuromuscular system helps people navigate their surroundings efficiently, effectively, and safely. Whether you are training for sport or for general health, this system is essential to maintaining balance, agility, coordination, and body awareness. Improving neuromuscular function may significantly reduce the risk for future falls and some musculoskeletal injuries (2, 15). Muscular fitness, cardiorespiratory endurance, and flexibility are important for long-term health and fitness; however, it would be difficult or even impossible to coordinate the thousands of muscle actions required to perform activities such as standing, walking, running, or jumping without a fully functional neuromuscular system. Fortunately, like the other body systems, the neuromuscular system can be trained to help the body respond more rapidly and economically to the physical demands faced in everyday life. The most effective means of training the neuromuscular system requires a targeted exercise strategy, which for the purposes of this chapter is referred to generally as neuromotor training. Neuromotor training, sometimes also referred to as functional fitness or sensorimotor training, involves specific exercises that challenge the neuromuscular system and are aimed at improving balance, agility, coordination, reaction time, and proprioception. This chapter outlines some of the important health and fitness benefits that can be derived from neuromotor training and details useful training tips to help you develop a personalized neuromotor training program based on your individual goals and needs.

Health and Fitness Benefits of Neuromotor Training

All movement requires a specific sequence of muscle actions, and the neuromuscular system coordinates and produces these muscle actions based on information learned from previous movement experiences. From infancy to adulthood, your neuromuscular system is continuously learning, processing, and storing new pieces of movement-related information that can be recalled at any time to help coordinate future motor tasks. Aging, deconditioning, musculoskeletal injury, and various neurological injuries and conditions can negatively affect neuromuscular function and movement quality. Neuromuscular function may begin to decline after the age of 30, resulting in diminished coordination and muscle control (24). Fortunately, emerging evidence suggests that neuromotor training can be an effective strategy for improving various skill-related components of fitness and may positively affect the structure and function of key brain and spinal centers involved in movement (1, 4, 27). The benefits of neuromotor training have been examined in aging and athletic populations and have been reported to improve balance, muscle strength, and agility and to reduce the risk of falls and some lower limb injuries (6, 11, 13, 14).

A number of underlying mechanisms have been attributed to neuromotor training including improved speed and efficiency of muscle recruitment, enhanced muscle force production, and improved reaction time in response to changes in environmental conditions and body position (12). In addition, because of the highly dynamic and multidimensional nature of neuromotor training, it is likely that this type of training may induce greater changes in the nervous system, resulting in improved skill acquisition and retention, when compared to more stationary, one-dimensional exercises (2).

Multifaceted physical activities such as tai chi and yoga involve varying combinations of neuromotor, resistance, and flexibility exercise and have become popular training methods for individuals ranging from professional athletes to the aging population. Tai chi and yoga provide individuals with low-impact and relatively safe forms of neuromotor exercise that can directly benefit balance, motor control, and proprioception (11, 25). In recent years, the term *functional training* has become popular within health, fitness, and athletic training settings and is used to refer to a specific form of exercise training. Historically, functional training was used as a rehabilitation strategy to engage patients in exercises that closely resembled, if not entirely replicated, normal activities of daily living. Over the past decade, functional training, as a form of neuromotor training, has become a very popular training method. Although the exercises prescribed for athletes and healthy adults may require greater function and skill compared to those used in clinical settings, the principles of functional training, when used among healthy adults, still retain their clinical roots by basing exercise strategies on movement patterns that mimic activities in daily life or athletic competition.

A more detailed description of some of these activities is provided later in this chapter. Some of the possible benefits of functional training are improved agility, reaction time, muscle force production, and body control (3). Improvements in these areas can directly affect how well people react to changes in their environment, especially when faced with rapidly changing conditions such as those experienced when one trips, stumbles, or loses balance.

Despite the potential value of participating in neuromotor training activities in non-clinical settings, much still needs to be learned about the optimal duration, frequency, and intensity of training for long-term, sustainable health and fitness benefits. Definitive exercise recommendations for neuromotor training across all ages and ability levels have not been established; however, it is likely that benefits exist for anyone participating in physical activities that require agility, balance, and other motor skills or anyone who may be deficient in any of these areas (11).

Neuromotor Assessments

Similar to developing training programs for other components of fitness, it is helpful to first establish baseline measures of neuromotor function. There are a number of assessments that have been developed and that can be used to establish your starting point. These assessments range from very sophisticated laboratory measures to tests you can perform in your own home with minimal equipment. This section provides simple assessments you can perform at home or with a qualified exercise professional, including the 4-stage balance test, standing reach test, Edgren side-step test, agility T-test, and the 8-foot up and go (this is typically used for older adults only). Additional assessments within this book, such as the chair-stand test for muscular fitness included in chapter 6, may also be helpful for older adults (16). A selection of two or three tests should be sufficient to track functional neuromotor improvements over time, including balance, agility, coordination, and body awareness.

The 4-Stage Balance Test

This test assesses static balance and proprioception (5). You will need a stopwatch. The test includes four progressively more challenging standing positions. The following steps outline the setup and results:

- Stand near a wall or by a fixed object in the event that you lose balance and need to support yourself using your hands. Start by standing with shoes off and feet together (see figure 8.1a).
- Stand and hold this position for 10 seconds without holding on to anything for support. If you are able to maintain the position without losing your balance, shift your feet so the instep of one foot is touching the big toe of the other foot (see figure 8.1b).
- Stand and hold this position for 10 seconds without holding on to anything for support. If you are able to maintain the position without losing your balance, shift your feet into the tandem position in which your feet are place heel-to-toe (see figure 8.1c). Repeat this until you are unable to balance for at least 10 seconds without moving your feet or needing to hold on to something for support.
- The goal is to advance to single-leg stance (see figure 8.1d).
- Once you are able to maintain the single-leg stance, use table 8.1 to determine your standing balance capacity (22). If you reach the "above average" range for your age group while standing with your eyes open, attempt the single-leg standing position with your eyes closed. Record the maximum time you can hold the single-leg stance position with eyes closed.

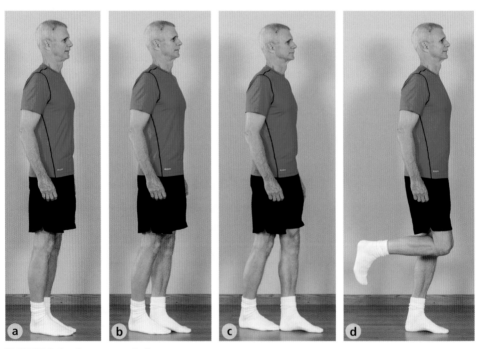

FIGURE 8.1   Four-stage balance test sequence.

TABLE 8.1   **Single-Leg Stance Time by Age Group**

	Age					
	18 to 39	**40 to 49**	**50 to 59**	**60 to 69**	**70 to 79**	**>80**
Eyes open (time in seconds)						
Above average	>43	>40	>37	>27	>15	>6
Average	43	40	37	27	15	6
Below average	<43	<40	<37	<27	<15	<6
Eyes closed (time in seconds)						
Above average	>9	>7	>5	>3	>2	>1
average	9	7	5	3	2	1
Below average	<9	<7	<5	<3	<2	<1

Adapted from B.A. Springer, R. Marin, T. Cyhan, et al., 2007, p. 11.

Standing Reach Test

This test assesses standing balance and postural control (7, 26). You will need a measuring stick and masking tape. The following steps outline the setup and results:

- Tape a leveled measuring stick on a wall horizontally at shoulder height.
- Stand with your right shoulder next to, but not touching, the measuring stick.
- Raise your arm to shoulder height (arm parallel to the ground), make a fist with your right hand, and note the number (in inches or centimeters) on the measuring stick that corresponds to the location of your knuckles (see figure 8.2a).
- When ready, with your arm outstretched, reach as far forward as you can without taking a step or losing balance (see figure 8.2b).

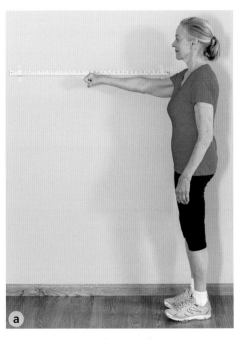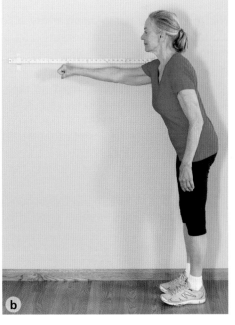

FIGURE 8.2   Standing reach test.

- Note the number (in inches or centimeters) on the measuring stick that corresponds to the location of your knuckles at the reaching position.
- Calculate the difference between the start and end reaching position.
- Use table 8.2 to determine your standing balance range (7). If you used a yardstick, convert your reach noted in inches to centimeters by multiplying by 2.54 (for example, a 6 inch reach would be 15 cm).A standing reach score less than 6 inches (15 cm) indicates a significant increased risk for falls, and a score of 6 to 10 inches (15-25 cm) indicates a moderate risk for falls.

TABLE 8.2   Normal Ranges for the Standing Reach Test for Males and Females in cm

	Age		
Males	**20 to 40**	**41 to 69**	**>70 years**
Above average	>19	>17	>15
Average	15 to 19	13 to 17	11 to 15
Below average	<15	<13	<11
	Age		
Females	**20 to 40**	**41 to 69**	**>70 years**
Above average	>17	>16	>15
Average	13 to 17	12 to 16	7 to 15
Below average	<13	<12	<7

Adapted from P.W. Duncan, D.K. Weiner, J. Chandler, and S. Studenski, 1990.

Edgren Side-Step Test

This test assesses sidestepping agility, quickness, and balance (8). You will need masking tape or cones, a tape measure, and a stopwatch. The following steps outline the setup and results:

- Find a flat, nonslip floor for your test location.
- Mark five lines using masking tape or place five cones in a line 3 feet (0.9 m) apart as illustrated in figure 8.3.
- Start the test standing at the center line or cone number 3.
- When ready, begin sidestepping to the right until your right foot touches or crosses the far right line or cone.
- Then, sidestep to the left until the left foot touches or crosses the far left line or cone.
- Continue to sidestep between lines or cones for 10 seconds and count the total number of lines or cones crossed when the test is complete.

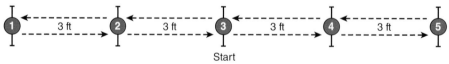

FIGURE 8.3   Edgren side-step test.

Adapted from H. Edgren, 1932.

- The test is scored based on the total number of line or cones crossed after 10 seconds. Since normal ranges are not available, use this assessment to track your score over time to see improvement. A better score is a higher number of lines or cones crossed during the 10-second period.

Agility T-Test

This test assesses agility in a forward, side, and backward direction (18). You will need a tape measure, cones, and a stopwatch. The following steps outline the setup and results:

- Set out four cones as illustrated in figure 8.4: 5 yards (4.6 m) and 10 yards (9.1 m) apart (21).
- Start at cone A.
- When ready, start the stopwatch and move as quickly as possible to cone B and touch the cone with your right hand.
- Then, sidestep left to cone C and touch the cone with your left hand.
- Then, sidestep to the right to cone D and touch the cone with your right hand.
- Sidestep to cone B, touch the cone with your left hand, and step backward to the start position at cone A. Stop the stopwatch and record the total time taken to complete the test.
- Use table 8.3 to compare results and track progress.

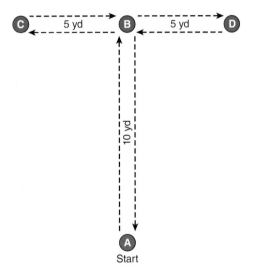

FIGURE 8.4   Agility T-test.

Adapted from K. Pauole, K. Madole, J. Garhammer, et al., 2000.

TABLE 8.3   **Ranges for Agility Fitness in Males and Females in Seconds**

	Males	Females
Excellent	<9.5	<10.5
Good	9.5 to 10.5	10.5 to 11.5
Average	10.5 to 11.5	11.5 to 12.5
Poor	>11.5	>12.5

Adapted from K. Pauole, K. Madole, J. Garhammer, et al., 2000.

8-Foot Up and Go Test for Older Adults

This test assesses agility and dynamic balance in older adults (19). You will need a standard-height chair (seat approximately 17 inches [43 cm] high) and a stopwatch. Steps to perform this test:

- Place the chair against a wall, and measure and mark a line 8 feet (2.4 m) away on the floor (see figure 8.5a).
- When ready, stand up from the chair.
- Walk to the line on the floor at a comfortable pace.
- Once both feet are past the line, turn around (see figure 8.5b).
- Walk back to the chair at a comfortable pace, and sit down again.
- Record the total time it takes you to stand from the chair, walk 8 feet (2.4 m), turn around, and sit back down.
- Normal ranges are found in table 8.4 (20). If your score is over the range listed, consider yourself above normal; if your score is below the range listed, consider yourself below normal. With this score, the shorter the time, the better (i.e., showing a faster completion of the test).

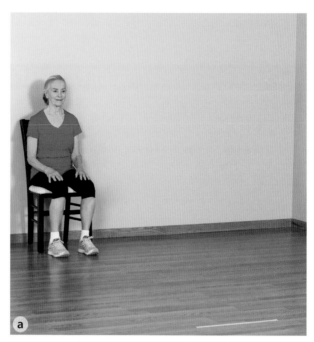

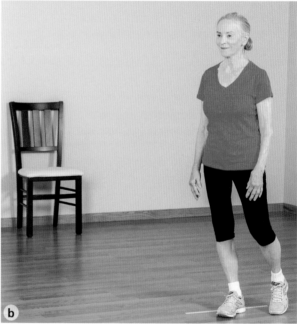

FIGURE 8.5   Eight-foot up and go for older adults.

TABLE 8.4   **Normal Ranges for the 8-Foot Up and Go Test for Older Adults in Seconds**

	Age						
	60 to 64	65 to 69	70 to 74	75 to 79	80 to 84	85 to 89	90 to 94
Males	3.8 to 5.6	4.3 to 5.9	4.4 to 6.2	4.6 to 7.2	5.2 to 7.6	5.5 to 8.9	6.2 to 10.0
Females	4.4 to 6.0	4.8 to 6.4	4.9 to 7.1	5.2 to 7.4	5.7 to 8.7	6.2 to 9.6	7.3 to 11.5

Adapted by permission from R.E. Rikli and C.J. Jones, 2013, pp. 89, 90.

Neuromotor Training Workout Components

Developing a safe and effective neuromotor training program requires consideration of the frequency, intensity, time, type, volume, and progression of exercises being performed. These training components vary depending on individual levels of physical conditioning, the presence of any preexisting injuries, and personal goals and needs. Because using exercise to specifically target the neuromuscular system in nonclinical populations is a relatively new training approach, there is no consensus concerning the optimal number of repetitions, intensity, or methods of progression for neuromotor exercise. This is due, in part, to the various types of training often included within neuromotor training. As a result, when research scientists and fitness professionals attempt to communicate the effectiveness of neuromotor training, it becomes difficult to identify whether improvements in health and function are associated with positive changes in neuromuscular function or are the result of improvements in some other body systems. However, there are some general exercise recommendations for frequency and duration that provide a good starting point for creating your own neuromotor training program (11). The general recommendations for neuromotor training presented in this chapter are based on the best and most recently available evidence.

Frequency

Neuromotor training exercise is recommended at least two to three days per week to improve balance and mobility (11). Note that this is only a suggested minimum; individuals who regularly participate in low-impact neuromotor training exercises such as tai chi, qigong, or yoga may be capable of performing these activities more frequently and may obtain additional health and fitness benefits without increasing the risk of injury (25). Neuromotor training exercises involving weighted resistance and explosive, high-impact activities (i.e., jumping, bounding, high-speed multidirectional agility) may place a greater physical stress on muscles, joints, and connective tissues. Under these training conditions, less frequent sessions of two or three days per week may be needed to allow for adequate recovery between sessions and to reduce risk of musculoskeletal injury. You may also consider fewer neuromotor training sessions if you are performing high-impact neuromotor exercises in conjunction with other forms of fitness training such as maximal strength training or high-volume aerobic training.

Intensity

The principle of overload states that in order to provide benefits from training, the intensity of exercise must be above and beyond that which is demanded of the body on a day-to-day basis. To date, the intensity prescription for many neuromotor exercises, especially those targeting balance, has not been clearly established or adequately measured in research studies (9). Attempts at increasing neuromotor training intensity for the purposes of overloading the neuromuscular system have included increasing the duration of training and increasing the difficulty of the exercises (i.e., single- versus double-leg stance, narrow versus wide base of support, unstable versus stable surface) (9). The challenge is that the way in which people experience the intensity of balance, agility, coordination, and proprioceptive exercise can vary greatly. Monitoring movement quality may be helpful for assessing how demanding an activity is on your neuromuscular system. For example, if you are unable to maintain good form on any given exercise, then the exercise may be too advanced or your neuromuscular system may have become overwhelmed by the demands of the activity. In either case, if you are unable to maintain proper posture, body segment alignment, or balance while exercising, this may be a good indicator that your body has been challenged above and beyond its normal capabilities, and a short rest period may be needed before continuing.

Time

Current recommendations suggest that approximately 30 to 45 minutes should be devoted to neuromotor training for each session throughout the week (17). This should provide you with enough time to perform between 6 and 10 exercises depending on the demands of the specific activities you choose. Keep in mind that the neuromuscular system responds best to high-quality repetitive movements, so as your training progresses you may need to increase your training time as long as movement quality and body control are not compromised.

Type

Because the neuromuscular system is so heavily involved in the body's capacity to learn new activities, the principle of specificity may be one of the most important components to consider when developing a neuromotor training program. To illustrate this point, consider the task of learning to ride a bicycle. Riding a bicycle requires the development and coordination of a specific set of skills. You may have used or heard the saying "It's like riding a bike." This comparison reflects the neuromuscular system's ability to adapt to the specific demands of an activity and to easily recall motor skills related to that activity at a later time. It may take many hours or even days to develop the skills needed to effectively ride a bicycle. Yet the more you challenge your neuromuscular system, the more proficient your body becomes at the task of riding. Eventually, your neuromuscular system commits to memory the specific muscle actions needed to pedal, balance, and steer; and what started off as a challenging activity becomes very easy. The neuromuscular system is so proficient at learning and retaining information that even after many months or years have passed, you can climb back onto a bicycle and begin riding as if no time had passed at all.

Adhering to the specificity principle is critical to the development of an effective individualized neuromotor training program. Improvements in neuromotor function are specific to the types of activities you perform. If you want to reduce your risk for falling, then you must perform activities that challenge your upright stability and balance. If your goal is to improve coordination and agility for athletic competition, then your training program must include sport-specific activities that challenge your neuromuscular system in this way. Lower extremity muscle strength can be improved through performance of repeated bouts of the seated leg press; however, improvements in seated leg strength may not translate to improved athletic performance if the neuromuscular demands of seated exercise are dramatically different from those experienced while evading tackles on the football field. Consequently, a multicomponent program involving task-specific neuromotor exercise may provide greater functional and performance benefit than one-dimensional exercise programs that focus on individual components of muscular strength, aerobic fitness, and flexibility (23). In addition, those forms of training that use various movements with and without visual feedback may be the most beneficial for improving specific components of neuromotor function such as proprioception and body awareness (2).

Volume

One of the most important aspects of neuromotor training is ensuring that you perform each exercise with the best form and technique possible. Your neuromuscular system learns from your repeated movement patterns. If you consistently perform an exercise incorrectly or in a way that does not engage the appropriate muscles in the right sequence or pattern, you may run the risk of "wiring" your neuromuscular system with the wrong series of muscle recruitment strategies. If you are new to exercise, knowing your physical limits and recognizing how your body responds to fatigue may be a challenge. Consulting a qualified exercise professional, even if only for a few sessions, may be helpful to guide you through proper exercise technique and form. This may better prepare you to recognize the signs of muscular fatigue and breakdown in movement performance and put you in a better position to optimize the benefits of your neuromotor training program.

Progression

Exercise progression and progressive overload are important concepts for all training. In order to maximize the potential benefits of neuromotor training, it is important to consistently and continuously challenge your neuromuscular system with activities that exceed the demands of your daily activities. For example, if sitting predominates in your day, then simple standing activities may be sufficient to challenge many neuromotor fitness domains. However, if your day involves significant time on your feet and possibly lifting, carrying, or moving objects, then it is likely that you will need to begin your neuromotor training program with more dynamic standing activities and possibly incorporate various standing surface conditions to optimize your benefits.

Although there is currently no clear consensus as to the most effective strategy for improving neuromuscular function through progressive neuromotor training, some logical progressions have been proposed. These progressions can be employed to ensure that your neuromotor training program effectively challenges your balance, coordination, agility, and proprioception (10). Table 8.5 provides a few examples of ways in which your neuromotor training program can be progressed through increasing degrees of difficulty. You can advance your neuromotor training program in almost an infinite number of ways, and no one way is necessarily better than another.

Progression of your exercise program will be based on your baseline level of physical conditioning and your personal comfort with performing different neuromotor exercises.

TABLE 8.5   **Sample Neuromotor Training Progressions**

Description	Sample levels of progression		
	Level 1	Level 2	Level 3
Change foot position and posture to gradually reduce the base of support.	Stand with feet side by side	Stand with feet in full-tandem position (heel to toe)	Stand on one leg
Vary dynamic movements that challenge the center of gravity.	Tandem walking	Braided walking (one foot crosses in front and then behind the other)	Backward walking
Challenge postural muscle groups.	Stand with feet flat on the ground	Stand with only heels touching the ground	Stand with only toes touching the ground
Gradually reduce sensory input.*	Stand with eyes open	Stand with one eye closed	Stand with both eyes closed
Complete exercises on progressively unstable surfaces.	Stand on a firm floor	Stand on a foam pad	Stand on a balance board or Bosu
Gradually increase movement speed.	Complete 20 side steps in 20 sec	Complete 20 sidesteps in 15 sec	Complete 20 sidesteps in 10 sec
Add weighted resistance to challenge balance and stability.	Stand in tandem while holding a single dumbbell by your side	Stand on one foot while holding a single dumbbell by your side	Stand on one foot while reaching down to pick up a kettlebell off the floor

*Note: Altering sensory input (such as with eyes closed) should be performed only while one is participating in stationary exercises. For safety, agility and multidirectional exercises should always be conducted with eyes open.

For example, you may find it more difficult to perform dynamic tasks (such as sidestepping or braided walking) and therefore need to begin your training with less dynamic stationary standing exercises. Likewise, you may find that stationary standing activities on firm, flat ground are very easy and therefore would need to begin with more difficult neuromotor activities like balancing on one foot while standing on an unstable surface. The focus of progression is to select exercises and levels of difficulty based on activities that are challenging but can be completed safely without increasing your risk of injury.

Your Neuromotor Training Program

A sample program for various levels is provided in figure 8.6. The time frame for the activities increases as the program is advanced. Sample exercises for each of the areas are provided in table 8.6 with pictures and descriptions later in this chapter.

Neuromotor Training Exercises

The neuromotor exercises you might wish to incorporate into your personalized training program are almost limitless. Your neuromotor training plan should be based on your individual needs and goals. Although these exercises are a great starting point, it is always helpful to consult a qualified exercise professional if you have any questions or concerns about developing a neuromotor training plan that is right for you.

FIGURE 8.6

Sample neuromotor training program.

	Exercises	Time per exercise	Total session time	Number of days per week
Beginner	You should remain at this stage until you feel comfortable performing your selected exercises with good form, body control, and balance.			
	Perform eight exercises in a circuit for time. Select two exercises from each of the following areas: agility, stationary balance, push, pull.	15 to 30 sec	20 min	2
Intermediate	You should remain at this stage until you feel comfortable performing your selected exercises with good form, body control, and balance.			
	Perform eight exercises in a circuit for time. Select two exercises from each of the following areas: agility, dynamic balance, push, pull.	30 to 45 sec	20 to 30 min	2 to 3
Advanced	At this stage, continue to incorporate the suggested neuromotor training progressions while ensuring that you maintain good form, body control, and balance.			
	Perform 8 to 10 exercises in a circuit for time. Select two or three exercises from each of the following areas: agility, dynamic balance, push, pull.	45 to 60 sec	30 to 45 min	2 to 3

TABLE 8.6 Neuromotor Training Exercise Guide

Category	Exercise
Stationary balance	Single-leg standing balance (p. 194) Single-leg forward reach (p. 194) Semi-tandem standing with diagonal reach (p. 195) Tandem standing balance (p. 196)
Agility	T-drill (p. 196) Lateral side step (p. 197) Braided side step (p. 198) 4-square agility (p. 199)
Push	Push-ups (various forms) (p. 107, 108, 135, 201) Prone plank (p. 143) Up–down prone plank (p. 200)
Pull	Rows (various forms) (p. 136-139) Push-up hold with dumbbell row (p. 201)
Dynamic balance	Step-over hurdle (p. 202) Lunge with forward reach (p. 203) Step-up with overhead reach (p. 204)

STATIONARY BALANCE EXERCISES

Your ability to maintain balance affects many routine aspects of daily life. These simple exercises provide a number of options to help improve balance.

Single-Leg Standing Balance

Stand near a wall or by a fixed object in the event that you lose balance and need to support yourself. Begin with both feet on the ground (a). When ready, lift one knee toward the ceiling in a marching position (b). Hold the lifted leg in the air with the upper thigh parallel to the ground. Hold this position, without holding on to anything for support if you can, for the desired time. Repeat on the other leg. Once you become proficient at standing on one leg without support for 30 to 45 seconds, increase the proprioceptive challenge by eliminating your sight perception by closing your eyes.

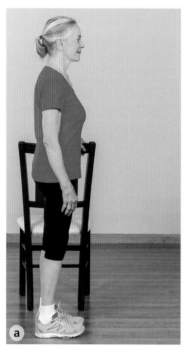 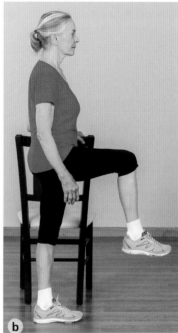

Single-Leg Forward Reach

Begin by standing with both feet on the ground; then lift your right foot in the air behind you (a). With your right foot in the air, slowly bend forward at the waist, maintaining your balance, and reach your right hand toward the ground while keeping the right foot in the air the entire time (b). Once the limits of your stability have been reached, stand back up while making sure to continue to balance on the left foot only. Repeat this movement for the desired time or number of repetitions. Alternate your feet, standing on the right foot and lifting the left foot in the air. Bend forward while reaching your left hand toward the ground, and then once again return to the starting standing position without placing the left foot on the ground.

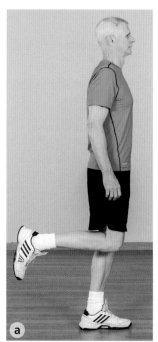

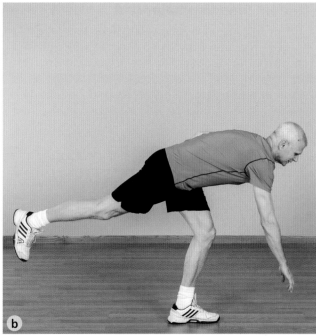

Semi-Tandem Standing With Diagonal Reach

Stand in a semi-tandem position with your left foot forward. Reach both arms in the direction of the back leg *(a)* and then reach up and across the body toward the direction of the forward leg *(b)*. Switch to the opposite side.

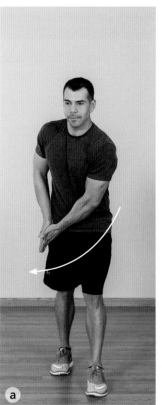

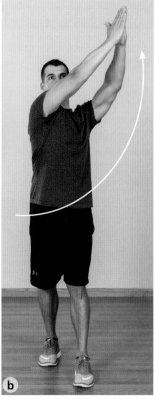

Tandem Standing Balance

Start in a standing position with feet together and arms by your side. Slowly step forward with your left foot so that you are standing heel to toe with your left foot in front. Hold this position for 30 to 45 seconds and then step back to the starting position with feet together. Repeat this same sequence but with the right foot forward and the left foot back. Repeat this exercise for the desired time or number of repetitions. You can advance this exercise by performing the same sequence with eyes closed.

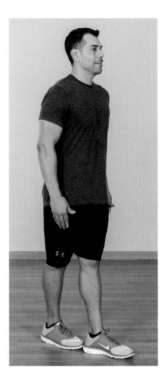

AGILITY EXERCISES

Agility exercises are used to challenge your body's ability to move and respond to changes in direction.

T-Drill

Follow the instructions for the Agility T-Test assessment earlier in this chapter. You will set up four cones in a T-shaped configuration (see figure 8.7) and then move from one cone to another by stepping forward, sideways, and backward. Complete as many circuits as possible following this movement pattern for the desired length of time.

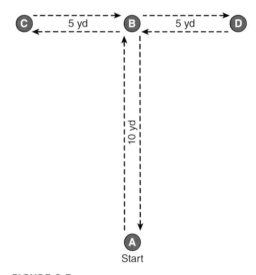

FIGURE 8.7

Adapted from K. Pauole, K. Madole, J. Garhammer, et al., 2000.

Lateral Side Step

Find a flat, nonslip floor for your exercise location. Mark two lines using masking tape or place two cones in a line, 15 feet (4.6 m) apart. You will sidestep toward your left *(a)* in order to touch or cross the line *(b)* and then repeat by sidestepping to your right *(c)*. Continue to sidestep, without crossing your feet, as quickly as possible, but safely, between the lines or cones for the desired length of time.

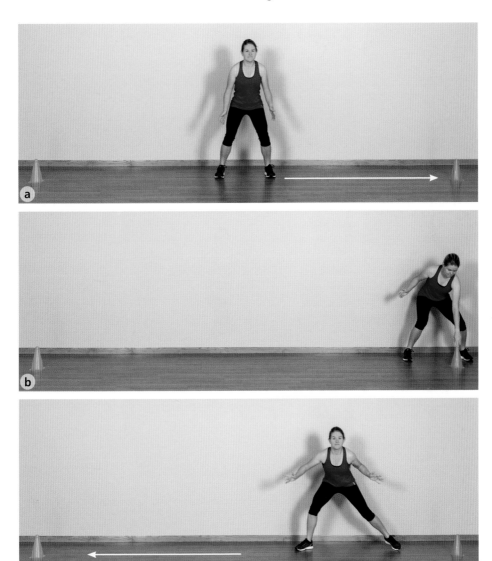

Braided Side Step

For the braided side step, follow the setup and execution as described in the lateral side-step exercise; the only difference is that your foot positions vary as you move from one line or cone to the other. In the braided side step, one foot crosses in front and then behind the other as you move from side to side (a and b). Move your feet as quickly as possible while still maintaining balance and body control.

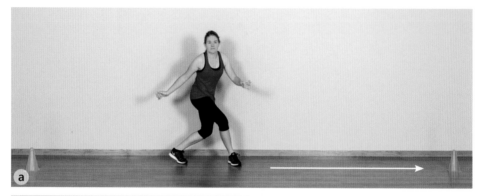

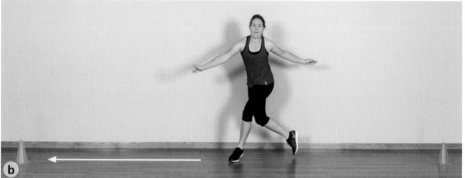

4-Square Agility

Begin by cutting two pieces of tape and placing them on the floor, one crossing the other through the center. Label the squares 1, 2, 3, and 4. Begin with both feet in square 1. When you are ready, work your way from square 1 to square 2 to square 4 to square 3 and back to square 1 by stepping with both feet to the side, backward, to the side, and forward, respectively *(a-d)*. Complete this sequence 10 times consecutively. Make it your goal to complete each circuit as quickly as you possibly can but safely. To increase the challenge of this exercise, transition from stepping to jumping from square to square, making sure not to touch the lines in the center with your feet. Additionally, you can an increase the challenge by varying the number sequence (e.g., 4-1-3-2, 4-2-3-1, 1-4-2-3, 1-3-4-2).

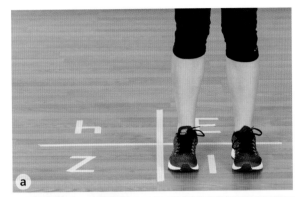

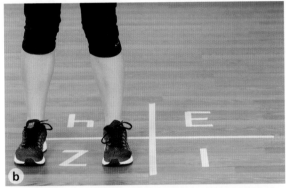

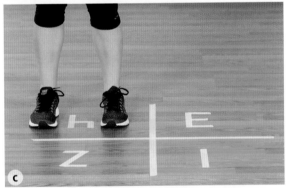

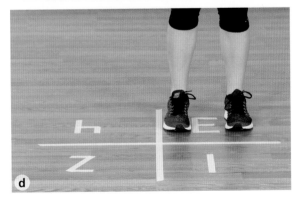

PUSH EXERCISES

The exercises in this section range from simple movements (e.g., push-ups) to more complex movements (e.g., up–down plank) that may be more appropriate once you have established a foundation of neuromotor training. Chapter 6 includes a number of these exercises (e.g., push-up options and prone plank).

Up–Down Prone Plank

This exercise combines and advances the full push-up and prone plank. Begin in the prone plank position *(a)*. Shift your body weight to the left elbow and shoulder while simultaneously transitioning: moving from your right elbow to your right hand *(b)*. Next, transition your weight to the right hand and shoulder, pushing up through the right arm and placing your left hand on the ground and pushing into full push-up position *(c)*. Repeat the steps in reverse until you return to the prone plank position on your elbows. Repeat the sequence for the desired number of repetitions or time. Be sure to alternate sides on which you are pushing up from the prone plank position so as not to work one arm and shoulder more than the other.

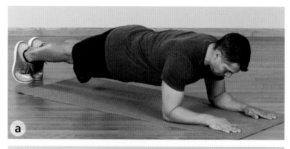

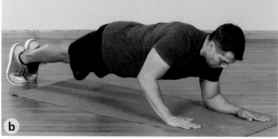

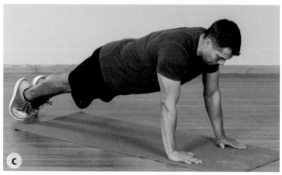

PULL EXERCISES

In addition to push exercises, the opposing movement—pulling—should be included in your neuromotor training program. Chapter 6 presents a number of options such as row exercises. Another option including the push-up position with the row movement is described in this section.

Push-Up Hold With Dumbbell Row

Assume a full push-up position but do so with hands holding two dumbbells *(a)*. Lower yourself down to the floor, and when the limits of your range of motion have been achieved, push up and lift one dumbbell off the floor toward your side *(b)*. Slowly lower the dumbbell back to the floor. Repeat this process for the desired amount of time or number of repetitions, remembering to alternate dumbbell lifts between the left and right arms.

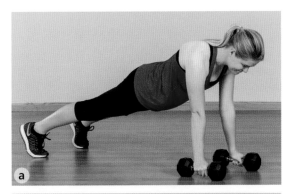

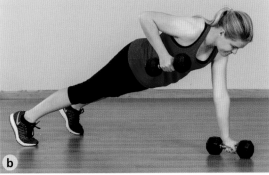

DYNAMIC BALANCE EXERCISES

In addition to the stationary balance exercises, dynamic balance exercises include the additional challenge of movement.

Step-Over Hurdle

Place a small box (e.g., shoe box) or taped line on the floor. Stand with your right shoulder facing the box *(a)*. When ready, lift your right knee toward the ceiling and step over the box to your right *(b)*. Place your right foot on the ground *(c)*, and lift your left foot over the box so that your left shoulder is now facing the box *(d* and *e)*. Repeat this exercise from side to side until the desired time or number of repetitions has been completed.

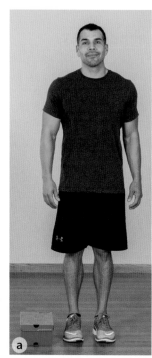

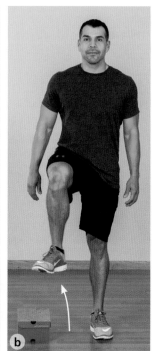

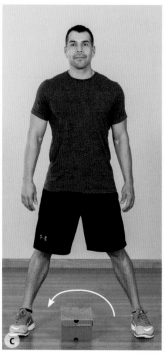

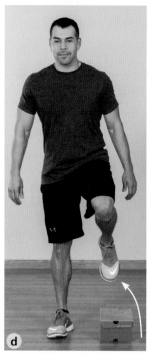

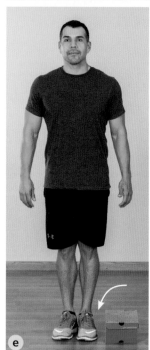

Lunge With Forward Reach

Begin in a standing position with both feet together and arms by your side *(a)*. Take a stride-length step forward with the left foot. In the lunge position, bend both knees so that the back knee moves downward toward the floor. As your knees bend, ensure that your trunk remains upright with the right shoulder, hip, and knee aligned. Once in this position, reach your arms out in front of you in order to further challenge your balance and limits of stability *(b)*. Once you have reached your maximum range of motion with the knees bent, push off the left foot, return to the start position with both feet together, and return your arms to your sides. Repeat this with your right foot stepping forward. Reach your arms out in front while maintaining your balance, and then return to the start position. Continue to alternate lunges between the left and right leg until the desired time or number of repetitions has been achieved.

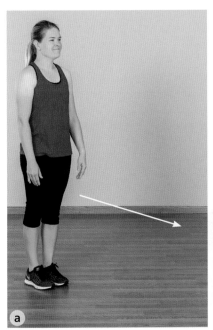 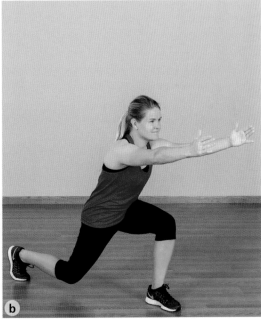

Step-Up With Overhead Reach

Stand in front of a step *(a)*. Begin by stepping up with the right foot *(b)*. Push yourself into a standing position on the step as you reach your arms overhead to the limits of your shoulder range of motion *(c)*. Step backward and down off the step, returning your arms to your side. Continue by stepping up with the left foot and reaching overhead as you come to a standing position on the step. Repeat until the desired time or number of repetitions has been reached. For an additional challenge when stepping up onto the bench with the right foot, keep the left foot elevated. Maintain this position with arms overhead for a moment before stepping back down with the left foot, followed by the right foot to return to the starting position. Continue, alternating feet.

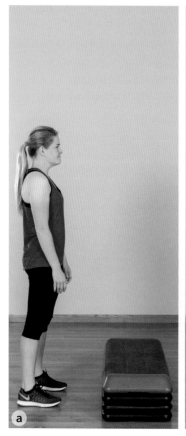
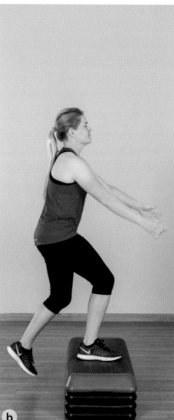
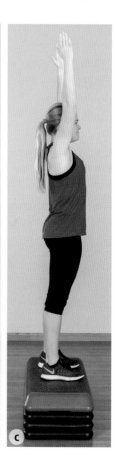

Although researchers are still seeking to identify the optimal frequency, intensity, time, type, and progression of neuromotor exercise, one thing is clear: Whether one is training for sport or for general health, neuromotor training is a recognized and necessary component of a comprehensive exercise training program. In the coming years, with advances in research and professional practice, exercise professionals and the broader exercise community will gain a much better understanding of the important role that neuromotor training plays in helping individuals of all ages and ability levels maintain optimal health, fitness, function, and quality of life.

Part III

Fitness and Health for Every Age

Regardless of your age, physical activity and nutrition are key factors in promoting health. Chapters 9 to 11 provide age-specific recommendations related to nutrition and exercise. You will see how it is never too early or too late to develop healthy habits.

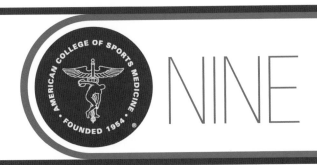

NINE

Children and Adolescents: Birth to Age 17

It is never too early in life to start developing healthy habits. Active youth have a better chance of growing into healthy adults. Risk factors for chronic diseases such as heart disease, high blood pressure, type 2 diabetes, and osteoporosis have their roots early in life (40). Regular physical activity and healthy dietary habits are two ways to lower the chance of developing risk factors for chronic lifestyle diseases (19).

Kids who are active on a regular basis display higher levels of aerobic and muscular fitness, decreased body fat, and stronger bones (13, 21, 33). Children and youth who regularly engage in physical activity also have better mental health and well-being (21, 33). Although the benefits of physical activity are well established, the activity levels of youth are below desired levels, with only about 25 percent of U.S. youth meeting recommended physical activity guidelines (37, 40). The percentage of children and youth who take part in health-producing physical activity also decreases with age (6). Similarly, a gap exists between recommended diets for youth and what the majority of youth actually consume (19). Thus, it is vital that adults provide opportunities for children and adolescents to be physically active and make good nutrition choices.

Because children and adolescents are not small versions of adults, this chapter specifically addresses healthy eating for youth, including how adults can encourage children and adolescents to make healthier eating choices. The chapter also lays out physical activity recommendations that are appropriate for youth, from infancy through late adolescence, and describes practical ways for youth to be active in home, school, and recreational settings.

Focus on Nutrition

As discussed in chapter 3, good nutrition is important for attaining optimal health and promoting growth and physical development (41). Children who are 2 years of age and older should eat a diet in which sufficient (but not excessive) calories come from a variety of nutrient-dense foods and beverages (including fruits and vegetables, dietary fiber, whole grains, fat-free and low-fat dairy products) while limiting the intake of solid fats, cholesterol, sodium, extra sugars, and refined grains. Motivating children to eat well can be challenging, and the majority of U.S. youth are falling short of meeting national dietary guidelines (7, 16, 31, 39).

Childhood is a pivotal time to encourage healthy dietary choices, and adults can play an important role in modeling a positive attitude toward nutrition and health (38). Children can watch parents and caregivers snacking on fruits, vegetables, and whole grains and including these foods in family meals. Shopping with your children can also serve as an opportunity to teach them about healthy foods, and you can team up with your child in the kitchen to tear lettuce for a salad, add veggie toppings to a pizza, develop a great-tasting fruit smoothie, or experiment by making a new type of trail mix.

Providing youngsters with a variety of foods at home enables them to obtain the nutrients they need from different food groups while building their food "repertoire." Healthy choices for protein include seafood, lean meat and poultry, eggs, beans, peas, soy products, and unsalted nuts and seeds. Serving a variety of fresh, canned, frozen, and dried fruits and colorful vegetables (dark green, red, and orange), along with peas and beans, can sustain healthy growth and development. Whole wheat bread, oatmeal, popcorn, quinoa, and brown or wild rice are healthy choices for nutrient-packed whole-grain foods, and low-fat milk and yogurt can provide essential nutrients while keeping calorie intake in check (41).

Although the "clean plate club" was used in the past to prompt kids to eat, the current recommendation is to encourage them to stop eating when they are full rather than when their plates are clean. Children who understand this concept are less likely to become overweight (38). Offering a number of healthy eating options and letting children make food selections allows them to decide what to eat while still allowing you to provide needed guidance. Because youngsters often don't eat enough at a meal to tide them over until the next meal, a good option is to plan for three meals, plus a couple of snacks, each day (38). Snacks should be nutritious and should not substitute for meals skipped. Whenever possible, try to avoid serving sugary snacks like soda and juice drinks, cakes, cookies, ice cream, and candy on a regular basis. Instead, have different types of fruits available for youngsters to eat in between meals and encourage children to create healthy snacks from ingredients like dry whole-grain cereal, dried fruit, and unsalted nuts or seeds.

Although younger children are influenced to a great extent by parents, caregivers, and other adults, older children and adolescents eat more meals and snacks outside of the home and make more personal decisions about what to eat. One factor that can have a strong impact on food choices is the media. Consider, for example, the number of television advertisements that focus on sugar-laden breakfast cereals, cookies, candy, and fast-food restaurants. Then count the number of advertisements for fruits and vegetables (if you can find any at all). Of course, there is no comparison! Because adolescents tend to consume more sweetened beverages, french fries, pizza, and other fast-food items, many older youth do not meet healthy eating recommendations for fruits, vegetables, dairy foods, whole grains, lean meats, and fish. This results in too much fat in the diet and insufficient intake of nutrients such as calcium and iron, as well as vitamins A, D, and C and folic acid. Unfortunately, many adolescents skip breakfast and actually consume about one-third of their calories from snacks, with sweetened beverages being a major contributor (19).

Making good nutrition choices is especially important for older boys and girls, as this is a time of active physical growth and development and a period in their lives when they begin to make personal decisions regarding dietary habits. It's important to remember that there are no magic foods that can increase health and fitness; from a nutrition perspective, eating vegetables, fruits, whole grains, protein foods, and fat-free and low-fat dairy foods is the ticket to good health (19). Learning how to prepare healthy meals and snacks can also help reduce the consumption of sweets and high-calorie snacks like candies, cookies, and ice cream. For older girls, eating smart includes consuming fat-free or low-fat milk, cheese, and yogurt to build stronger and denser bones, as well as engaging in weight-bearing physical activities like walking, running, and skating (38).

Areas of the Diet to Increase for Youth

The dietary intake of some nutrients, including calcium, potassium, fiber, magnesium, and vitamin E, appears to be low for many youth (41). The low intake of fiber may be linked to underconsumption of whole grains, fruits, and vegetables. Also, low magnesium and potassium intake is reflected by insufficient fruit and vegetable intake. Low calcium intake usually results from inadequate consumption of milk and milk products. Vitamin E intake can be improved through the consumption of fortified cereals, as well as various nuts and oils.

Replacing less nutritious items with more nutritious ones can improve the diets of youth (42). Making some simple substitutions in dietary choices can help to strengthen these areas of deficiency and improve the nutrient content of children's diets. The following are some practical ways to address these nutrition concerns:

- Substitute whole fruit for fruit juice.
- Replace starchy vegetables (e.g., white potatoes) with dark green vegetables (e.g., broccoli) and orange vegetables (e.g., carrots, sweet potatoes).
- Increase the consumption of low-fat or skim milk in place of soda.
- Eat breakfast on a daily basis, including cereals fortified with vitamin E.

Areas of the Diet to Reduce for Youth

Although experts promote the consumption of fruits, vegetables, and whole grains for optimal health, the top sources of calories for U.S. youth are grain desserts (e.g., cakes, cookies, doughnuts, pies, and granola bars), pizza, and sugar-sweetened beverages (soda and fruit drinks). Consequently, the amount of added sugar and fat consumed is excessive. Children need to reduce their consumption of solid fats and added sugars (SoFAS is a common abbreviation used for these dual targets). Nearly 40 percent of the calories youth consume are SoFAS (41)! For example, on average, youth consume 171 calories each day from sugar-sweetened beverages (soda and fruit drinks combined). SoFAS are overconsumed by youth and often result in excessive intake of calories with little nutritional value. Reducing the consumption of SoFAS may be one of the most important steps in stemming the growing prevalence of obesity in youth.

Because of the high calorie content but limited nutrient value of the foods youth often consume (e.g., soda and high-fat fried foods), the overall caloric intake of youth is higher than desired. When the number of calories consumed is not offset by physical activity, this can lead to overweight and obesity. Foods with a high fat content are considered calorie dense, meaning that, per gram, the calorie content is high and the nutrient content is relatively low. Ideally, foods should be high in nutrients (i.e., nutrient dense) relative to the number of calories they contain. Table 3.4 gives examples of reduced-calorie, lower-fat alternatives to foods with a higher fat content. In addition to making simple substitutions, adults can make other changes that can address overweight and obesity in youth, such as the following (41, 42):

- Limit fast-food meals.
- Limit screen time (TV, computer).
- Don't let youth skip breakfast.
- Keep a check on portion size.

Taken together, these are action-oriented steps that can help address the growing problem of overweight and obesity in youth.

Dietary Focus for Youth

Improving the diets of children and adolescents requires greater attention to making nutritious choices at home, at school, and in community settings. Promoting good nutrition early in life and providing positive role models for healthy eating are two important ways of improving the eating patterns of youngsters. The purpose of making healthy dietary choices is not just to avoid chronic disease (although the benefits related to heart disease and other chronic conditions are clear), but also to meet nutrient requirements that lead to the best possible level of function and the ability to engage in physical activity. Food is the fuel for physical activity, and selecting high-grade fuels provides

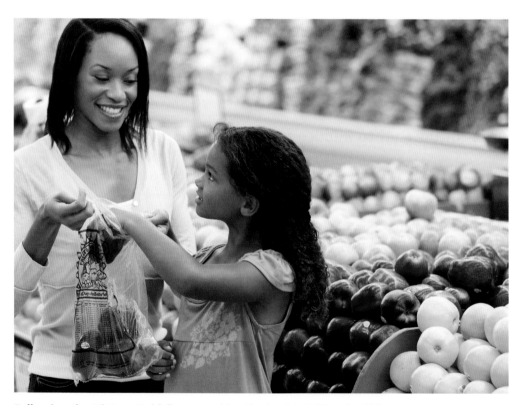

Following the *Dietary Guidelines* provides the best nutrition for kids.

the nutrients needed to power routine daily activities, moderate and vigorous physical activity, and sport performance.

Normal growth requires good nutrition (38). As with adults, children's weight in relation to height can be assessed easily via the body mass index (BMI). However, use of BMI is a bit more complex for youth because weight and height change with age, and the relationship between body fatness and weight and height also varies with age. Consequently, BMI charts that are specific for age and sex must be used for youth between the ages of 2 and 20 (see figure 9.1 or go to www.cdc.gov/growthcharts/

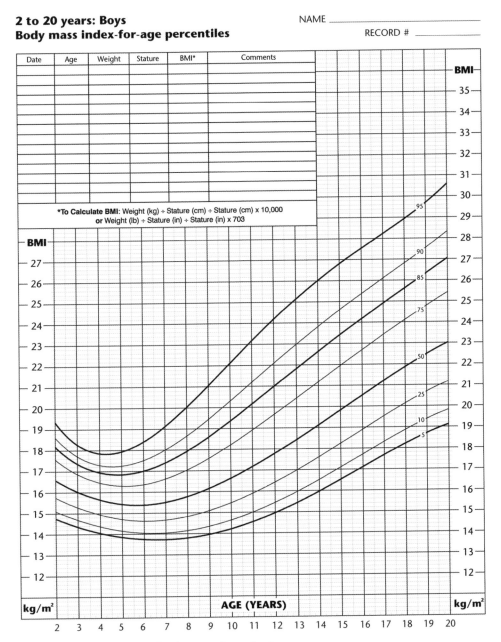

FIGURE 9.1a Body mass index for age charts for boys.

From ACSM, 2017, *ACSM's complete guide to fitness & health,* 2nd ed. (Champaign, IL: Human Kinetics). Developed by the National Center for Health Statistics and the National Center for Chronic Disease Prevention and Health Promotion, 2000.

2 to 20 years: Girls
Body mass index-for-age percentiles

NAME _____

RECORD # _____

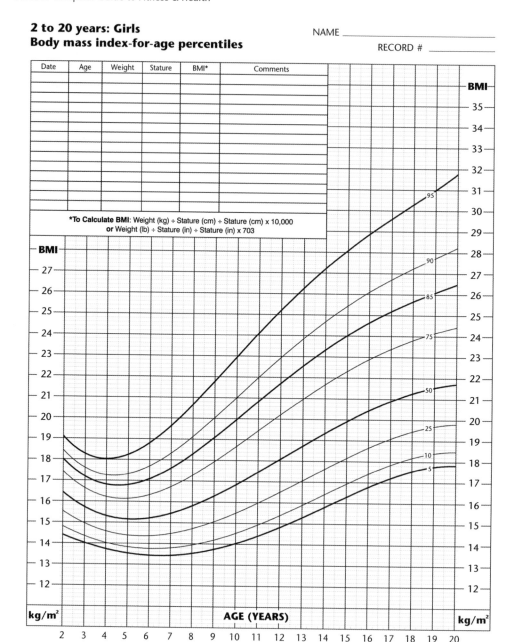

FIGURE 9.1b   Body mass index for age charts for girls.

From ACSM, 2017, *ACSM's complete guide to fitness & health*, 2nd ed. (Champaign, IL: Human Kinetics). Developed by the National Center for Health Statistics and the National Center for Chronic Disease Prevention and Health Promotion, 2000.

and enter "BMI calculator" into the search window for an easy online calculator and individualized interpretation of BMI) (11). Once the child's BMI has been calculated (see figure 18.1), follow the horizontal line matching the BMI value until it intersects with the vertical line for the child's age, and note the percentile line closest to this point of intersection.

Based on guidelines established by the Centers for Disease Control and Prevention, a BMI value between the 5th percentile and less than the 85th percentile is considered to fall within the healthy weight category (10). The BMI range for being classified as overweight is between the 85th and less than the 95th percentile, and a classification of obesity is indicated if BMI is equal or greater than the 95th percentile. A BMI that is less than the 5th percentile indicates underweight. As BMI does not take into account body composition (i.e., the relative contribution of fat and lean tissue to overall body weight), it is appropriate to schedule a visit with a health care provider for further evaluation and consultation for a child who is classified as overweight, obese, or underweight using the BMI calculation.

Consuming an appropriate number of calories and foods from various categories results in optimal nutrition. Table 9.1 provides age-specific daily calorie and serving size recommendations for grains, fruits, vegetables, and milk and dairy items for boys

TABLE 9.1   Daily Estimated Calories[1] and Recommended Servings for Children and Adolescents

	1 year	2 to 3 years	4 to 8 years	9 to 13 years	14 to 18 years
Calories[2]	900 kcal	1,000 kcal	1,400 kcal for males; 1,200 kcal for females	1,800 kcal for males; 1,600 kcal for females	2,200 kcal for males; 1,800 kcal for females
Fat	30 to 40% kcal	30 to 35% kcal	25 to 35% kcal	25 to 35% kcal	25 to 35% kcal
Milk, dairy[3]	2 cups[6]	2 cups	2 cups	3 cups	3 cups
Lean meat, beans	1.5 oz	2 oz	4 oz for males; 3 oz for females	5 oz	6 oz for males; 5 oz for females
Fruits[4]	1 cup	1 cup	1 1/2 cups	1 1/2 cups	2 cups for males; 1 1/2 cups for females
Vegetables[4]	3/4 cup	1 cup	1 1/2 cups for males; 1 cup for females	2 1/2 cups for males; 2 cups for females	3 cups for males; 2 1/2 cups for females
Grains[5]	2 oz	3 oz	5 oz for males; 4 oz for females	6 oz for males; 5 oz for females	7 oz for males; 6 oz for females

[1]Calorie estimates are based on a sedentary lifestyle. Increased physical activity will require additional calories: By 0 to 200 kilocalories/day if moderately physically active and by 200 to 400 kilocalories/day if very physically active.

[2]For youth 2 years and older; adopted from Table 2, Table 3, and Appendix A-2 of the *Dietary Guidelines for Americans* (2005), https://health.gov/dietaryguidelines/2005.asp. Nutrient and energy contributions from each group are calculated according to the nutrient-dense forms of food in each group (e.g., lean meats and fat-free milk).

[3]Milk listed is fat-free (except for children under the age of 2 years). If 1 percent, 2 percent, or whole-fat milk is substituted, this will use, for each cup, 19, 39, or 63 kilocalories of discretionary calories and add 2.6, 5.1, or 9.0 grams of total fat, of which 1.3, 2.6, or 4.6 grams are saturated fat.

[4]Serving sizes are 1/4 cup for 1 year of age, 1/3 cup for 2 to 3 years of age, and 1/2 cup for >4 years of age. A variety of vegetables should be selected from each subgroup over the week.

[5]Half of all grains should be whole grains.

[6]For 1-year-old children, calculations are based on 2 percent fat milk. If 2 cups of whole milk are substituted, 48 kilocalories of discretionary calories will be used. The American Academy of Pediatrics recommends that low-fat or reduced fat milk not be started before 2 years of age.

Reprinted with permission from S.G. Gidding et al., 2005.

and girls. Because the calorie recommendations in this table are for an inactive child, about 200 calories would need to be added for a moderately active child, and 200 to 400 calories per day would need to be added for a very physically active child (19).

While table 9.1 can be helpful in providing guidelines for caloric intake for children from 1 to 18 years of age, the number of calories that youth need for healthy growth and development depends on various factors, such as age, sex, physical activity levels, and genetics (43). Nonetheless, it is possible to create sample meals that are healthy, composed of foods from each major food category, and also cater to your child's tastes and food preferences. One way of planning a healthy meal is to select a food item from each food group listed in table 9.2 (note that these are examples of items in amounts that might commonly be consumed and do not necessarily reflect a defined serving size).

Based on the information presented in table 9.2, here are examples of meals for breakfast, lunch, and dinner:

- *Breakfast:* One banana, a slice of whole-grain bread with peanut butter, and low-fat milk
- *Lunch:* Turkey sandwich with cheese, dark leafy lettuce, tomato, and red peppers on whole wheat bread, 6-ounce yogurt snack pack, bottle of water

TABLE 9.2 **Healthy Meal Planning**

Fruits and veggies	Grains	Protein	Dairy
1 banana or apple	1/2 cup oatmeal or whole-grain cereal	1 scrambled or hard-boiled egg	1 cup fat-free or low-fat milk
1 handful of fresh berries or grapes	2 DVD-sized whole-grain or buckwheat pancakes	1 tablespoon peanut butter	6- to 8-oz yogurt pack
1 cup romaine lettuce or spinach	1 slice whole wheat bread	1 small handful walnuts or almonds	1 cup low-fat cottage cheese
1 handful baby carrots, strips of peppers, or celery sticks	1 small whole-grain muffin	1 tablespoon hummus	1 slice of Swiss or provolone cheese
1 cup tomato, vegetable, apple, or orange juice	1 whole wheat tortilla	1 piece sliced, lean turkey or ham	1 stick string cheese
1 snack pack of fruit salad in natural juices (not syrup)	1/2 cup brown rice	1/3 can tuna	1 handful shredded, low-fat mozzarella cheese
1 medium sweet potato (baked)	2 cups popcorn	1 soy or bean burger patty	1 snack pack of pudding made from milk
1/2 cup steamed broccoli, green beans, or other veggie	1/2 cup whole-grain pasta	1 portion of lean beef, grilled chicken, tofu, or baked fish (size of the palm of your hand)	1 cup non-fat frozen yogurt

Data from USDA Center for Nutrition Policy and Promotion.

- *Dinner:* One whole wheat tortilla with chicken, low-fat cheese, chopped tomato, and romaine lettuce

As you can see, many combinations of foods in the four major food groups can be put together in creative ways to make healthy, tasty meals for youth of all ages.

Importance of Family Meals

While it can sometimes be challenging for family members to eat together, doing so provides a daily opportunity not only to enjoy a communal meal but also to talk about what's going on in each person's life and strengthen family bonds. From a nutrition point of view, eating meals as a family unit has been linked to increased fruit and vegetable consumption, higher intakes of nutrients such as dietary fiber, calcium, vitamins B_6, B_{12}, C, and iron, and less intake of fried foods and soda (29). Moreover, a greater frequency of eating dinner as a family is associated with a positive sense of the future, positive values and identity, higher levels of motivation and involvement in school, and a greater commitment to learning (18). In addition, research has shown that younger children (younger than 13 years old) who eat breakfast on a regular basis demonstrate greater on-task behavior in the classroom and higher school grades and achievement test scores (2).

The U.S. Department of Agriculture My Plate for kids is an excellent nutrition resource. The website www.choosemyplate.gov/kids includes resources for younger age groups, including games, activity sheets, and recipes.

Children begin to establish dietary habits and preferences during the first years of life. Working together, parents and caregivers can guide, educate, and motivate youngsters to make wise nutrition choices. Developing healthy eating habits during childhood and adolescence is a foundational life skill that can help prevent the genesis of diet-related diseases later in life.

■ Q&A

What are ways a family can develop healthy eating patterns?

The following tips can help a family eat well (38):

- *Make half your grains whole.* Select whole-grain foods more often (e.g., whole wheat bread, brown rice, oatmeal, low-fat popcorn).
- *Vary your veggies.* Eat a variety of vegetables, and in particular, seek out dark green and orange vegetables (e.g., spinach, broccoli, carrots, sweet potatoes).
- *Focus on fruits.* Fruits can be part of meals or snacks, whether they are fresh, frozen, canned, or dried.
- *Eat calcium-rich foods.* Low-fat and fat-free milk and other milk products should be consumed several times a day to help build strong bones.
- *Go lean with protein.* Protein can be found in lean or low-fat meats, chicken, turkey, and fish, as well as dry beans and peas.
- *Change your oil.* Good sources of oil are fish, nuts, and liquid oils (e.g., corn, soybean, canola, and olive oil).
- *Don't sugarcoat it.* Check labels and choose foods and beverages that do not have sugar and sweeteners as one of their primary ingredients.

Focus on Physical Activity

From 1960 to 2010, the prevalence of obesity in American youth increased in dramatic fashion. Based on current estimates, nearly one out of three youth in the United States is overweight, while more than one in six is obese (12, 32). Not surprisingly, children who are overweight and obese do not typically meet current physical activity guidelines for youth (12).

Budget-related cutbacks in physical education and increased time spent in sedentary activities have led to an escalation in the overweight status of youth and have contributed to a substantial reduction in childhood physical activity. Over half of young boys and three out of four young girls do not participate in daily physical activity (9). Moreover, children and youth spend more than 7 hours a day in sedentary pursuits, and inactivity increases with age (6). The long-term consequences of high levels of body weight and physical inactivity include a greater risk of early death and the presence of chronic health conditions, such as heart disease, high blood pressure, diabetes, and certain forms of cancer (17, 26, 35).

Benefits of Physical Activity for Children and Adolescents

Involvement in regular physical activity during childhood and adolescence can enhance cardiovascular and musculoskeletal health, can produce beneficial changes in blood lipid (cholesterol) levels, and has been tied to higher levels of physical self-concept and better cognitive and academic performance (4, 33, 36). Because youth who are overweight are more likely to become overweight adults (15), adopting a physically active lifestyle early in life can play a key role in establishing good health and avoiding unhealthy weight gain (28). Inactivity and low physical activity patterns tend to be harder to modify with age (34); this reality further emphasizes the need to encourage youth to develop and maintain an active lifestyle.

Right From the Start

How early is too early to encourage children to be active? This is an issue the National Association for Sport and Physical Education (NASPE) addressed for children up to 5 years of age in a recent book titled *Active Start* (24). Now in its second edition, *Active Start* highlights the role that parents, child care providers, and teachers can play in

■ Q&A

Do all children and adolescents need a medical screening before engaging in physical activity?

Most healthy children and adolescents can begin a physical activity program without a visit to a physician or health care provider (3). However, if a preexisting condition exists (e.g., asthma, diabetes, or obesity), or if there are any other special circumstances or concerns, then consulting with a physician or health care provider before increasing activity is warranted. Often, simple adjustments can be made to the activity program, such as starting out with a lower amount of activity and progressing more slowly. For youth involved in competitive sports, a sport physical is typically required to ensure that no health conditions exist that could limit the ability to endure the rigors of a particular sport.

motivating very young children to be active, which includes serving as active role models and creating environments that facilitate play and movement exploration. The overall position of NASPE is that all children from birth to age 5 should engage daily in physical activity that promotes movement skillfulness and a foundation in health-related fitness (24).

Increasing physical activity levels to 20 to 30 minutes three or more days a week has been shown to improve bone health, motor skills, aerobic fitness, and some aspects of self-esteem in children 2 to 5 years of age (36). Based on evidence that physical activity behavior tends to track during early childhood (30) and that a sizable portion of preschool-aged boys and girls do not meet current activity recommendations to improve physical fitness and competency in performing motor skills (23), it is important to provide a wide range of opportunities for children to be active during the earliest years of life.

Physical Activity Guidelines From Birth to Late Adolescence

The next section presents physical activity guidelines for each developmental phase of the child relative to the frequency, intensity, time, and type (i.e., FITT profiles) of recommended physical activity. The intensity range of physical activity varies from moderate to vigorous. Moderate-intensity physical activities (such as briskly walking to school) can be performed and maintained easily, whereas vigorous-intensity activities (such as running on the playground) feature substantial increases in heart rate, breathing rate, and sweating and often require more rest periods (40).

Infants (Birth to 1 Year)

From the first days of life, the ability to move and explore allows infants to begin to understand and make sense of their surroundings. During the first year, infants start to develop and repeat movement patterns as their muscles learn to respond to information sent from the brain. Consequently, infants need numerous opportunities to participate in a variety of physical activities that promote skill development and movement competency. The acquisition of new movement skills also helps newborns adapt to unfamiliar physical surroundings (1).

FITT Profile for Infants   Parents and caregivers should play with infants several times a day during waking hours, especially when infants are alert and happy. Although parents and caregivers should engage infants in active play, the intensity level of physical activity is determined by the child. When infants are not interested in engaging in active play, they typically communicate this by crying or looking away. A variety of positive facial and other nonverbal and verbal expressions can be used to motivate infants to be active.

Infants should be encouraged to participate on a daily basis in a variety of activities that promote the development of basic movement skills, such as reaching, grasping, holding, squeezing, pushing, pulling, crawling, sitting, standing, and moving their arms and legs. Examples of activities include playing games such as patty cake and peek-a-boo; placing objects of different sizes, textures, colors, and shapes within or just beyond their reach; and assisting with movement skills such as sitting, crawling, standing, and stepping. Infants may also enjoy banging objects and moving to music, crawling across a surface decorated with brightly colored objects, bouncing in a baby seat, lying or sitting in a supported position while reaching out and manipulating a suspended mobile, and playing and moving while taking a bath. Many toys and objects used for play by infants can be found at home or can be purchased inexpensively.

Recommended Activity Settings for Infants   Infants should be placed in settings during the day that are safe and promote movement and exploration of their surroundings. If the play environment is too small, or if the infant is placed in a sedentary or restrictive setting (e.g., a baby seat or playpen) for extended periods, a delay may occur in learning and practicing fundamental behaviors such as rolling over, sitting, crawling, creeping, and standing. Play equipment should be nontoxic, should contain no sharp edges or points, and should be free of pieces that can be swallowed. Playing, rolling, and crawling activities can be performed on a rug or blanket in a floor-based setting that is at least 5 feet by 7 feet (1.5 by 2.1 m) (24).

Toddlers (1 to 3 Years)

Once a child can walk, a new vista of physical activity choices emerges. Learning to stand and walk in an upright, hands-free posture allows the toddler to acquire and refine fundamental movements (e.g., walking, running, jumping, leaping, throwing, catching, kicking, bouncing) that form the basis of many sport, fitness, and dance activities. Although the ability to perform these core movement patterns is a partial by-product of physical growth, an environment that is supportive and stimulating and that provides opportunities for the toddler to safely engage in structured and unstructured physical activity is also essential. Regular exposure to age- and developmentally appropriate physical activities helps toddlers become more confident in their attempts to master their physical environment while developing cardiorespiratory endurance, strength, balance, and flexibility.

FITT Profile for Toddlers   When alert and awake, toddlers should engage in multiple bouts of short-burst, moderate to vigorous physical activity in indoor and outdoor settings. Although the length of these bouts will vary depending on the age and developmental stage of the child, at least 30 minutes of structured physical activity and at least 60 minutes (and up to several hours) of unstructured physical activity should be accumulated each day. Toddlers should not be sedentary for longer than 60 minutes at a time except when sleeping (24). Structured physical activities for toddlers are planned and directed by a parent or caregiver and can include activities such as action-oriented follow-along songs, dancing to rhythms of taped music or music videos, moving through an obstacle course that provides opportunities to employ manipulative or movement skills, and simple chase games. Unstructured physical activity is initiated by the toddler during exploration of the surrounding environment. Examples might include playing on and around playground structures, moving on a variety of riding toys (e.g., tricycles, scooters) while wearing a safety helmet, and digging and building in a sandbox. A toddler's interest in being physically active can be enhanced through the use of age-appropriate toys and equipment in a variety of movement environments.

Recommended Activity Settings for Toddlers   Indoor and outdoor play areas for toddlers should meet or exceed recommended safety standards and be large enough to facilitate large-muscle activities. Play environments should also be childproof, accessible, and inviting. Each toddler should have a minimum indoor activity space of 35 square feet (3.3 sq m) of activity room and an outdoor activity space of at least 75 square feet (7 sq m) (24).

Preschoolers (3 to 5 Years)

The preschool years are an optimal time to learn and refine fundamental movements and locomotor activities in a variety of settings so that the child can develop motor skill proficiency before entering kindergarten. Performing a gross motor skill is the result of a learned sequence of movements that allow preschoolers to complete physical tasks in a smooth and coordinated fashion. Promoting the development of needed movement patterns at this stage of life will carry forward into the future. The period from 3 to 5 years of age is also a good time to help children develop good nutrition habits; expend enough calories to ward off excessive weight gain; and increase heart fitness, muscular strength, flexibility, and bone density. The physical activity profile of a preschooler depends on a number of factors, including age, maturity, ability, and previous exposure to motor learning and development, as well as their natural activity patterns, which feature spontaneous and intermittent movement (36). Parents and caregivers should also keep in mind that at a given age, preschoolers can exhibit varying degrees of proficiency in performing motor tasks.

FITT Profile for Preschoolers   Parents and caregivers of preschoolers should plan structured physical activity sessions that are moderate to vigorous in intensity and that last between 6 and 10 minutes. A minimum of 60 minutes of structured physical activity should be accumulated daily (24). Although preschool children have the capacity to sustain structured, developmentally appropriate physical activity for longer durations (e.g., 30 to 45 minutes), they should also be encouraged to accumulate multiple shorter bouts of structured activity spread throughout the day. In addition to engaging in structured activity, preschoolers should participate in inside and outside unstructured physical activity lasting at least 60 minutes to several hours a day at self-selected intensity levels. With the exception of sleeping, periods of sedentary activity lasting more than 1 hour should be avoided (24).

Preschoolers can enjoy an array of structured physical activities, including obstacle courses that promote movement and manipulative skills, mimicking animal

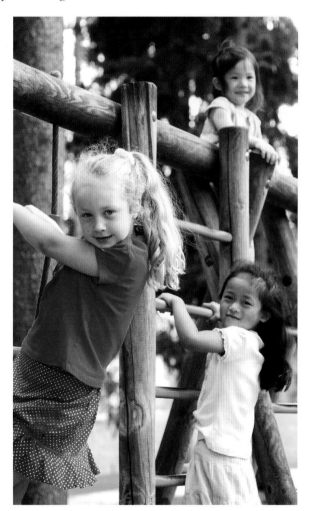

Climbing on playground structures is fun and also helps to build muscular fitness.

movements to develop strength and flexibility, and cardiorespiratory activities that improve aerobic fitness. Playing imitative games (such as Simon Says) using a variety of movement patterns, dancing to music of various tempos and rhythms, and receiving formal instruction in various motor skills are other structured forms of physical activity that are appropriate for preschool children. Unstructured physical activities for 3- to 5-year-olds include climbing on playground structures; playing with bats and balls; running up and down inclined surfaces; riding a variety of wheeled riding toys (while wearing a safety helmet); and chasing bubbles, balls, and hoops. Active play is another less formal activity option for the preschool child and might involve "dressing up," going on treasure hunts, or performing specific movement patterns (e.g., galloping like a horse) while another child or other children mimic the activity.

Recommended Activity Settings for Preschoolers   Activity spaces for preschoolers should be large enough to accommodate child-directed play or physical activities supervised by adults. The play environment should be one that can be modified or reconfigured to allow for different types of activity. Ideally, each child should have a minimum indoor space of 35 square feet (3.3 sq m) for structured movement activities and a minimum of 75 square feet (7 sq m) of outdoor play space (24). Larger play areas may be required to accommodate activities such as running, skipping, and kicking.

Children and Adolescents

The association between physical activity and good health in school-aged youth is well established (21, 25, 33, 40). Regular physical activity during childhood and adolescence has beneficial effects on cardiovascular and musculoskeletal health, body composition, bone mineral density, blood lipid levels, and blood pressure (21, 33). In addition, a positive influence of physical activity and fitness on mental health (e.g., anxiety, depression, self-concept), academic performance, and classroom behavior has been observed in schoolchildren (8, 33).

Current guidelines indicate that school-aged youth (ages 6 to 17) should accumulate a minimum of 60 minutes, and up to several hours, of age-appropriate physical activity of at least moderate intensity on all, or most, days of the week (21, 25, 33, 40). However, because some improvement in health-related fitness can be achieved by being active for an average of just 30 minutes a day (21), accumulating even less than the recommended amounts of physical activity on a daily basis would appear to be beneficial, especially for children and adolescents who are relatively inactive. Experts recommend that children and adolescents avoid extended periods (over 2 hours) of sedentary behavior (e.g., screen time) each day (27).

■ Q&A ■

What type of physical activity should children and adolescents do?

The physical activity profile of children and adolescents should feature activities that stimulate the aerobic system, increase muscular fitness, and produce stronger bones. School-aged youth should also participate in activities that are enjoyable and appropriate for their age, developmental status, and personal preferences. A variety of physical activities, games, and sports can be used to meet the recommended guidelines.

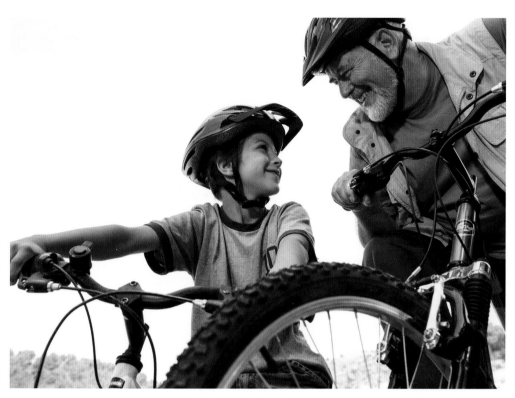

Kids of all ages enjoy bike riding, which is a great way to increase aerobic fitness.

FITT Profile for Aerobic Fitness The majority of children's daily 60-minute activity period should incorporate rhythmic, large-muscle, moderate to vigorous aerobic physical activities. Moderate-intensity activity can be considered a level 5 or 6 on a 10-point scale of effort (in which 0 is sitting at rest and 10 is the highest level of effort possible) (40). Vigorous-intensity aerobic activity (level 7 or 8 on the 10-point scale) should also be performed at least three days a week (40). Youth frequently engage in short bursts of activity interspersed with brief rest intervals; any time spent in moderate or vigorous aerobic activities can be counted toward meeting the aerobic guidelines. However, a majority of the 1-hour target time should be spent being active. For example, during a 20-minute recess, a child might accumulate 12 minutes of physical activity in periods lasting between a few seconds and several minutes and 8 total minutes of rest. Some activities, such as bicycling, can be classified as either moderate or vigorous depending on how intensely energy is being expended. Table 9.3 lists aerobic activities for children and adolescents that can be performed at moderate or vigorous intensities.

FITT Profile for Muscular Fitness and Bone Strengthening Current recommendations are that a portion of the 60-minute period of daily physical activity of children and adolescents include muscle-strengthening activities at least three days a week (40). The primary targets of strengthening should be the major upper and lower body muscle groups (legs, hips, back, abdomen, arms, chest, shoulders). Table 9.4 lists games and resistance training exercises that promote muscle strengthening and can be included as part of indoor or outdoor play activity. An example of a properly aligned weight machine is shown in figure 9.2.

TABLE 9.3   Examples of Aerobic Activities for Children and Adolescents

	Children	Adolescents
Moderate intensity	• Active recreation such as hiking, skateboarding, and rollerblading • Bicycle riding • Brisk walking	• Active recreation such as canoeing, hiking, skateboarding, and rollerblading • Riding a stationary or road bike • Brisk walking • Housework and yardwork, such as sweeping and pushing a lawn mower
Vigorous intensity	• Active games involving running and chasing, such as tag • Bicycle riding • Jumping rope • Martial arts, such as judo and karate • Running • Sports such as soccer, ice or field hockey, basketball, swimming, and tennis • Cross-country skiing	• Active games involving running and chasing, such as flag football • Bicycle riding • Jumping rope • Martial arts, such as judo and karate • Running • Sports such as soccer, ice or field hockey, basketball, swimming, and tennis • Cross-country skiing • Vigorous dancing

Adapted from U.S. Department of Health and Human Services, 2008.

TABLE 9.4   Examples of Muscle- and Bone-Strengthening Activities for Children and Adolescents

	Children	Adolescents
Muscle strengthening	• Games such as tug-of-war • Push-ups (knees on floor) • Resistance exercises using body weight or resistance bands • Rope or tree climbing • Sit-ups, curl-ups, or crunches • Swinging on playground equipment or bars	• Games such as tug-of-war • Push-ups or pull-ups • Resistance exercises using resistance bands, free weights, and weight machines • Climbing wall • Sit-ups, curl-ups, or crunches
Bone strengthening	• Games such as hopscotch • Hopping, skipping, jumping • Jumping rope • Running	• Hopping, skipping, jumping • Jumping rope • Running • Sports such as gymnastics, basketball, volleyball, and tennis

Adapted from U.S. Department of Health and Human Services, 2008.

The ACSM supports the use of resistance training for youth provided that the training program is properly designed and competently supervised (14). Myths still abound regarding resistance training for youth, including the idea that growth plates can be injured, resulting in stunted growth, or that strength gains are not possible in younger kids. In reality, resistance training improves muscular strength and endurance in youth, helps strengthen bones while having no negative effect on physical growth, and confers no greater injury risk than other childhood sports or recreational activities (14). In addition, resistance training, rather than causing injury, can potentially decrease the incidence and severity of injury (5).

To maximize safety during resistance training, adults must ensure that children and adolescents are mature enough to follow directions. Sessions should also be supervised by a knowledgeable adult who understands standard safety guidelines. Youth should be instructed to start with relatively light loads, gradually increase resistance as strength develops, and use controlled movements for all resistance training activities. Using proper technique is a key requirement, and emphasis should be placed on improvement of personal performance rather than on how much weight is lifted. Warm-up and cool-down periods should also be part of each resistance training session.

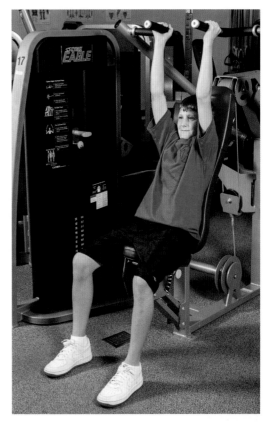

FIGURE 9.2 Ensure correct alignment when using weight machines.

The guidelines for resistance training outlined in chapter 6 can be modified for children and adolescents by having them do one to three sets of 8 to 15 repetitions of a given exercise (3). Resistance training can occur two to three days a week, with one day between sessions to allow the muscles to respond and recover. The intensity of training should not be maximal (i.e., to the point of muscle failure). Rather, training intensity should be moderate and should focus on learning and performing resistance exercise with good technique (14).

Muscle-strengthening activities that generate high-impact forces, such as running, jumping, and basketball, also cause bones to become stronger and denser. Because the

■ Q&A ■

How young is too young to start resistance training?

Strength training has been used with boys and girls as young as 7 to 8 years of age (13). Options include using rubber tubing or weight machines designed specifically for children. Younger children may also be able to engage in muscle-strengthening activities such as push-ups (either regular or modified) or sit-ups. The goal of resistance training is to improve musculoskeletal strength as part of a well-rounded fitness program that also features the development of endurance, flexibility, and agility.

greatest gains in bone mass occur just before and during puberty (22, 40), engaging in weight-bearing activities during the childhood and adolescent years can have a positive impact on bone health later in life (22). As with muscle-strengthening activities, bone fitness activities should be performed at least three days a week as part of the 60-minute period of daily physical activity (20). Table 9.4 identifies various activities that can be used to increase bone strength in school-aged youth.

Children and adolescents who do not meet the aforementioned guidelines should gradually raise their physical activity levels over time by initially aiming to be active more frequently, for longer time periods, or both (40). As levels of physical activity start to improve, the activity intensity can also be raised gradually as well. Youth who are following the physical activity recommendations should consider becoming even more active, especially in view of recent research suggesting that additional health benefits can be realized when minimum recommended levels of physical activity are exceeded (20). Lastly, youth who exceed the recommended activity guidelines should continue to maintain their level of performance and vary their physical activity routines to avoid overtraining, boredom, or injury (40).

Although children and adolescents can meet the recommended physical activity guidelines by participating in the activities listed in tables 9.3 and 9.4, they should also look for opportunities to be active throughout the day. Examples of lifestyle physical activity include walking or riding a bicycle with friends, taking a "physical activity break" from studying or playing video games, or helping with active household chores such as vacuuming and washing the family car. Having a posted checklist is one way to visually promote these lifestyle activities. After all the items have been checked off, a small reward may be given (e.g., gift card, tickets to a sporting or fitness event, new exercise clothes). An even simpler approach to promoting physical activity in youngsters is to maximize outside time and minimize inside time (it's much harder to be sedentary when you're outdoors and very easy to be sedentary when inside). Parents,

Meeting the Physical Activity Guidelines for Children and Adolescents

An endless number of routines that combine aerobic activity with muscle-strengthening and bone-building activities can be created to meet current physical activity recommendations for school-aged youth. Some youth may be involved in competitive sports while others enjoy various play and general activities. Parents and children can work together to come up with a weekly "physical activity menu" that lists several activities from which to choose, providing variety and promoting creativity. These are some examples:

- Active chores: washing the car, mowing the grass, doing yardwork
- Fun games: tag, kickball, Frisbee golf
- Playground activities: swinging on monkey bars, climbing on playground equipment, jumping rope, playing hopscotch
- Team sports: soccer, basketball, flag football, volleyball
- Other activities: swimming, tennis, dancing, lifting weights

family members, and teachers who participate in regular physical activity can also be real-life models of how to integrate activity and movement into everyday living.

Promoting Active Living and Healthy Eating in Youth

The use of the FitnessGram program to assess various components of health-related fitness is discussed in chapters 5, 6, and 7. FitnessGram is a part of the Presidential Youth Fitness Program (PYFP), which provides a model for educating school-aged youth about fitness within the context of a quality school-based physical education program. Children in kindergarten through third grade can participate in the PYFP Fitness Club and receive recognition for learning about various fitness components, while youth in 4th through 12th grade complete the FitnessGram assessment to determine whether their fitness scores fall within the Healthy Fitness Zone (HFZ). To track scores, use figure 9.3.

Families are encouraged to make healthy eating and active living a regular part of their lives. One way to promote these behaviors is to pledge to be a MyPlate Champion. This program encourages the following:

- *Eat more fruits and veggies.* Make half your plate fruits and vegetables every day.
- *Try whole grains.* Ask for oatmeal, whole-wheat breads, or brown rice at meals.
- *Re-think your drink.* Drink fat-free or low-fat milk or water instead of sugary drinks.
- *Focus on lean protein.* Choose protein foods like beans, fish, lean meats, and nuts.
- *Slow down on sweets.* Eat sweets, like cakes or cookies, once in a while and in small amounts.
- *Be active your way.* Find ways to exercise and be active for at least 1 hour a day like walking to school, riding your bike, or playing a sport with friends.

Kids that pledge to take these healthy actions can print a personalized certificate (see https://www.choosemyplate.gov/kids-become-myplate-champion).

FIGURE 9.3

Fitness assessment progress chart for youth*.

	Current	6-month assessment	1-year assessment
One-mile run	____ HFZ or above ____ Needs improvement	____ HFZ or above ____ Needs improvement	____ HFZ or above ____ Needs Improvement
Curl-up	____ HFZ or above ____ Needs improvement	____ HFZ or above ____ Needs improvement	____ HFZ or above ____ Needs improvement
Push-up	____ HFZ or above ____ Needs improvement	____ HFZ or above ____ Needs improvement	____ HFZ or above ____ Needs improvement
Sit-and-reach	____ HFZ or above ____ Needs improvement	____ HFZ or above ____ Needs improvement	____ HFZ or above ____ Needs improvement
BMI for age	____ Percentile	____ Percentile	____ Percentile

*HFZ = Healthy Fitness Zone.

From ACSM, 2017, *ACSM's complete guide to fitness & health*, 2nd ed. (Champaign, IL: Human Kinetics).

When looking at ways to encourage activity, the PYFP suggests some ways that family members can become more active:

- Provide children with toys and play equipment (e.g., balls, kites, jump ropes) that can be used during play and physical activity.
- Encourage youngsters to learn or try to perform a new physical activity.
- Limit time spent watching television and don't place a TV in a child's bedroom. Children and youth who are 2 years of age and older should limit TV viewing to a maximum of 2 hours daily.
- Spend time together as a family performing an activity that requires moving, like going to the park, exploring trails, or biking on a greenway.

See what other activities are enjoyed by the family and make ongoing plans to be active together.

■ Q&A

What are some practical ways to encourage activity and healthy eating for a child who is overweight?

Developing a plan in consultation with the child's pediatrician along with talking over options with the child is key. The following are some ideas:

- Create an activity chart on which the child tracks physical activity (e.g., walking to school, taking the dog for a walk around the neighborhood park, riding a bike), and create a chart for the parents as well. The first one to reach 300 minutes of activity chooses the next weekend family outing (e.g., window shopping at the mall, a picnic at a local park, a day at the beach). At that point, everyone starts over and again works up to 300 minutes. This encourages each family member to find ways to increase activity, and the low-level competition can create a fun atmosphere of encouraging more activity.
- Limit TV viewing to one program per night. Replace television viewing with physical activity such as shooting baskets, playing Frisbee golf, or doing dance videos together. Replacing screen time with fun activities not only provides more physical activity, but also cuts down on the consumption of unneeded calories from snacking that often goes along with TV viewing.
- Commit to decreasing the number of visits to fast-food restaurants. Preparing some bulk meals on the weekend allows the family to quickly and easily prepare workday and school-day meals.
- Eat breakfast together. Setting the alarm clock to go off 20 minutes earlier allows time for breakfast together.
- Replace soda with low-fat milk for the child at breakfast and dinner. Water flavored with a lemon can be substituted at other meals and snacks.

All of these changes are steps toward helping the family increase physical activity and create a more nutritious diet.

Changes Over Time

Movement exploration and the acquisition of basic motor skills start early and continue during the first years of life. Once children enter school, their exposure to movement possibilities expands and motor skill patterns undergo further refinement. The school years are also a time when youth receive specialized instruction in physical education and gain familiarity with playing various games and sports. With the onset of adolescence, greater emphasis can be placed on using physical activity to improve and maintain cardiovascular and musculoskeletal health. Figure 9.4 illustrates how the relative contributions of motor skill development and physical activity as an agent for improving health and fitness change from birth to age 18 (33).

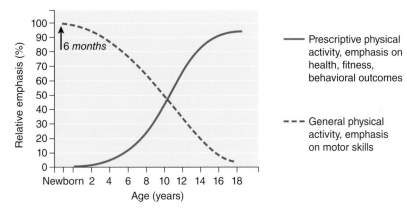

FIGURE 9.4   Relative contributions of motor skill development and prescriptive physical activity during childhood and adolescence.

Reprinted by permission from Strong, Malina, Blimkie, et al., 2005, p. 736.

With a balanced nutrition plan to complement a well-rounded physical activity program, children and adolescents can reap numerous health and fitness benefits and positive behavioral outcomes that can improve the ability to perform daily living activities and successfully engage in recreational and sport pursuits. Healthy youth also have a better chance of growing into healthy adults. It is never too early, or too late, to develop habits that promote healthy eating and active living.

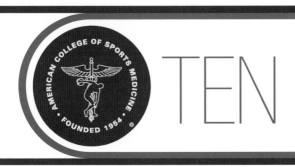

Adults:
Ages 18 to 64

If you are a healthy adult between the ages of 18 and 64 years, this chapter is for you. (If you are between the ages of 50 and 64 years and have a chronic condition or functional limitation, then chapter 11 provides more appropriate guidance.) Adulthood should be a time of experiencing life to the fullest. With robust health and fitness, you can fully embrace your diverse roles within your family, community, and workplace. Unfortunately, throughout this age span, a shift toward sedentary behavior tends to occur (6). The tendency is to become more inactive in leisure time rather than pursue active recreational options (see figure 10.1). In addition, although ideally 100 percent of adults would engage in both aerobic activity and resistance training, the percentage

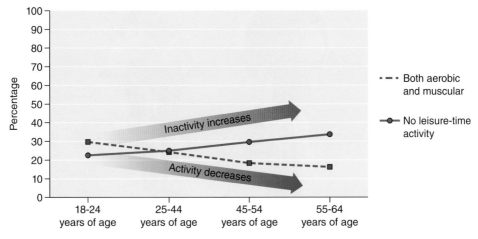

FIGURE 10.1 Percentage of American adults engaging in moderate aerobic activity and resistance training and those who are inactive in their leisure time.

Source: U.S. Department of Health and Human Services Office of Disease Prevention and Health Promotion.

of adults engaging in these activities decreases with age (6). Even though this is a bit discouraging, let's focus on the positive side—and on you! By reading this book and applying the recommendations, you are taking steps to change your personal health path. By focusing on nutrition and physical activity, you can claim a healthier and more active life.

Focus on Nutrition

Nutrition is the process of taking food into your body so your body can use that food to provide energy for daily activities and exercise. Too often the word "nutrition" brings to mind unappealing foods without taste. Healthy eating does not mean surviving on dry toast and celery sticks. A balanced diet should include a variety of appetizing foods that provide needed nutrients, as described in chapter 3. Food can have non–nutrition-related functions as well. For example, social celebrations, holiday get-togethers, and expressions of support for a family facing an illness or tragedy often include food. Food is part of everyday life. Rather than seeing nutrition as an obstacle, you can focus on positive food choices as part of your emphasis on a healthy lifestyle.

You may be asking yourself, does nutrition really have much of an impact? To drive home the importance of nutrition, consider that an estimated 16 percent of deaths in men and 9 percent of deaths in women have been attributed to missing the mark with regard to nutrition (4). The following sections will help sharpen your focus on optimizing your diet.

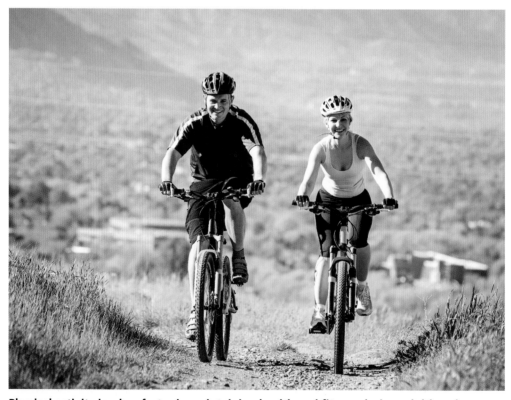

Physical activity is a key factor in maintaining health and fitness during adulthood.

Areas of the Diet to Increase

American adults consume sufficient amounts of most nutrients but are lacking in others (8, 9). Underconsumption of a number of nutrients has been highlighted as a particular public health concern; these include calcium, potassium, vitamin D, and dietary fiber. Iron is also underconsumed by women between the ages of 19 and 50 years (8). Fortunately, many foods contain these vitamins and minerals (7, 8). Table 10.1 lists some examples of good sources. Reflect on your own eating habits and consider small changes you can make to ensure that you consume adequate amounts of these nutrients.

Falling short in regard to these nutrients as well as others (e.g., magnesium, choline, vitamins A, E, and C) is likely related to an inadequate consumption of vegetables, fruits, whole grains, and dairy (8). Take a second look at table 10.1 to identify a couple of items in each row that you could substitute for another less nutritious item in your diet. To ensure adequate iron status, premenopausal women should consume foods with heme iron (e.g., lean meats, poultry, seafood) as well as non-heme sources (e.g., legumes, dark green vegetables, fortified products). When consuming non-heme sources

TABLE 10.1   Examples of Food Sources for Nutrients and Fiber Often Lacking in the Adult Diet

Nutrient	Examples of food sources
Calcium	Milk, yogurt, cheese
	Spinach, kale, broccoli
	Fish with soft bones that are consumed (e.g., sardines, salmon)
	Other calcium-fortified products (e.g., cereals, some orange juice)
Potassium	Potato or sweet potato, baked with skin
	Tomato paste, puree, juice, and sauce
	Milk, yogurt
	Clams, halibut, yellowfin tuna, salmon, snapper
	Cooked lima beans, soybeans, Swiss chard, acorn squash
	Banana
Vitamin D	Fatty fish (e.g., salmon, tuna, mackerel)
	Fish liver oils
	Fortified products (e.g., milk, many breakfast cereals)
	Also can form in the body through the interaction of sunlight on the skin
Fiber	Beans (navy, kidney, black, white, pinto, lima, great northern)
	Bran or oat bran cereal
	Whole wheat pasta
	Apple, pear, raspberries, blackberries, dates
	Hazelnuts, pecans, pistachios, almonds
Iron	Lean meats, poultry, seafood
	Legumes (beans and peas)
	Dark green leafy vegetables
	Other iron-fortified products (e.g., breads, cereals)

Sources: U.S. Department of Health and Human Services Office of Dietary Supplement and Office of Disease Prevention and Health Promotion.

■ **Q&A** ■■

What is the recommended intake of folic acid?

Folate is one of the B vitamins found naturally in many foods (e.g., beans and peas, fruits, dark green leafy vegetables, dairy products, poultry and meat). Folic acid is a synthetic form of the vitamin found in fortified foods and supplements (9). Fortification of grain products with folic acid was implemented in the United States to reduce the incidence of neural tube defects. It is recommended that all women capable of becoming pregnant consume 400 micrograms of folic acid daily (from fortified foods, supplements, or both) in addition to the amount of folate consumed as part of a healthy eating pattern (8).

---

of iron, include foods rich in vitamin C (e.g., orange juice along with fortified cereal), which enhances the body's ability to absorb the iron (8).

Areas of the Diet to Reduce

Although adults may underconsume some nutrients, they often overconsume other nutrient and dietary components. The *Dietary Guidelines* reveals that most Americans exceed recommended intakes for added sugars, saturated fats, and sodium. In addition, caloric intake is higher than needed, resulting in weight gain over time. The key is to make shifts in the composition of current foods and beverages consumed in order to ensure adequate intake of needed nutrients within the caloric requirements and personal preferences for each individual (8).

Dietary sodium intake is recommended to be less than 2,300 milligrams per day (8, 10). Salt (or more technically, sodium) intake is linked with higher blood pressure (see chapter 12 for more information on how sodium can be related to high blood pressure). To decrease the risk of developing high blood pressure, keep a handle on your sodium intake and also ensure adequate intake of potassium (10) by checking on sources noted in table 10.1. Both naturally occurring sodium and added salt within the cooking process or at the table account for some of your total intake (12 and 11 percent, respectively). Most salt consumption (77 percent), however, is related to packaged and restaurant food (10). Snack favorites that typically are high in sodium include pretzels, potato or tortilla chips, and salsa. Some items vary in their sodium content among manufacturers. Soup is a good example of a product that can be very high in sodium or reasonable, in the case of some new lower-sodium options. Keep an eye on product labels. Low-sodium products have less than 140 milligrams of sodium, or less than 5 percent of the Daily Value for sodium (10).

Saturated fat should account for less than 10 percent of total calories. Only about 29 percent of the U.S. population meets this target. Common sources of saturated fats include mixed dishes, especially those containing meat or cheese (e.g., burgers, sandwiches, pizza, pasta or rice dishes), as well as snacks and sweets, protein foods, and dairy products. Shifting from consuming food items high in saturated fats to products high in polyunsaturated and monounsaturated fats is recommended (8). Monounsaturated fat sources include olive and canola oils. Polyunsaturated fat sources include foods (e.g., nuts, fish) as well as various oils (e.g., soybean, corn, sunflower).

Among adults, intake of added sugars is also too high (8). Some common sources of added sugars are snacks and sweets (e.g., cakes, cookies, dairy desserts, candies, sweet toppings). A major source of added sugars is beverages, accounting for almost half of

■ **Q&A**

What can I do to reduce salt in my diet?

Consider the following ways to reduce salt consumption (10):

- Check the Nutrition Facts label and select lower-sodium options.
- Prepare your own food without salting during cooking, and limit adding salt at the table.
- Substitute herbs and spices for salt to flavor food (e.g., no-salt seasoning blends, pepper, rosemary, basil).
- Select fresh rather than processed products when possible.
- Examine sodium content of condiments like ketchup and salad dressings; select low- or no-sodium options and watch portions.

---

added sugars consumed by Americans. Consider how shifting from sugar-sweetened beverages such as soft drinks and sweetened fruit drinks to water or low-fat or fat-free milk provides benefits for calorie reduction (with water) or improved nutrient content (e.g., milk) (8).

Substitutions can be made in many aspects of one's diet. Replacing refined grains with whole grains is recommended. Refined grains are found in breads, tortillas, mixed dishes using rice and pasta, snacks, chips, and crackers. Some examples of whole-grain products are whole-grain bread, whole wheat cereal, brown rice, and wild rice. In situations when a substitution is not available or desired, decreasing portion size could be considered as a way to reduce added sugars in the diet.

When considering areas of your diet that might be improved, focus on some areas to modify, making shifts in your diet where needed. Keep a healthy dietary pattern in mind rather than becoming solely focused on restriction. These are some suggestions (8):

- Adjust recipes, mixed dishes, and even sandwiches to reflect greater emphasis on fruits, veggies, and whole grains.
- Focus on including foods providing underconsumed nutrients (e.g., vegetables, fruits, whole grains, seafood, nuts, and dairy products).
- Replace saturated fats with polyunsaturated and monounsaturated options.
- Make water a preferred beverage choice.

One last area to think about related to overconsumption is caloric intake. To maintain body weight, the number of calories consumed in foods and beverages must equal the number of calories the body uses for basic functions as well as to provide energy for work, activities of daily living, and exercise. Shifts in this balance as a result of even small amounts of extra calories on a daily basis may contribute to the gradual increase in body weight often seen throughout adulthood. One of the benefits of a physically active lifestyle is the additional calories used on a daily and weekly basis. For more detailed information on weight management, see chapter 18.

Dietary Focus

Adults should focus on an adequate intake of all vitamins and minerals and, in particular, those listed previously as often being underconsumed. The foods and beverages you consume create your eating pattern and should reflect your cultural and personal preferences (8). Meeting nutrient needs while staying within limits in some areas (e.g., saturated fats, added sugars, sodium, calories) is the focus. An example of the Healthy U.S.-Style Eating Pattern (2,000-calorie level) is shown in table 10.2.

To keep a positive viewpoint on nutrition, focus on dietary patterns rather than a list of "good foods" and "bad foods." Recommendations include these (9):

- Focus on a dietary plan that is rich in vegetables, fruit, whole grains, seafood, legumes, and nuts.
- Keep your dietary plan moderate for low- and nonfat dairy products.
- Dietary patterns should be lower for red and processed meat and low in sugar-sweetened foods and beverages as well as refined grains.

TABLE 10.2   Healthy U.S.-Style Eating Patterns at the 2,000-Calorie Level

Food group	Amount[a] in the 2,000-calorie level pattern
Vegetables	2 1/2 c-eq/day
Dark green	1 1/2 c-eq/week
Red and orange	5 1/2 c-eq/week
Legumes (beans and peas)	1 1/2 c-eq/week
Starchy	5 c-eq/week
Other	4 c-eq/week
Fruits	2 c-eq/day
Grains	6 oz-eq/day
Whole grains	>3 oz-eq/day
Refined grains	<3 oz-eq/day
Dairy	3 c-eq/day
Protein foods	5 1/2 oz-eq/day
Seafood	8 oz-eq/week
Meats, poultry, eggs	26 oz-eq/week
Nuts, seeds, soy products	5 oz-eq/week
Oils	27 g/day
Limit on calories for other uses (% of calories)[b]	270 kcal/day (14%)

[a]Food groups are shown in cup-equivalents (c-eq) or ounce-equivalents (oz-eq), and oils are shown in grams. The equivalents for the food groups are as follows:

- Vegetables and fruits: 1 cup-equivalent is 1 cup raw or cooked vegetable or fruit, 1 cup vegetable or fruit juice, 2 cups leafy salad greens, 1/2 cup dried fruit or vegetable.
- Grains: 1 ounce-equivalent is 1/2 cup cooked rice, pasta, or cereal; 1 ounce dry pasta or rice; 1 medium (1 ounce) slice bread; 1 ounce of ready-to-eat cereal (about 1 cup of flaked cereal).
- Dairy: 1 cup-equivalent is 1 cup milk, yogurt, or fortified soymilk; 1 1/2 ounces natural cheese such as cheddar cheese or 2 ounces of processed cheese.
- Protein foods: 1 ounce-equivalent is 1 ounce lean meat, poultry, or seafood; 1 egg; 1/4 cup cooked beans or tofu; 1 Tbsp peanut butter; 1/2 ounce nuts or seeds.

[b]Assumes that food choices to meet food group recommendations are in nutrient-dense forms. Calories from added sugars, added refined starches, solid fats, alcohol, and eating more than the recommended amount of nutrient-dense foods are accounted for under this category.

Source: U.S. Department of Health and Human Services and U.S. Department of Agriculture, 2015.

▪ Q&A

Does alcohol have any place in the dietary pattern of adults?

Alcohol should be consumed only by adults of legal drinking age, and there are situations in which alcohol is not recommended (e.g., during pregnancy, when one is taking certain medications, before driving). The *Dietary Guidelines* does not recommend that individuals start to drink alcohol; if they do, moderation is recommended (i.e., up to one drink per day for women and up to two drinks per day for men) (8). Alcohol contains about 7 calories per gram and thus should be accounted for within one's overall dietary intake.

Simple changes can have an impact over time. Bringing an apple, orange, or a container of cut vegetables to work may help you avoid grabbing a less nutritious, high-calorie item from a vending machine. Ideally, food selections should be nutrient dense. This simply means that the food item packs the biggest punch possible with regard to vitamins, minerals, and fiber for the least number of calories (8). Compare 100 calories of jelly beans to 100 calories from orange slices. First, the orange offers a greater quantity (over a cup's worth) for the same 100 calories (see figure 10.2). Second, the orange provides calcium, potassium, vitamin C, and folic acid among other vitamins and minerals. In contrast, 100 calories of jelly beans (about 25 pieces) provides some potassium and sodium along with added sugar. The potassium in the orange slices is over 375 milligrams compared to 10 milligrams in the jelly beans. This simple example clearly demonstrates the benefits of consuming natural, nutrient-dense foods.

With these guidelines in mind, you may realize that your current diet is right on track, or you may see that changes are needed. If some changes are desired, consider a series of substitutions rather than a sudden overwhelming overhaul. Food should be enjoyed, and with some attention, it can also be good for your health.

Focus on Physical Activity

Incorporating an exercise program into your busy day may seem impossible. Adulthood is full of responsibilities at home as well as at work. Time spent on exercise may feel frivolous or even selfish. In reality, a regular exercise program is one of the

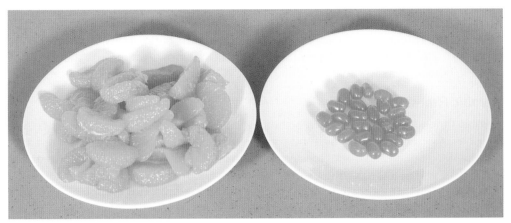

FIGURE 10.2   Nutrient density: Compare 100 calories of jelly beans to 100 calories of orange slices.

most important investments you can make for your future and that of your family. If you have been reading from the beginning of this book, you are aware of the impressive list of benefits from exercise—physical as well as mental. Your personal health is valuable, but it requires attention on a regular basis.

Each day you have the opportunity to make investments in your future health. As with a financially solid retirement plan, you need to start early and continue for the greatest benefit. You don't need to spend hours per day to be healthy, but it does require a time commitment. Take a moment to reflect on the reasons you can benefit from including exercise in your weekly plan. This reflection is a process you will want to repeat in the future because your areas of focus will likely change over time. Chapters 2 and 4 offer additional guidance about formulating your personal expectations and goals, as well as hints for fitting exercise into your busy schedule.

The benefits of exercise for adults of all races and ethnicities, both males and females, have been clearly documented (1, 3, 5). As discussed in more detail in chapter 1, physical activity reduces the risk of premature death from heart disease as well as some cancers. If you improve your fitness with regular aerobic exercise, you can reap the rewards of lower blood pressure, better cholesterol levels, and a decreased risk of both heart disease and stroke. Regular exercisers can also lower the risk of developing type 2 diabetes, colon cancer, and breast cancer. In addition, adults who engage in a regular activity regimen have a healthier body weight and body composition as well as other benefits such as increased bone strength, improved sleep quality, and lower risk of depression. These benefits are impressive—and are yours for the taking!

In view of the numerous health benefits of regular exercise, it is surprising how many people are not active. Although the reasons vary widely, for some, fear of being injured or having a heart attack during physical activity overrides any potential benefits they might gain from being active. Risks of adverse events during physical activity are real, but for most people they are outweighed by the benefits (5).

To help minimize risks, begin at a low to moderate intensity and build your fitness slowly over time (1). Complete the preparticipation screening provided in chapter 2. If needed, consult with your physician or health care provider to determine whether you need to modify any general exercise guidelines because of your personal health history and current activity status.

Physical Activity Guidelines for Adults

Adults need to move beyond the usual light or even sedentary daily activities to include physical activity focused on aerobic fitness, muscular fitness, flexibility, and neuromotor fitness (1). The American College of Sports Medicine strongly supports the inclusion of these components to provide a complete and balanced physical activity program.

Aerobic Fitness

Aerobic fitness refers to your body's ability to take in and use oxygen during physical activities. Assessment of aerobic fitness can require complex laboratory measurements, but chapter 5 outlines two simple ways to estimate your fitness (for more details on the one-mile walking test and the 1.5-mile run test). The final score from whichever test you complete is an estimate of your $\dot{V}O_{2max}$, or the maximal amount of oxygen your body can use during activity. The higher the value is, the better your aerobic fitness is. You can compare your score to those of others of your sex and age in table 5.1.

As you may have noted when looking up your score, $\dot{V}O_{2max}$ tends to decrease with age. Loss of fitness occurs as a result of the physical changes associated with aging, but it also is influenced by activity level. Sedentary, or inactive, lifestyles speed up the age-related decline in fitness. In contrast, maintaining a physically active lifestyle with focused attention on aerobic activities can help you retain your fitness. Although a balanced exercise program isn't the elusive fountain of youth, maintaining (or beginning) an exercise program will provide a better quality of life.

The U.S. government's *Physical Activity Guidelines for Americans,* as well as ACSM, recommends that adults engage in regular aerobic physical activity (1, 5). The following provide substantial health benefits:

- Moderate-intensity aerobic activity at least 30 minutes per day five days per week (or a weekly total of at least 150 minutes), or
- Vigorous-intensity aerobic activity at least 20 to 25 minutes per day three days per week (or a weekly total of 75 minutes), or
- A combination of moderate-intensity and vigorous-intensity aerobic activity at least 20 to 30 minutes per day three to five days per week

Moderate intensity refers to activities that noticeably increase your heart rate and breathing. An example is brisk walking. Vigorous-intensity activities substantially increase heart rate and breathing. Examples are jogging and running. For more details on aerobic fitness, see chapter 5.

For additional health benefits such as lowering the risk of colon and breast cancer, the Physical Activity Guidelines suggests a greater amount of physical activity, which can be achieved by one of the following targets (5):

- 300 minutes of moderate-intensity activity per week, or
- 150 minutes of vigorous-intensity activity, or
- A combination of moderate- and vigorous-intensity activity (e.g., approximately 40 to 60 minutes per day three to five days per week)

Exceeding these levels may provide even more benefits (e.g., a lower risk of premature death), although scientists have not yet determined what the upper limit is above which no additional health benefits accrue (5).

Muscular Fitness

Muscular fitness includes muscular strength (how much you can lift in one maximal effort), muscular endurance (maintaining a muscle contraction or contracting a muscle repeatedly without tiring), and power (rate of muscular action) (1). Muscular fitness is a vital component of an exercise program (5). Loss of muscle is a common result of aging and is technically referred to as sarcopenia. As muscle function is lost, the ability to generate force declines (2). This loss of muscle translates into difficulty lifting, pushing, pulling, and other activities of daily living. In addition, muscular fitness is vital for full participation in most recreational and sporting activities.

The *Physical Activity Guidelines for Americans* and ACSM both suggest resistance training a couple of days per week to maintain muscular fitness or improve your current fitness level (1, 5). You should resistance train each of the major muscle groups two to three times per week, ensuring that you have at least 48 hours of recovery time between these sessions (i.e., don't resistance train the same body part two days in a row). Each session should include two to four sets of 8 to 12 repetitions and a rest between sets of 2 to 3 minutes (1). For more details on resistance training, see chapter 6, which includes assessments of muscular fitness and activity suggestions.

Flexibility

Flexibility is a fitness attribute that can influence your ability to perform activities in your day-to-day life. The ability to reach, bend, and turn provides freedom of motion. Many recreational activities and sports also benefit from a full range of motion (e.g., golf, tennis, and swimming). Therefore, stretching is recommended for all adults.

Stretching should target all of the major joints in the body and should be done when the muscles are warm in order to be most effective (1). ACSM recommends that adults stretch at least two to three days per week. When using static stretching, hold the stretch for 10 to 30 seconds and repeat this in order to complete a total of 60 seconds of stretching for each activity. For example, if you hold the stretch for 15 seconds, you would repeat this four times (i.e., $15 \times 4 = 60$). For dynamic stretching, be sure to use controlled movements and bring the targeted body part through its range of motion. More complete details on flexibility and stretching are found in chapter 7.

Neuromotor Fitness

Neuromotor fitness includes balance, coordination, gait, agility, and proprioception (this refers to your sense of body position as you move in your environment) (1). Although neuromotor training is more often a focus for older adults for fall prevention, younger adult athletes may find help with injury reduction due to improved balance and agility (1). Few research studies have examined benefits in adults, but consider the potential benefit for movements you engage in every day (3). Neuromotor fitness affects your ability to effectively function during routine physical activities—thus the alternative term often used is *functional fitness* (1). Unlike the situation with other components of fitness, precise recommendations are not yet established. You may want to consider including some of the activities from chapter 8 a couple of days per week.

Programs to Meet and Exceed the Physical Activity Guidelines for Adults

Chapters 5, 6, 7, and 8 provide detailed information on activities to promote aerobic fitness, muscular fitness, flexibility, and functional (neuromotor) fitness. Now it is time to put these components together into a weekly program.

As you begin an exercise program, be realistic. Reflect on the type of program that will work with your schedule. Remember, you can split your activity into several shorter bouts over the course of the day (each should be at least 10 minutes long). Including 10 minutes of brisk walking in the morning, at noontime, and in the evening is a way to meet the target for moderate-intensity aerobic activity. For others, one 30-minute period may work better. No one pattern is right or wrong. The best exercise program is one you enjoy and continue to follow for years to come.

Easing into your exercise program is recommended to decrease your risk of injury and avoid muscle soreness, which can lead to discouragement. Figures 10.3, 10.4, and 10.5 offer sample activity programs for beginning exercisers, intermediate-level exercisers, and more established exercisers, respectively. Note that each program includes aerobic activity, resistance training, stretching, and optional neuromotor activity. You

■**Q&A**

Can fitness be achieved on a budget?

Cost doesn't need to be a barrier. You can include exercise for little to no cost. If your employer provides a fitness facility at the workplace, you may be able to adjust your schedule to take advantage of this opportunity. Outdoor activities like walking or hiking can provide great aerobic benefits. If the outdoors isn't an option due to weather or safety concerns, consider walking at a shopping mall. Your own residence is another potential exercise location. You can include body weight exercises (e.g., push-ups, sit-ups) for free. For another no-cost option, check out workout DVDs at your local library to try some new activities like aerobic dance or power yoga. You could also purchase some inexpensive resistance bands to focus on muscular fitness.

---

may find that you are able to easily progress through the levels of the program, or you may need to take an extra couple of weeks at each level. The ACSM recommends the following (1):

- *Aerobic activity:* Typically three to five days per week depending on the intensity of the activity
- *Resistance training:* Typically two to three days per week
- *Stretching for flexibility:* A minimum of two to three days per week
- *Neuromotor training:* Two to three days per week suggested

Each activity in figures 10.3 through 10.5 presents a range of days to match your goals as well as your strengths and weaknesses. The simple fitness assessments in chapters 5 through 8 can provide some insight into areas in which you may need to spend some additional time. Repeating the fitness assessments periodically (e.g., every three to six months) can be helpful for charting your progress. This is covered in the next section on tracking your progress.

Tracking Your Progress

No matter where you start (beginner, intermediate, established), advancing your fitness can provide additional health and fitness benefits. You can progress by manipulating the FITT components (frequency, intensity, time, and type of activity) in the sample activity programs in figures 10.3, 10.4, and 10.5. For aerobic activity, you could increase the number of days per week (frequency) or the number of minutes you spend in each exercise session (time). How hard you exercise (intensity) is another factor. Keep in mind that both moderate- and vigorous-intensity activities are ways to improve your health. If you find moderate-intensity activity more attractive, you will have to spend more time exercising than if you did vigorous-intensity activity. Similarly, you can improve your muscular fitness by manipulating the number of resistance training sessions you do per week, the amount of weight or resistance you use, and even the type of resistance activities you do.

As you adjust these FITT components, you can gauge your body's response in a number of ways. If you are a beginner or intermediate exerciser, you can use the fitness assessments every two to four months. If you are an established exerciser, assessing

FIGURE 10.3

Sample beginner exercise program for adults*.

Weeks	Aerobic	Resistance	Stretching and neuromotor activities**	Comments
1-2	Three days per week; 10 to 20 min per day; light intensity (level 3 or 4)	Two days per week; one set, 8 to 12 reps of six exercises***	Two days per week; 10 min of stretching activities with additional option for agility and balance exercises	An easy beginning aerobic activity is walking. Select a comfortable pace. If you haven't been very active, target 5 to 10 min at a time for your aerobic activity. Include some stretching activities (see chapter 7) after your walk. For resistance training, see chapter 6 for details on what activities to include.
3-4	Three days per week; 20 to 30 min per day; light to moderate intensity (level 4 or 5)	Two days per week; one or two sets, 8 to 12 reps of six exercises***	Two days per week; 10 min of stretching activities with additional option for agility and balance exercises	The focus for the next couple of weeks will be getting comfortable with at least 20 min of aerobic exercise at least three days per week. Continue with your resistance training program.
5-7	Three or four days per week; 20 to 30 min per day; moderate intensity (level 5)	Two days per week; two sets, 8 to 12 reps of six exercises***	Two days per week; 10 min of stretching activities with additional option for agility and balance exercises	For the next three weeks, get comfortable with at least 30 min of moderate-level aerobic exercise at least three days per week. Continue with your resistance training program, completing two sets per exercise and adding more weight if the 12 repetitions for a given exercise now feel easy.
8-10	Three or four days per week; 30 to 45 min per day; moderate intensity (level 5 or 6)	Two days per week; two sets, 8 to 12 reps of six exercises***	Two days per week; 10 min of stretching activities with additional option for agility and balance exercises	Over the past couple of months you have been developing a good aerobic fitness base. For some variety, you can consider other activities such as biking or swimming (for more ideas, see chapter 5). If you like walking, you can also keep doing that. For your resistance training program, consider adding some variety and trying some other exercises (see chapter 6 for details).

*All activity sessions should be preceded and followed by a 5- to 10-minute warm-up and cool-down.

**Include stretching activities after aerobic exercise to improve flexibility. For specific stretches to target the major muscle groups, see chapter 7. You may also want to include some additional activities for agility and balance (i.e., neuromotor training) as shown in chapter 8.

***Resistance training is more fully outlined in chapter 6. Beginners should select one exercise for each of the following body areas: hips and legs, chest, back, shoulders, low back, and abdominal muscles.

FIGURE 10.4

Sample intermediate-level exercise program for adults*.

Week	Aerobic	Resistance	Stretching and neuromotor activities**	Comments
1-2	Three or four days per week; 30 to 45 min per day; moderate intensity (level 5 or 6)	Two days per week; one or two sets, 8 to 12 reps of 8 to 10 different exercises***	Two or three days per week; 10 min of stretching activities with additional option for agility and balance exercises	You should be doing aerobic activity for a total of 100 to 150 min per week (moderate-intensity activity). For resistance training, include exercises for biceps and triceps (in addition to the body areas previously targeted) and add exercises for the quadriceps and hamstrings in the second week, so you will have included a total of 10 exercises (see chapter 6 for details).
3-5	Three to five days per week; 30 to 50 min per day; moderate intensity (level 5 to 6)	Two days per week; one or two sets, 8 to 12 reps of 10 different exercises***	Two or three days per week, 10 min of stretching activities with additional option for agility and balance exercises	The focus for the next three weeks is to increase the time you spend in aerobic exercise or to increase the intensity, but don't do both at the same time. If you feel more comfortable with moderate-intensity activity, 150 min per week is appropriate. If you feel ready to increase intensity (e.g., jogging rather than walking), you can cut back the time to 20 to 30 min per day and still realize the same benefits (note that the target for vigorous-intensity activity is 75 min per week). You may want to consider a mix of moderate- and vigorous-intensity activity as well (see chapter 5 for more details). Continue with your resistance training program.
6-10	Three to five days per week; 30 to 60 min per day; moderate intensity (level 5 or 6)	Two or three days per week; two sets, 8 to 12 reps of 10 exercises***	Two or three days per week, 10 min of stretching activities with additional option for agility and balance exercises	For your aerobic activity, you can either increase the time spent per day or increase the number of days per week. Ultimately, you want your weekly total to be 150 to 200 min of moderate-intensity activity or 75 to 100 min of vigorous-intensity activity (recall that 2 min of moderate activity equals 1 min of vigorous activity) or a combination of moderate and vigorous activity. For your resistance training, consider trying some different exercises this week while still targeting the same muscle groups (see chapter 6 for details).

*All activity sessions should be preceded and followed by a 5- to 10-minute warm-up and cool-down.

**Include stretching activities after aerobic exercise to improve flexibility. Target all the muscle groups, holding each stretch for 10 to 30 seconds, repeated for a total of 60 seconds. For specific stretches to target the major muscle groups, see chapter 7. You may also want to include some additional activities for agility and balance (i.e., neuromotor exercises) as shown in chapter 8.

***Resistance training is more fully outlined in chapter 6. Select one exercise for each of the following body areas: hips and legs, chest, back, shoulders, low back, and abdominal muscles. As you progress, you will expand the number of body areas you target by adding quadriceps and hamstrings as well as biceps and triceps. This provides 10 body areas to target. Examples of exercises you can include for each body area are found in table 6.6.

FIGURE 10.5

Sample established exercise program for adults*.

Weeks	Aerobic	Resistance	Stretching and neuromotor activities**	Comments
1-2	Five days per week for moderate exercise Or: Three days per week for vigorous exercise Or: Three to five days per week for a mix of moderate and vigorous exercise	Two or three days per week; two sets, 8 to 12 reps of 10 different exercises***	Two or three days per week, minimum; 10 min of stretching activities with additional option for agility and balance exercises	Congratulations on your ongoing commitment to exercise. To find specific aerobic activities, see chapter 5. Ultimately, you want your weekly total to be 150 to 300 min of moderate-intensity activity or 75 to 150 min of vigorous-intensity activity (recall that 2 min of moderate activity equals 1 min of vigorous activity) or a combination of moderate and vigorous activity. See chapter 6 for details on resistance training activities to include.
3-4	Two or three days per week of moderate activity and one or two days of vigorous activity	Two or three days per week; two sets, 8 to 12 reps of 10 different exercises***	Three days per week, minimum; 10 min of stretching activities with additional option for agility and balance exercises	For the next couple of weeks, try mixing up your activities. Try a new aerobic activity or change the intensity of an activity you already do on a regular basis. Continue with your resistance training program.
5-7	Five days per week for moderate exercise Or: Three days per week for vigorous exercise Or: Three to five days per week for moderate and vigorous exercise	Two or three days per week; two sets, 8 to 12 reps of 10 exercises***	Three days per week, minimum; 10 min of stretching activities with additional option for agility and balance exercises	Continue with your aerobic training program. For your resistance training, consider trying some different exercises (see chapter 6 for details). If you typically use machines, try a couple of new exercises using dumbbells to provide your muscles with a new challenge. Be sure to maintain good form when trying new activities.
8-10	Five days per week for moderate exercise Or: Three days per week for vigorous exercise Or: Three to five days per week for moderate and vigorous exercise	Two or three days per week; three sets, 8 to 10 reps of 10 exercises***	Three days per week, minimum; 10 min of stretching activities with additional option for agility and balance exercises	Continue with your aerobic training program. For your resistance training, consider doing three sets rather than two (see chapter 6 for details). You may need to cut back on your reps to add the additional set.

*All activity sessions should be preceded and followed by a 5- to 10-minute warm-up and cool-down.

**Include stretching activities after aerobic exercise to improve flexibility. For specific stretches to target the major muscle groups, see chapter 7. You may also want to include some additional activities for agility and balance (i.e., neuromotor exercises) as shown in chapter 8.

***Resistance training is more fully outlined in chapter 6. Select one exercise for each of the following body areas: hips and legs, chest, back, shoulders, low back, abdominal muscles, quadriceps, hamstrings, biceps, and triceps. Examples of exercises you can include for each body area are found in table 6.6.

every four to six months would likely provide sufficient feedback because changes will likely be less dramatic. The rate of improvement will naturally slow down the more fit you become because you will be getting closer to your maximal capacity. At this point, increasing the time between assessments to six months will still help you gauge your status without becoming an undue burden. Figure 10.6 is a chart for recording your scores or rankings.

By tracking your workouts, you can watch for signs of improving fitness. Between fitness assessments, you can note your progress in less objective ways, including the following for aerobic conditioning:

- Your resting heart rate is lower.
- When doing the same activity, your heart rate and perception of effort are lower.

FIGURE 10.6

Fitness assessment progress chart for adults.

	Assessment 1 (baseline)	Assessment 2*	Assessment 3**
Body composition assessments			
Body mass index			
Waist circumference			
Cardiorespiratory fitness assessments			
Rockport One-Mile Walking Test ($\dot{V}O_{2max}$ estimate) or 1.5-mile run test ($\dot{V}O_{2max}$ estimate)			
Muscular fitness assessments			
1-repetition maximum (for strength)			
Push-up test (for endurance)			
Flexibility assessments			
Sit-and-reach test			
Back scratch test			
Neuromotor fitness assessments			
4-stage balance test			
Single-leg stand time			
Standing reach test			
Edgren side-step test			

*From baseline: Two months for a beginner, three months for an intermediate exerciser, and four months for an established exerciser

**From baseline: Four months for a beginner, six months for an intermediate exerciser, and eight months for an established exerciser

From ACSM, 2017, *ACSM's complete guide to fitness & health*, 2nd ed. (Champaign, IL: Human Kinetics).

- Your heart rate returns to resting levels faster following your workout.
- You are able to complete the same number of minutes of activity, but at a higher intensity.
- You are able to continue longer at the same intensity.
- You are increasing the total time you spend exercising each week.

For resistance training, you may observe the following as evidence of improvements:

- You are able to lift the same weight 12 times rather than just 8 before becoming fatigued.
- You are able increase the weight lifted or the resistance you overcome.
- You are able to complete more body weight exercises (e.g., push-ups, curl-ups).
- You increase the number of sets completed targeting a particular muscle group.

For flexibility, you may observe that you are able to reach farther or hold a position with less tension than you could earlier in your stretching program. With neuromotor fitness training, you may find that you are more stable when moving or have improved ability to respond to challenges to your balance or agility.

As you progress from week to week, ask yourself a couple of simple questions:

- Is the same workout easier than it was last week?
- Are you able to complete longer workouts or add additional exercises?
- Do you find you feel energized by your exercise program?

If you answer yes to the questions, you are right on track. If you answer no to any of the questions, you may need to slow the pace of your progress or adjust your workouts to ensure that your body has sufficient time to adapt. Because each person is unique, a cookie-cutter approach to exercise does not work. To improve, you need to provide your body with a new challenge, but you also need to allow your body enough time to respond and improve. This is why increases in time or intensity are done slowly over a number of weeks. When assessing the success of your exercise program, don't forget the real key to a successful exercise program—enjoyment! Continue to look for activities that you enjoy doing so you can maintain your activity.

To keep an eye on your progress, consider tracking your weekly workouts. Figure 10.7 is a summary chart that may be helpful. Writing down your workouts can be helpful so you can look back on them. An activity chart provides a weekly accounting of how many sessions have targeted aerobic fitness, muscular fitness, flexibility, and neuromotor fitness (see figure 4.3 for an example).

Regardless of your current fitness level, recording your exercise and reflecting on your progress allow you to check off short-term goals (e.g., increasing the number of minutes per week, increasing the intensity, including different resistance training exercises) as you continue to move to your long-term goals (e.g., reaching the "good" category for aerobic fitness, losing weight, improving your flexibility).

FIGURE 10.7

Fitness progress chart for adults.

	Total time spent in aerobic exercise (min of moderate and vigorous activity per week)	Number of resistance training sessions per week	Number of resistance training exercises per session	Number of reps per set	Number of sessions per week of stretching activities
Week 1	Moderate: ____ min Vigorous: ____ min				
Week 2	Moderate: ____ min Vigorous: ____ min				
Week 3	Moderate: ____ min Vigorous: ____ min				
Week 4	Moderate: ____ min Vigorous: ____ min				
Week 5	Moderate: ____ min Vigorous: ____ min				
Week 6	Moderate: ____ min Vigorous: ____ min				
Week 7	Moderate: ____ min Vigorous: ____ min				
Week 8	Moderate: ____ min Vigorous: ____ min				
Week 9	Moderate: ____ min Vigorous: ____ min				
Week 10	Moderate: ____ min Vigorous: ____ min				

From ACSM, 2017, *ACSM's complete guide to fitness & health, 2nd ed.* (Champaign, IL: Human Kinetics).

Adulthood can be a hectic and busy time. Too often, personal health and fitness take a back seat just when you can least afford it. Taking charge of your diet and physical activity will provide many benefits (e.g., lower risk of heart disease and type 2 diabetes), as well as a better quality of life. Within your diet, keep a focus on fruits, vegetables, whole grains, and low-fat dairy products while avoiding the overconsumption of fat (especially saturated and trans fats), sodium, and sugar. Physical activity along with a solid nutritional plan will help you maintain your desired body weight as well as promote your overall fitness. Aerobic activities, resistance training, and stretching together provide a comprehensive program to maximize the benefits to your health.

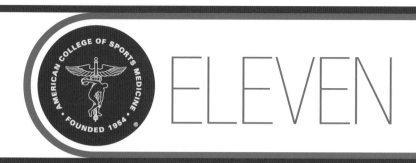

Older Adults:
Ages 65 and Older

If you remember one message from this chapter it should be this: *It is never too late to reap the health and functional benefits from regular participation in physical activity.* The health benefits relate to the reduction in risk factors associated with a number of diseases, including heart disease, diabetes, cancer, and osteoporosis. The functional benefits include improvements in stamina, strength, flexibility, and balance. The risk of falling will also be reduced as you enhance your muscle strength and balance. These adaptations contribute to your ability to maintain an independent lifestyle and a high quality of life in the later years. You will be able to continue to participate in activities associated with daily living such as shopping, gardening, and playing with your grandchildren without limitations. These are just a few of the many benefits that accompany regular involvement in a physical activity program.

Remaining sedentary or physically inactive actually contributes to many well-documented health risk factors that have generally been attributed to the "aging process." Additionally, other physiological and psychological factors such as a reduction in cardiovascular and skeletal muscle function, as well as declines in cognitive performance, were thought to be a normal part of the aging process. However, recent studies suggest that, while a portion of these changes may be due to growing older, a significant factor is an increase in sedentary behavior associated with older populations (24). Chronic sedentary behavior is associated with increased risk for at least 35 chronic diseases and clinical conditions (6) and increased mortality (death) rates (27). In addition, chronic sedentary behavior contributes to a reduction in aerobic capacity, muscle strength, and overall metabolic function.

To achieve these many benefits from regular physical activity, you do not need to exercise as intensely or for as long as competitive athletes. Many older adults resist starting an exercise program for fear of injury, falling, or soreness from an intense bout of exercise. The good news is that you can participate in moderate-intensity exercise such as walking, swimming, and bicycling and still receive both the health and the functional benefits from your time spent being physically active. As you will

■ Q&A

Can declines in health over the years be attributed to the normal aging process?

The decline in health and functional capacity previously attributed to the aging process is more likely a result of a chronic sedentary lifestyle. Many negative age-related changes can be significantly avoided or delayed by regular physical activity. Getting active is the best choice to make to promote health and fitness.

see throughout this chapter, the rewards from participation in a physical activity program, including the maintenance of an independent lifestyle, lower health risks, and overall improved quality of life, clearly outweigh any risks associated with engaging in regular physical activity. To promote safety when starting to become more physically active or when increasing your exercise program, refer to the screening process outlined in chapter 2.

Focus on Nutrition

Having a healthy diet is important regardless of your age. Eating well contributes to good health and vitality. The recommendations in the *Dietary Guidelines for Americans* (26), put forth by the U.S. Department of Health and Human Services, provide general guidelines for people of all ages. The core recommendations can be summarized as follows:

- Follow a healthy eating pattern across the lifespan. This includes maintaining energy (caloric) balance to keep your body weight stable. Control caloric intake to match calories burned through daily activities and exercise while ensuring adequate nutrient intake.

- Choose a variety of nutrient-dense foods, including a variety of fruits and vegetables, whole grains, low-fat milk and proteins (fish, lean meat, eggs, nuts, and beans), grains, and oils.

- Decrease consumption of foods and beverages that are higher in trans fats, saturated fats, salt (sodium), and refined sugar.

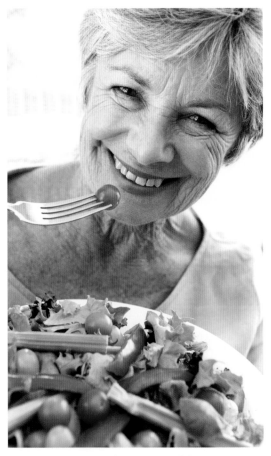

A diet consisting of a variety of fruits and vegetables is essential for healthy aging.

However, a few dietary modifications may be needed to further promote healthy aging. The reasons for these adjustments range from changes in metabolism and muscle and bone mass to a reduction in activity levels and exposure to sunlight. Older adults may benefit from these particular adjustments (18).

Ensuring Consumption of the Proper Amount of Calcium and Vitamin D on a Daily Basis

Calcium is required for many functions of the body but, importantly for the older adult, is one of the major building blocks for bone. Maintaining healthy bones also requires getting sufficient amounts of vitamin D. Vitamin D assists your body in absorbing calcium and also plays a role in other bodily functions such as the nervous and immune systems. Your skin can use exposure to sunlight to form vitamin D; however, older adults may get less exposure to the sun (to protect against skin cancer), and the process of forming vitamin D is less efficient. Dietary sources of vitamin D include dairy products such as milk, cheese, and yogurt. Vitamin D can also be found in leafy green vegetables and saltwater fish. If you are having difficulty getting the proper amount of vitamin D each day (800-1,000 IU per day), you may consider taking a vitamin D supplement to ensure that you meet the daily requirements. Good food sources for calcium include low-fat and nonfat milk, cheeses, and yogurt. Other food products such as cereals, breads, and bottled water can have calcium added. If you are not getting enough calcium through your diet (1,000-1,200 milligrams per day), calcium supplements are available and may be considered. Consult with your health care provider regarding supplementation of calcium, vitamin D, or both.

Ensuring Consumption of the Proper Amount of Vitamin B_{12} on a Daily Basis

Vitamin B_{12} plays an important role in metabolism, red blood cell formation, and nerve function. A vitamin B_{12} deficiency can result in tingling feelings in legs or hands, memory problems, personality shifts, fatigue, and anemia (shortage of red blood cells). Dietary sources of vitamin B_{12} include meat, eggs, milk, shellfish, and cereals fortified with vitamin B_{12}. Your ability to digest and absorb vitamin B_{12} may be impaired as you get older or due to a side effect from certain medications (such as metformin used to treat diabetes). In these cases, supplements may be prescribed by your health care provider.

Ensuring Consumption of the Proper Amount of Fiber

Dietary fiber is important in that it plays a role in stomach or digestive health and may prevent problems such as constipation. Fiber has been shown to lower the "bad" cholesterol levels in your blood as well as blood sugar, thereby reducing your risk for both heart disease and diabetes. There is evidence to suggest that dietary fiber may lower your risk for colon cancer. In addition, fiber adds bulk to your diet, giving you a feeling of fullness that prevents hunger and helps with overall weight control. Sources of fiber can be found in plant foods—fruits, vegetables, whole grains, beans, and nuts. Leaving the skin on the fruits (e.g., peaches) and vegetables (e.g., baked potatoes) will increase the fiber content of your meal. Add fiber slowly to prevent gas and bloating.

Avoiding Excess Salt (Sodium), Certain Fats (Trans and Saturated Fats) and Simple, Refined Sugar

These substances increase your risk for high blood pressure, heart disease, and diabetes. As salt is a component of fresh foods as well as added to many prepared foods, try to avoid adding salt while cooking or at the dinner table. Your goal should be to consume only about 2/3 of a teaspoon of salt per day. Saturated fats found in red meats and trans fats added to products such as microwave popcorn, cookies, margarine, and crackers contribute to your risk of heart disease. You should minimize the intake of these types of fats. Finally, too much sugar can affect your body's ability to respond to the hormone insulin, which is the initial step leading to the development of type 2 diabetes. Reduce the amount of sweets consumed in candies, cakes, cookies, and so on. Also, carefully read the label on products, as many prepared food items have added sugar (e.g., ketchup).

Understanding the Need for or Lack of Need for Specific Supplements

Advertisements for supplements are abundant and pop up in many venues including television, the Internet, and magazines. Dietary supplements, which come in a variety of forms (pills, powders, extracts, liquids), are substances to be used if your diet is deficient in key nutrients. Supplements may also be taken to improve your health by lowering your risk for a disease (e.g., heart disease, arthritis). These products may contain vitamins, minerals, antioxidants, fiber, proteins, or herbs. The National Institute on Aging recommends that to get the proper amount of needed nutrients, you should eat a variety of healthy foods (18). If you do so, you will not require the use of supplements that can be expensive as well as harmful in some cases. However, some dietary supplements can help older adults who do not meet specific nutrient needs within their daily diet. These special circumstances generally involve calcium, vitamin D, or vitamin B_{12}. Thus, taking supplements containing these nutrients may be recommended by your health care provider, as mentioned earlier.

Eating habits and requirements may change as one ages, but enjoying the foods and beverages consumed is key to making nutritious choices a lifelong habit. Healthy eating can be individualized through consultation with a Registered Dietitian or through resources available from MyPlate tailored specifically for older adults (for more information, see www.choosemyplate.gov/older-adults).

Focus on Physical Activity

As already highlighted in this chapter, regular physical activity can favorably affect a broad range of body systems and thus may be a lifestyle factor that discriminates between those who experience successful aging and those who do not. A complete exercise program for older adults includes aerobic exercise, muscle-strengthening exercises, and flexibility exercises. In addition, balance exercises are recommended (11).

Physical Activity and Its Impact on Daily Function

Physical activity has many benefits related to chronic disease, but also can affect two areas that can be a concern with advancing years—a good night's sleep and cognitive function. Both sleep and brain activity are foundational to one's ability to fully embrace life experiences. The benefits of physical activity in these areas are discussed in the following sections.

Physical Activity and Sleep for the Older Adult

You may have noticed that the quality of your sleep is not quite what it used to be. Recent scientific studies support this observation and suggest that the "sleep" centers located in the brain are altered with age. As a result, sleep is lighter and more frag-mented (less continuous periods of sleep; rather, episodes broken up into shorter blocks, including daytime sleeping) (4, 28). Also, the total sleep time for a given day may be reduced. You may find that you are going to sleep earlier as well as awakening earlier compared to the pattern in your younger days. You may also find yourself falling asleep during the daytime while watching TV or reading. Over time, these types of sleep disruptions can be associated with depression and anxiety disorders, cognitive and memory impairment, fatigue, and an increased risk for falls (12).

However, there is good news regarding the benefits of regular physical activity on overall sleep quality. Regular endurance exercise appears to be an effective treatment to significantly improve sleep quality in older adults who suffer from chronic sleep problems, including insomnia (15, 19). In addition to improving the quality of your sleep, regular exercise can reduce the time it takes you to fall asleep as well as reduce the need for or the dosage of sleep aids you may be currently taking. This is impor-tant, as these drugs, frequently used to help with sleep problems (sedative hypnot-ics), are often associated with side effects such as sleepwalking, daytime drowsiness, and dizziness (21). Other types of exercises, such as tai chi and yoga, have also been shown to be beneficial in reducing sleep problems in older adults (9). These benefits can be realized in as little as one month's time after the beginning of such an exercise program but are generally observed after three to six months. In order to continue to receive these benefits you will need to stick with your exercise program, as any long-term stoppage will result in a reversal of these sleep benefits. Regular exercise is a simple, nonpharmacologic treatment that can be safely implemented to improve both the quality of sleep and overall quality of life in older adults.

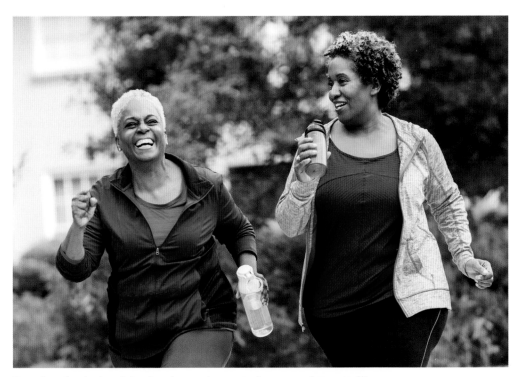

Regular physical activity has been shown to improve sleep quality.

Physical Activity and the Cognitive Function in Older Adults

Advancing age is associated with a decrease in cognitive function as well as an increase in risk for developing some form of dementia. It is estimated that one-third of adults over the age of 65 die with Alzheimer's disease or some other form of dementia (1), and the risk of developing Alzheimer's doubles every five years after the age of 65. These adverse alterations in brain function clearly have a negative impact on the quality of life. Although concerning, a positive aspect is the impact of regular aerobic exercise on your brain. This holds true for prevention in healthy individuals as well as for treatment in people who already have mild memory impairment, as well as early stages of Alzheimer's disease (10). Various factors associated with exercise may be involved, including increased blood flow and nerve activity. If you exercise on a regular basis, this chronic stimulation of brain blood flow and activity can reduce the risk of vascular dysfunction (poor blood vessel responsiveness) in the brain as it ages. In addition, recent studies have shown that aerobic exercise lowers the amount of toxic proteins in the brain that are associated with Alzheimer's disease (3). Thus, the combination of the reduction in these toxic proteins and improved blood vessel function has led experts in the study of Alzheimer's disease to conclude that no currently available medications can approach the beneficial effects of exercise in the treatment and prevention of this age-associated disease.

There is also accumulating evidence suggesting that regular exercise can help you maintain or even improve your cognitive function and memory as you age (3). These studies indicated that higher levels of cardiovascular fitness were associated with better performance on a variety of tasks testing cognitive function (7). It appears that participation in different modes of exercise (aerobic, strength, balance, flexibility), as described in this chapter, can result in an even better outcome when one examines the role that exercise has in improving cognitive function and memory. Such benefits of exercise have also been reported in people already suffering from mild cognitive impairment (22).

Finally, regular physical activity can improve symptoms of other mental maladies such as anxiety and depression even in individuals already afflicted with Alzheimer's disease and dementia (10). While the mechanisms responsible for the effect that exercise has on depression and anxiety remain unclear, regular physical activity clearly lessens the symptoms, leading to greater feelings of well-being. Additionally, the psychological and emotional benefits resulting from regular physical activity are worth noting; these include improving your ability to cope with stressful situations, enhanced confidence, empowerment, extended social interaction, improved mood states, and overall relaxation.

■ Q&A

What type of activities should be included to promote cognitive function?

A complete exercise program that includes aerobic activity, muscle-strengthening activity, and balance and flexibility exercises appears to provide the most benefits. The good news is that the advantages possible for cognitive function and memory are in addition to the myriad of other health and fitness benefits.

Physical Activity Guidelines for Older Adults

Physical activity for older adults should focus on aerobic fitness, muscular fitness, flexibility, and functional fitness (neuromotor exercise training). Including each of these areas in a comprehensive program is discussed in the following sections.

Aerobic Fitness

Endurance or aerobic activities will improve your stamina and allow you to engage in a variety of activities for a longer period of time. For example, you will be able to work in the garden or yard much longer before you feel tired or fatigued. Similarly, improvements in your aerobic fitness will allow you to go on hikes, play with your grandchildren for an extended period of time, or play several sets of tennis. Endurance exercise produces these benefits by enhancing the health and function of your heart, lungs, and circulatory system. Additionally, regular participation in endurance activities greatly improves your health by lowering several risk factors associated with a variety of diseases. This will result in the reduction or prevention of a number of diseases that are common in older adults, including heart disease, type 2 diabetes, and certain types of cancers (11, 23). The health and functional benefits associated with regular participation in an endurance exercise program are numerous.

Key risk factors related to the development of heart disease are significantly improved with endurance exercise (23). These include cardioprotective adaptations such as a reduction in the "bad" cholesterol (low-density lipoprotein [LDL]-cholesterol), an increase in the "good" cholesterol (high-density lipoprotein [HDL]-cholesterol), lower

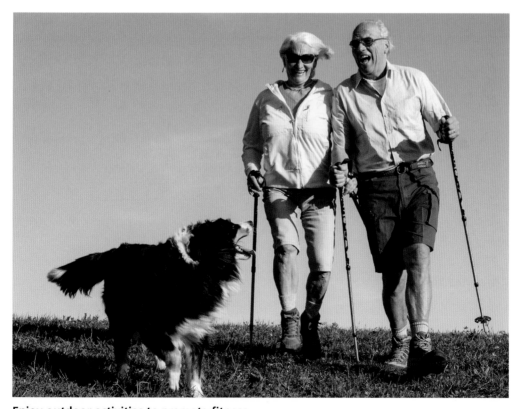

Enjoy outdoor activities to promote fitness.

triglycerides (a fat that contributes to coronary heart disease), improvements in resting blood pressure, and a reduction in total body fat.

Importantly, endurance exercise is well documented to improve your sensitivity to insulin. This is critical for several reasons. First, a decrease in insulin sensitivity or an increase in insulin resistance is the primary cause for the development of type 2 diabetes, which is the most common type of diabetes (90-95 percent of people with diabetes are type 2). Second, as you get older, you are at a greater risk of developing type 2 diabetes; thus, regular aerobic exercise is an ideal preventive strategy as well as a treatment for this disease. Regular endurance exercise may be beneficial for certain types of cancers including breast, prostate, and colon cancers. These benefits relate to both lowering the risk for these specific cancers and aiding in the rehabilitation and recovery from cancer treatment. Finally, the weight-bearing component of activities such as walking, running, and tennis helps to maintain bone health (bone mineral density), thereby reducing your risk for bone fractures and breaks. This is particularly important for postmenopausal women, who have a much higher incidence of osteo-porosis (weak and brittle bones) than others.

In order to reap the optimal benefits from your exercise program, ACSM recom-mends paying attention to the frequency, duration, and intensity of your exercise session (11, 13). The exercise session should involve large-muscle groups (such as the legs) in a continuous, rhythmic fashion. Examples include walking, biking, and swim-ming. Older adults should try to avoid high-impact activities that put excessive strain on joints, muscles, and ligaments.

Ideally, you should engage in endurance exercise three to five days per week. The lower the exercise intensity, the more often the exercise should be done. For example, if you enjoy walking, at least five days per week is recommended for this moderate-intensity exercise. However, if you are doing more strenuous exercise, such as biking or singles tennis, three days per week will be sufficient to provide the desired benefits. The recommended duration, or amount of time you spend in an exercise session, is at least 30 minutes for moderate-intensity exercise and at least 20 minutes for more strenuous activities. If you prefer, you can divide these sessions into 10-minute seg-ments throughout the day. Try to accumulate at least 150 minutes each week.

The final component of your endurance exercise program is the exercise intensity. The greater the exercise intensity, the shorter the exercise duration required. Strenuous or vigorous exercise will cause you to breathe heavily, perhaps to the point where it is difficult to talk. On a scale of 0 to 10, with 0 equal to sitting at rest and 10 represent-ing your maximal possible exertion, a strenuous exercise bout would be in the range of 7 or 8. A moderate exercise intensity session would be in the range of 5 or 6. You may want to track your daily movements with a commercial activity tracker or with a smartphone app.

Muscular Fitness

Muscular fitness training has many rewards beyond stronger muscles. These rewards range from making it easier for you to get into and out of your car, climb stairs, and carry objects to improving your balance and reducing the risk of falls and broken bones.

Strength training should be performed at least two times per week focused on the major muscle groups (legs, arms, shoulders, chest, abdominal muscles, and back). For a given muscle group, find a weight that you can lift ~8 to 12 times (repetitions) before fatiguing (if you are just starting with resistance training, a range of 10 to 15 repeti-tions might be preferable). For example, when doing an arm curl to strengthen your biceps, you may find that you can lift a 5-pound (2.3-kg) dumbbell 10 times but not 11. Thus this would be a good weight for this exercise. After resting for a few minutes, repeat the same exercise. Do the same routine for the other major muscle groups. Do not hold your breath while performing your strength exercises. Lift the weight slowly (about 2 seconds) and return the weight slowly (about 3 seconds). Over time, as you become stronger, you should increase the weight you are using to continue to challenge your muscles and remain in the 8- to 12-repetition range. If you do not have access to handheld weights, you can use common kitchen items such as soup cans or water bottles. Also, the use of resistance bands may make certain exercises easier for you to perform.

In addition to increasing your strength, a resistance training program will help you maintain and possibly increase your muscle mass. This is critical for enhancing your quality of life at many levels. A common problem among older adults in the United States today is a significant loss in muscle mass (known as sarcopenia). Connected with this loss in muscle mass is a loss in strength, which has direct implications for your ability to go about activities associated with daily living. Maintaining your muscle mass and strength will enhance your quality of life by improving your mobility, balance, and overall independence. Finally, strength training is extremely valuable in promoting healthy bones. The mechanical stress placed upon your bones while you are doing resistance exercises stimulates the bone to become stronger, thereby lowering the risk of age-associated osteoporosis (a disease that makes bones brittle). This is especially important for the bones in your upper body, as they receive little stimulation and benefit from endurance exercises that rely primarily on the legs.

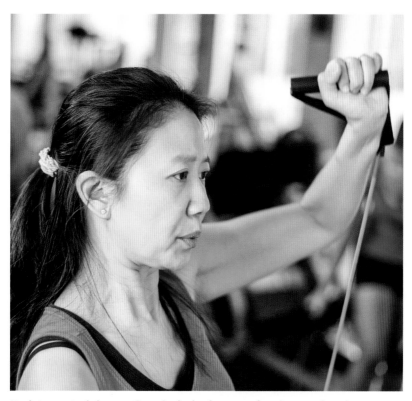

Resistance training options include the use of resistance bands.

Flexibility

Flexibility, or limberness, is defined as the ability to move joints and muscles through their full range of motion. Unfortunately, an individual's flexibility generally declines with age. However, with regular and proper stretching exercises, your flexibility can be well maintained throughout life. The significance of achieving proper flexibility will translate into an enhanced quality of life and safety by maintaining a good range of motion in all joints.

Ideally, stretching should occur when your muscles are warm and your body temperature is raised. Many people combine their stretching program with their endurance exercise session. A good time for stretching is after an endurance workout, while the muscles and joints are still warm. For best results, you should stretch at least two days per week for a minimum of 10 minutes. Each stretch should be accomplished to a degree of mild tightness in the muscles. Do not stretch to the point of pain or discomfort. Try to do each particular stretch three or four times per session. Static stretches, in which you hold the stretched position, should be done for 30 to 60 seconds (13). Remember to keep breathing while the stretch is being held. Also, it is important to slowly initiate the stretched position, avoiding any bouncing or jerking motions.

Key areas to focus on, where flexibility generally decreases with age, include the neck, shoulders, back, and legs. Chapter 7 includes a number of activities that can be included in your stretching program. The benefits of maintaining and improving your flexibility are many. As a result of the loss of flexibility in the neck and back associated with aging, some older individuals have difficulty turning around to look behind them (e.g., when backing out of a parking space). This, of course, can be dangerous as it limits full visibility. Other benefits associated with improved flexibility include bending over to tie your shoes or to pick objects up off the floor, reaching objects located a little bit higher, as in kitchen cabinets or closets, and twisting or achieving range of motion when executing a golf or tennis swing.

Neuromotor Training

Balance is defined as your ability to move or to remain in a stable position without losing control or falling. It is essential to maintain your balance as you age. Millions of older Americans are rushed to emergency rooms each year as a result of fall-related injuries. Consequences of these falls can be severe, resulting in fractures of the arms, legs, and hips as well as serious head traumas. These injuries may result in permanent disability and in some cases are life threatening. Hip fractures alone account for about 260,000 hospital visits per year among individuals 65 years and older (8). Approximately 95 percent of these hip fractures are caused by falling, frequently leading to long-term functional impairment, nursing home admission, and increased mortality (5). Physical limitations may result in a lack of ability to perform activities of daily living (16). Women, who are more prone to age-related osteoporosis, have up to 75 percent of all hip fractures (25). A number of people who fall develop a fear of falling. This frequently causes them to limit their activities, contributing to reduced mobility, loss in leg strength, and poor balance, which in turn actually increases their risk of falling (17).

The best results for balance and stability are seen when coupled with improvements in strength (as discussed previously) and, in particular, leg strength. Stronger leg muscles provide superior support for both forward–backward motions and lateral or side-to-side movement and balance. The motions are common components of activities associated with daily living such as shopping, gardening, and playing with small children. To help promote balance, various exercises can be performed two to three days per week, each exercise lasting 10 to 30 seconds. Examples of balance (neuromotor) exercises are included in chapter 8. The benefits in maintaining and improving your balance are well worth the time spent. The most important benefits are the reduction in the rate of falls and subsequent injuries related to such falls.

Optimal Program Progression to Promote Safety

The majority of older adults can safely participate in the activities described in this chapter, which focuses on a moderate-intensity level. If you are starting an exercise program for the first time or if you have not engaged in regular physical activity for a number of years, begin slowly at the lower recommended exercise intensities. This will give you the opportunity to determine your exercise tolerance, limitations, and any potential orthopedic problems that may affect your ability to exercise. Over time, as you progress and improve your fitness, you can gradually increase exercise intensity or duration, or both, so that you can optimize the benefits from your training. If you have any existing medical conditions, such as high blood pressure, diabetes, or hip and knee pain, you should have a discussion with a health care provider regarding what types of exercise you should avoid and which activities are best suited for your condition. Actually, regular physical activity is often prescribed, as it is known to be beneficial, when done properly, in individuals with existing conditions such as heart disease and diabetes—but you must be aware of your limitations.

Engaging in a 5- to 10-minute warm-up before your exercise session is important to help prevent injury and the consequences of an abrupt start. The warm-up will increase muscle temperature as well as gradually prepare your heart and lungs for the more intense exercise to come. While exercising, particularly when you are outside on a warm day, be sure to drink fluids to keep your body hydrated. You may not feel thirsty even if your body is low on fluids. If it is extremely hot outside, you should find an indoor location (such as a gym, shopping mall, or swimming pool) that has climate control where you can exercise safely.

Once you have completed your exercise session, a 5- to 10-minute cool-down is recommended to gradually lower your heart rate, blood pressure, body temperature, and breathing rate. As with the warm-up phase, the cool-down should be performed at very low exercise intensities. The cool-down prevents any negative effects on the heart and on blood pressure that may be associated with abruptly stopping the physical activity. After the cool-down, while your muscles are still somewhat warm, is a good time to do stretching exercises to improve your flexibility.

Generally, it is not a good idea to exercise when you are sick or suffering from an infection. This is particularly true if you have a fever and muscle aches. A small amount of light exercise can be tolerated if you are suffering from a head cold or an upper respiratory tract infection, but ideally, you should rest and give your immune system a chance to fight the infection. Finally, reasons to stop exercising and seek medical attention include chest pain or pressure, feelings of nausea or dizziness, or pain in your joints and extremities.

Remember that it is always smart to take the proper safety precautions when exercising, and that the health benefits from a program of regular physical activity greatly outweigh the risks. Many older adults are reluctant to begin an exercise program at this stage of their life for fear of negative consequences (falling, joint pain, cardiac events). However, remaining sedentary or physically inactive is a much greater health risk than participation in regular physical activity (2, 14).

Programs to Meet and Exceed the Physical Activity Guidelines for Older Adults

If you are beginning an exercise program for the first time or have been physically inactive for an extended period of time, here are a few guidelines to get you started. First, complete the health screening described in chapter 2. Maintaining good communication with your health care provider is recommended, especially if you have any current health limitations. Second, it is important to know your starting point or initial level of fitness. Chapters 5, 6, 7, and 8 address a number of techniques and exercises to assess your aerobic fitness, muscular fitness, flexibility, and neuromotor fitness. For a number of areas, specific assessments are available for older adults, including the 6-minute walk test for aerobic capacity, the chair stand and the arm curl test for muscular fitness, the chair version of the sit-and-reach for flexibility, and the 8-foot up and go test for neuromotor fitness (20). Regular and accurate performance feedback can assist you in developing realistic expectations of your own progress.

Knowing your current level of fitness in the areas of endurance, strength, and flexibility will better allow you to more accurately determine the optimal intensity, duration, and frequency at which to begin or advance your exercise program. A sample tracking form is shown in figure 11.1. This can serve as a motivational tool as well as a way to monitor your progress. Repeating the assessments periodically can ensure you are staying on track with your exercise program.

Once you have established your initial fitness level, it is recommended that you set both short- and long-term goals. A sample of a beginner exercise program is shown in figure 11.2, and a sample for a regular exerciser is in figure 11.3. Your goals should be realistic such that they can be accomplished in the time frame you have set. Setting unrealistic goals that cannot be met will lead to disappointment and a lower desire to continue with your exercise program. Examples of short-term goals might include being able to walk around the block without feeling fatigued or being able to lift your grandchild without discomfort and strain. Long-term goals might include regaining control of your blood sugar levels to within a normal range by your next doctor's appointment or being able to ride your bike to a friend's house.

Tracking Your Progress

In order to reap the many benefits from physical activity, you must be active on a regular basis. Here are a few tips to help incorporate exercise into your daily routine and lifestyle. Choose activities that you enjoy and find appealing. Also, adding some variety to your activities will keep things fun and interesting. For example, if you like to walk or hike, try exploring new neighborhoods or trails. Also, consider new activities, such as joining a bowling league or signing up for a yoga class. Activities that have a social component can promote regular participation. If you prefer tennis or golf, find a regular group of like-minded individuals for weekly matches. When exercising in your home, listen to music or watch your favorite TV show when you are doing your balance and flexibility exercises.

FIGURE 11.1

Fitness assessment progress chart for older adults.

	Assessment 1 (baseline)	Assessment 2*	Assessment 3**
Body composition assessments			
Body mass index			
Waist circumference			
Aerobic fitness assessment			
6-min walk test			
Muscular fitness assessments			
Chair stand test			
Arm curl test			
Flexibility assessments			
Sit-and-reach test			
Back-scratch test			
Neuromotor assessments			
4-stage balance test			
Standing reach test			
8-foot up and go test			

*From baseline: Two months for a beginner, three months for an intermediate exerciser, and four months for an established exerciser.

**From baseline: Four months for a beginner, six months for an intermediate exerciser, and eight months for an established exerciser.

From ACSM, 2017, *ACSM's complete guide to fitness & health,* 2nd ed. (Champaign, IL: Human Kinetics).

Importantly, do not get discouraged during the first few weeks of starting your physical activity program. Initially, your muscles may feel sore or may ache. This is natural, and these sensations will disappear as you continue with your activity level. In sticking with your program you will see some rewards relatively soon (weeks to months) and others that may not be as obvious. For example, any benefits relating to your blood sugar levels or blood pressure will not be recognized until your next checkup with your doctor. Keeping track of your progress can be a useful motivational tool. Figure 11.4 provides a simple chart whereby you can track your fitness progress over the course of 10 weeks.

Finally, life can get busy. Unfortunately, it seems that being physically active is the agenda item frequently put on the back burner. Please remember how important being active is to your health and well-being. Make it a high priority in your daily routine.

FIGURE 11.2

Sample beginner exercise program for older adults*.

Weeks	Aerobic**	Resistance	Stretching***	Neuromotor exercise	Comments
1-3	Three days per week; 10 to 20 min per day; light intensity (level 3 or 4)	Two days per week; one set, 10 to 15 reps of six different exercises****	Two days per week; 10 min of stretching activities	Two days per week; 10 min of balance activities	Walking is an easy beginning aerobic activity. Select a comfortable pace. If you haven't been very active, target 10 min at a time for your aerobic activity. Include some stretching activities (see chapter 7) after your walk. For resistance training, see chapter 6 for details on what activities to include. For balance training, see chapter 8 for details on what activities to include.
4-6	Three days per week; 15-25 min per day; light to moderate intensity (level 4 or 5)	Two days per week; one or two sets, 10 to 15 reps of six different exercises****	Three days per week; 10 min of stretching activities	Two or three days per week; 10 min of balance activities	The focus for the next three weeks will be getting comfortable with at least 20 min of aerobic exercise at least three days per week. Gradually increase your intensity to a moderate level by the sixth week. Continue with your resistance training program and add an additional set by week 5. Add an additional session of balance training by the sixth week.
7-9	Three or four days per week; 20-30 min per day; moderate intensity (level 5)	Two days per week; two sets, 10 to 15 reps of six different exercises****	Three days per week; 10 min of stretching activities	Three days per week; 10 min of balance activities	For the next three weeks, try to increase your total time spent in moderate aerobic activity (either 40 min per day three days per week or 30 min per day four days per week). Continue with your resistance training program, completing two sets per exercise and adding more weight if you are able to do 15 repetitions relatively easily.
10-12	Three or four days per week; 25-35 min per day; moderate intensity (level 5 or 6)	Two days per week; two sets, 10 to 15 reps of six different exercises****	Three days per week; 10 min of stretching activities	Three days per week; 10 min of balance activities	Over the past couple of months you have been developing a good aerobic and muscular fitness base. For some variety, you can consider other activities such as biking or swimming (for more ideas, see chapter 5). If you like walking, you can also keep doing that. For your resistance training program, consider adding some variety and trying some other exercises (see chapter 6 for details).

*All activity sessions should be preceded and followed by a 5- to 10-minute warm-up and cool-down.

**Intensity is based on a 10-point scale with 0 being rest and 10 your highest effort level. Moderate intensity is a level 5 to 6.

***Include stretching activities after your aerobic exercise to improve flexibility. For specific stretches to target the major muscle groups, see chapter 7.

****Resistance training is more fully outlined in chapter 6. Beginners will select one exercise for each of the following body areas: hips and legs, chest, back, shoulders, low back, and abdominal muscles.

From ACSM, 2017, *ACSM's complete guide to fitness & health,* 2nd ed. (Champaign, IL: Human Kinetics).

FIGURE 11.3

Sample established exercise program for older adults*.

Weeks	Aerobic**	Resistance	Stretching***	Neuromotor exercise	Comments
1-3	Five days per week for moderate exercise (level 5 to 6) Or: Three days per week for vigorous exercise (level 7 to 8), Or: three to five days per week for a mix of moderate and vigorous exercise	Two days per week; two sets, 8 to 12 reps of 10 different exercises****	Two or three days per week; 10 min of stretching activities	Three days per week; 10 to 15 min of different neuromotor exercises	Congratulations on your ongoing commitment to exercise. To find specific aerobic activities, see chapter 5. For resistance training, see chapter 6, and for stretching and neuromotor exercise training, refer to chapters 7 and 8.
4-6	Two or three days of moderate activity and one or two days of vigorous activity	Two days per week; two sets, 8 to 12 reps of 10 different exercises****	Two or three days per week; 10 min of stretching activities	Three days per week; 10 to 15 min of different neuromotor exercises	For the next couple of weeks, try mixing up your activities. Try a new aerobic activity or change the intensity of an activity you already do on a regular basis. Continue with your resistance training program and balance training.
7-9	Five days per week for moderate exercise Or: Three days per week for vigorous exercise Or: Three to five days per week for a mix of moderate and vigorous exercise	Two or three days per week; two sets per exercise, 8 to 12 reps of 10 different exercises****	Two or three days per week; 10 min of stretching activities	Three days per week; 10 to 15 min of different neuromotor exercises	Continue with your aerobic training program. For resistance training, consider trying some different exercises (see chapter 6 for details). If you typically use machines, try a couple of new exercises using dumbbells to provide your muscles with a new challenge. Be sure to maintain good form when trying new activities.
10-12	Five days per week for moderate exercise Or: Three days per week for vigorous exercise Or: Three to five days per week for a mix of moderate and vigorous exercise	Two or three days per week; two or three sets per exercise, 8 to 12 reps of 10 exercises****	Two or three days per week; 10 min of stretching activities	Three days per week; 10 to 15 min of different neuromotor exercises	Continue with your aerobic training program. Consider doing three sets instead of two during one of your resistance training sessions (see chapter 6 for details). You may need to cut back on your reps to add the additional set.

*All activity sessions should be preceded and followed by a 5- to 10-minute warm-up and cool-down.

**Intensity is based on a 10-point scale with 0 being rest and 10 your highest effort level. Moderate intensity is a level 5 to 6 and vigorous is a level 7 to 8.

***Include stretching activities after your aerobic exercise to improve flexibility. For specific stretches to target the major muscle groups, see chapter 7.

****Resistance training is more fully outlined in chapter 6. Select one exercise for each of the following body areas: hips and legs, chest, back, shoulders, low back, abdominal muscles, quadriceps, hamstrings, biceps, and triceps. Examples of exercises you can include for each body area are found in table 6.6.

From ACSM, 2017, *ACSM's complete guide to fitness & health,* 2nd ed. (Champaign, IL: Human Kinetics).

FIGURE 11.4

Fitness progress chart for older adults.

	Total time spent in aerobic exercise (min of moderate and vigorous activity per week)		Number of resistance training sessions per week	Number of resistance training exercises per session	Number of sessions per week of stretching activities	Number of sessions per week of balance exercises
Week 1	Moderate: ____ min	Vigorous: ____ min				
Week 2	Moderate: ____ min	Vigorous: ____ min				
Week 3	Moderate: ____ min	Vigorous: ____ min				
Week 4	Moderate: ____ min	Vigorous: ____ min				
Week 5	Moderate: ____ min	Vigorous: ____ min				
Week 6	Moderate: ____ min	Vigorous: ____ min				
Week 7	Moderate: ____ min	Vigorous: ____ min				
Week 8	Moderate: ____ min	Vigorous: ____ min				
Week 9	Moderate: ____ min	Vigorous: ____ min				
Week 10	Moderate: ____ min	Vigorous: ____ min				

From ACSM, 2017, *ACSM's complete guide to fitness & health, 2nd ed.* (Champaign, IL: Human Kinetics).

Healthy aging involves making a number of sound decisions and commitments on lifestyle factors. The scientific evidence is very clear on the role of nutrition and exercise in promoting healthy aging. The benefits for both body and mind go a long way toward maintaining independence and quality of life in your later years. The scientific evidence is just as clear as to the deleterious effects of remaining sedentary or physically inactive. An inactive lifestyle contributes to an elevated risk for the development of many chronic, life-threatening diseases that become more common and prevalent with advancing years. The choice to be active or not seems obvious.

Part IV

Fitness and Health for Every Body

Various circumstances can affect your health and fitness journey, including medical conditions. Chapters 12 to 20 highlight how opportunities remain in these situations to optimize health through physical activity and nutrition. Benefits of regular physical activity and a healthy diet are well documented for those with heart disease, diabetes, and osteoporosis. In addition, evidence of benefits of physical activity and nutrition is found for arthritis, Alzheimer's disease, depression, and cancer. Other areas affected by physical activity and nutrition are weight management and pregnancy. Personalizing your fitness program will allow you to reap health and fitness benefits.

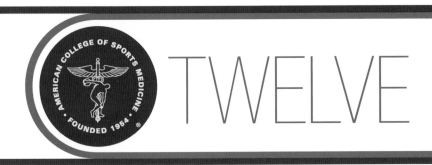

Cardiovascular Health

Cardiovascular disease (CVD) is one of the leading causes of death in industrialized countries such as the United States. Cardiovascular disease includes medical conditions and diseases such as heart attacks, chronic chest pain, stroke, and heart failure. While the number of deaths attributable to CVD has declined over the last decade in the United States, the overall public health burden of CVD remains unacceptably high, and both men and women are affected. According to the American Heart Association (AHA), the overall death rate linked to CVD in 2011 was 229.6 deaths per 100,000 Americans, or a total of 786,641 deaths (15). Stated another way, more than 2,150 Americans die of CVD every day, which means that 1 death occurs every 40 seconds. Moreover, this is not a disease that affects only older adults—approximately 155,000 of the deaths were in adults younger than 65 years of age. The costs associated with CVD are astronomically high. In 2011, the annual costs for CVD and stroke were estimated at approximately $320 billion (15).

What causes CVD? Cardiovascular disease often starts with damage to the cells lining the inside of blood vessels, and inflammation plays a key role in CVD progression (13). The disease process is known as atherosclerosis. As one example, blood vessels in the heart that are partially or fully blocked with plaque can impair blood flow. In some cases, a partially blocked vessel causes chest pain with exertion; this is known as angina. In other cases, the plaque that blocks the blood vessel can rupture, cause a blood clot inside the blood vessel, and therefore cut off the blood supply (14). If the blood flow is not immediately restored, the heart muscle will be damaged; this is referred to as a myocardial infarction or, simply, heart attack. A heart attack can weaken the heart muscle, sometimes leading to heart failure, which is associated with symptoms such as shortness of breath, fatigue, and fluid retention.

Fortunately, CVD is largely preventable. Lifestyle management through proper diet and regular physical activity underlies CVD prevention and treatment (11).

Risk Factors for Cardiovascular Disease

It is important to emphasize that CVD prevention includes preventing the development of risk factors, treatment of risk factors, and prevention of recurrent CVD events. Risk factors for CVD include several that cannot be altered such as increasing age, having a family history of CVD, race, and sex (men are at greater risk then women). More importantly, there are many risk factors that can be altered through lifestyle modifications; these include cigarette smoking, high blood pressure, high cholesterol, physical inactivity, obesity, and diabetes (7). These risk factors are highlighted in table 12.1 and discussed in the following sections. In addition, other factors such as excessive alcohol consumption and stress can contribute to the development of CVD. Consistent with the overall theme of this book, this chapter focuses on proper diet and physical activity in relation to CVD. In particular, lifestyle choices that lead to optimal cardiovascular health and improved quality of life are emphasized.

As you can see, many risk factors for CVD can be altered with lifestyle changes. Focusing on modifiable aspects is a positive step you can take to promote heart health.

TABLE 12.1   Risk Factors for Cardiovascular Disease

Nonmodifiable risk factors	Sex	Men have a greater risk of CVD than women, and men also have heart attacks earlier in life. CVD risk increases after menopause for women.
	Age	The risk for CVD increases with age. Men 45 and older and women 55 and older are at increased risk.
	Race	CVD is higher among Mexican Americans, American Indians, native Hawaiians, and African Americans.
	Family history	CVD often runs in families, so if your parents had heart disease, you are at increased risk.
Modifiable risk factors	Smoking	Smoking dramatically increases your risk of developing CVD.
	High blood pressure	High blood pressure makes your heart work harder and causes your heart muscle to thicken and become stiffer over time.
	High cholesterol	As your cholesterol increases, so does your CVD risk. Cholesterol can also be affected by age, sex, heredity, and diet.
	Physical inactivity	A sedentary lifestyle is a risk factor for CVD.
	Obesity	Excess body weight, particularly around the waist, increases your risk of developing CVD.
	Prediabetes, diabetes	Diabetes increases the risk for CVD even if your blood glucose levels are under control, but the risk is much greater in poorly controlled diabetes.
	Diet	The foods you eat can affect other risk factors for heart disease such as your blood cholesterol, blood pressure, weight, and diabetes.

Source: American Heart Association.

Cigarette Smoking

While tobacco use has declined in the United States, there are still far too many people who smoke. In 2013, approximately 18 percent of adults and 16 percent of high school students smoked. The AHA estimates that nearly one-third of heart disease deaths are attributable to smoking and exposure to secondhand smoke (15). Of recent concern is the use of e-cigarettes and the possibility that they may serve as a gateway to traditional cigarettes. If you are a smoker, quitting immediately is one of the most important things you can do to improve your overall health. Many smokers require assistance before quitting—consult your health care provider for additional information.

High Blood Pressure

Known as the "silent killer," high blood pressure (or hypertension) is a major contributing factor to the development of CVD (19). The word "silent" highlights that there are often no outward signs or symptoms of high blood pressure. Blood pressure recordings include the systolic blood pressure (top number) and diastolic blood pressure (bottom number), and the unit used is millimeters of mercury (mmHg). An optimal blood pressure is a systolic blood pressure less than 120 mmHg and diastolic blood pressure less than 80 mmHg. Systolic pressures between 120 and 139 or diastolic pressures between 80 and 89 are classified as *prehypertensive* blood pressures, and generally signal that an individual is at greater risk for higher blood pressures in the future. However, when the systolic pressure exceeds 140 mmHg or the diastolic pressure exceeds 90 mmHg, a diagnosis of hypertension is usually made by a health care provider (10). It is important to note that values must be confirmed on at least two separate occasions before a diagnosis is made.

Among all U.S. adults, nearly one-third have hypertension, which represents approximately 80 million people (15). Hypertension rates are especially high in African Americans. Blood pressure values usually increase with age. There are many treatment options for hypertension, and lifestyle modifications such as proper diet and exercise, as discussed in this chapter, are key to achieving optimal blood pressure values (18).

High Cholesterol

Elevated levels of cholesterol in the blood contribute to the development of CVD. Values above 200 milligrams per deciliter (mg/dL) increase risk for CVD. Unfortunately, nearly 31 million U.S. adults have cholesterol values above 240 mg/dL (15). In addition to the importance of assessing the total amount of cholesterol in the blood, it is common to check for levels of low-density lipoprotein (LDL) cholesterol, which is often referred to as "bad" cholesterol, and high-density lipoprotein (HDL) cholesterol, which is often referred to as "good" cholesterol. Low-density lipoprotein values below 100 mg/dL and HDL values above 60 mg/dL are desirable. Individuals with CVD should strive for even lower LDL values to decrease their risk of having a cardiovascular event (21). While proper nutrition and regular exercise are important lifestyle modifications to help reach optimal cholesterol levels, many adults with CVD also require medication to get their LDL levels down to an acceptable range. If your cholesterol is too high, you should work with your health care provider to take steps to lower your levels to recommended ranges in to order decrease your risk of having a cardiovascular event.

The most common class of medications used is known as statins. In rare situations, statin use can lead to rhabdomyolysis (skeletal muscle protein is abnormally released into the blood, with subsequent damage to the kidneys). When someone taking a statin performs exercise, muscle discomfort or pain could be a result of the medication rather than the exercise. People in this situation should report any uncommon muscle discomfort or pain to their health care provider.

Physical Inactivity

Having a sedentary lifestyle is major risk factor for CVD. Nearly 31 percent of adults in the United States do not engage in any leisure-time physical activity (15). This is a major public health issue. Having a high level of habitual physical activity has its own independent health benefits, but high activity levels also favorably influence several other risk factors such as obesity, prediabetes, high cholesterol, and high blood pressure. Exercising regularly also helps to maintain mobility in old age and to prevent frailty. Quality of life measures are higher in adults who exercise regularly. The standard recommendation is for adults to get at least 150 minutes of moderate-intensity aerobic activity per week, which can be accomplished with brisk walking, or 75 minutes of vigorous-intensity exercise per week (25). Additional details regarding exercise recommendations are provided later in this chapter.

Obesity

Excess body weight is a leading cause of death and disability in the United States. Being overweight or obese makes it more likely that you will have other cardiovascular risk factors. In particular, people who are overweight or obese are far more likely than others to have type 2 diabetes. Sixty-nine percent of adults in the United States are classified as overweight or obese, and these high rates are viewed as a public health crisis. Unfortunately, far too many children are classified as overweight or obese; approximately 32 percent of children between 2 and 19 years of age fall into this category. Sadly, obese children usually become obese adults (15).

Prediabetes and Diabetes

Fasting blood glucose (i.e., sugar) should be less than 100 mg/dL for children and adults. Values higher than this suggest prediabetes or diabetes. The latest statistics suggest that 21 million adults have diagnosed diabetes, 8 million have undiagnosed diabetes, and 81 million have prediabetes (15). Those with prediabetes have fasting blood glucose values between 100 and 125 mg/dL; those with diabetes have fasting blood glucose values greater than or equal to 126 mg/dL (2). Having diabetes dramatically increases your chances of developing CVD. Fortunately, regular exercise and proper nutrition can help prevent the development of diabetes.

Diet

A healthy diet provides many potential benefits for health and for risk factor reduction. The relationships between nutrition choices and cholesterol levels, blood pressure, and heart disease highlight the value of heart-healthy eating (as discussed in greater detail in the next section).

Healthy Approaches to Managing CVD

Diet and physical activity are two important lifestyle factors that promote cardiovascular health (11). These are two lifestyle factors over which you have control. Nutrition and exercise can contribute to optimizing the health of your heart and blood vessels, as well as your overall fitness.

Focusing on Nutrition

Nutrition plays an important role in cardiovascular health. Poor nutrition is considered a risk factor for elevated cholesterol levels, high blood pressure, and heart disease. Unfortunately, the average American diet increases risk for all of these conditions. The typical American diet is high in refined grains, added sugars, and red and processed meats while falling short in key food groups such as vegetables, fruits, whole grains, and dairy (22). In particular, you should thoughtfully review the composition of your diet and consider changing the types of fats you eat and lowering your sodium intake and the calories you consume while increasing whole grains, lean proteins, fruits, and vegetables to promote optimal heart health. Indeed, research has shown that a healthy dietary pattern is beneficial for reducing CVD risk (22).

Heart-Healthy Dietary Recommendations

Consuming a heart-healthy diet is not as difficult as it sounds if you carefully consider the types of foods you should include. For instance, selecting whole grains over refined grains is a great first step. Whole grains are found in many foods, including cereals, grains, pasta, and brown rice (e.g., look for the word "whole" in front of the type of grain). Aim for at least three servings of whole grains a day. Further, whole grains provide fiber, which includes two types: soluble and insoluble. Soluble fiber can help to lower LDL-cholesterol levels. Good sources of soluble fiber include oatmeal, fruits, vegetables, and kidney beans. Total fiber intake should be in the range of 20 to 30 grams, with 10 to 25 of those grams coming from soluble fiber sources (12). When it comes to fruits and vegetables, aim for five servings a day. Select a variety of colorful fruits and vegetables to increase your intake of nutrients. Sources can include fresh, frozen, or dried fruit and fresh, frozen, or canned vegetables without added fat or salt. Remember, sodium is often added to canned vegetables. For protein, select lean protein sources, options include both animal and plant based foods. Lean cuts of beef and pork (loin, leg, round, extra-lean ground beef), skinless poultry, fish, and venison are good animal-based choices, while dried beans and peas, nuts and nut butters, egg whites, or egg substitutes constitute great plant-based sources of protein. Adequate protein is important in the diet, although too much can be detrimental as it provides excess calories that are stored as fat.

■ **Q&A** ▬▬▬▬▬▬▬▬▬▬▬▬▬▬▬▬▬▬▬▬▬▬▬▬▬▬▬

Are fruit juices an ideal source to meet serving recommendations for fruit consumption?

While fruit juices do come from fruit, they also provide a lot of calories and contain no fiber, so it is best to get fruit from whole sources.

Fat and Cholesterol Recommendations   While most people have heard the recommendation to eat a low-fat, low-cholesterol diet, or a heart-healthy diet, you may not know that the source of fat in your diet is the most important consideration as opposed to overall content. Health agencies such as the Academy of Nutrition and Dietetics (AND) and the AHA recommend keeping dietary fat between 25 and 35 percent of your daily caloric intake. While this may not seem low enough to you, the type of fat you consume is very important to heart health. Several types of dietary fat exist, as discussed in chapter 3. Saturated fats contribute to the blocking of your arteries by increasing LDL-cholesterol levels. Several large research studies have revealed that for every 1 percent increase in calories from saturated fatty acids as a percent of the total calories consumed, LDL-cholesterol levels rise about 2 percent in individuals who have high blood cholesterol levels (12). For every 1 percent reduction in saturated fatty acid intake, serum cholesterol is reduced by approximately 2 percent. Therefore, AHA and the American College of Cardiology both recommend that less than 7 percent of your daily calories come from saturated fats (11). Saturated fat is predominantly found in animal sources such as meat and dairy products including fatty beef, lamb, pork, poultry with skin, beef fat, lard, and cream, butter, and cheese (5). Another type of fat called trans fat should be consumed as little as possible because it tends to increase LDL-cholesterol similarly to saturated fatty acids (11), as well as decrease HDL cholesterol (6). If you see the words "hydrogenated" or "partially hydrogenated" on the ingredient list for a food, that food item contains trans fats. Examples of foods containing trans fat include stick margarine, shortening, some fried foods, doughnuts, cookies, crackers, muffins, pies, and cakes. You should limit your intake of these types of products. Finally, your cholesterol intake is still important to consider. Cholesterol not only comes from the foods you eat but can also be produced by the body. Limiting your body's production of cholesterol and reducing blood cholesterol levels are best achieved by reducing your cholesterol and dietary saturated fat intake. Cholesterol is found in foods such as meat (particularly those with lots of visible fat); processed meats such as sausage, bologna, salami, and hot dogs; egg yolks; whole milk; cheeses; shrimp; lobster; and crab. You can easily lower the cholesterol content of your diet by choosing lean cuts of meat with minimal visible fat and leaner cuts of beef such as round, chuck, sirloin, or loin.

So, if saturated and trans fats as well as cholesterol are the types of fat you should limit, what should you consume? Unsaturated fats are recommended to make up most of the fat you consume (as covered in chapter 3). These fats are known as monounsaturated and polyunsaturated fats. Monounsaturated fats can be found in oils such as canola, peanut, and olive oil. Polyunsaturated fats are generally found in vegetable oils but also include the omega-3 fats. Omega-3 fats are found in several types of fish including salmon, tuna, mackerel, herring, lake trout, albacore tuna, and sardines but can also be found in oils including canola and soybean. Omega-3 fats are thought to decrease your risk of heart disease; adding two servings of baked or grilled fish (about 3.5 ounces or about 100 grams) to your diet each week is one way to increase your intake of healthy fats such as the omega-3 fats and is recommended by the AHA (4). If you are unable to get your omega-3s from fish, your health care provider may recommend fish oil supplements. The AHA recommends that people with heart disease get 1 gram of omega-3 fatty acids from a combination of EPA and DHA (two types of omega-3 fats) daily (9).

Dietary Sodium Recommendations   While lowering your intake of foods such as saturated fat that increase cholesterol levels in the body is important, lowering sodium intake

■ Q&A

What are some ways to reduce sodium consumption?

If you add table salt to your food, a great place to start is to get rid of the salt shaker, though this will not be enough. Shopping wisely and reading labels are very important. Looking for labeling on packages that say "very low sodium," "low sodium," "lite in sodium," "reduced sodium," "sodium-free," or "salt-free" is a great way to reduce sodium consumption.

---

is equally so. Most Americans consume far too much sodium. The U.S. Department of Agriculture estimates that the current average intake for both men and women is ~3,300 milligrams of sodium (23). Many organizations recommend sodium reduction, including AHA, AND, and the World Health Organization. The *Dietary Guidelines for Americans* recommends 2,300 milligrams of sodium or less per day; and for those with established hypertension, a lower target of 1,500 milligrams per day is the aim (22). These recommendations are based on research studies that have documented a decline in blood pressure with dietary sodium restriction (9, 20). More recently there has been a push to recommend the 1,500 milligrams per day level for most Americans. So, where does all this sodium come from? Well, 75 percent of typical sodium intake comes from processed, prepackaged, and restaurant foods. Most food items found in a box or a can contain sodium (even breakfast cereals!). Therefore, looking closely at food labels and comparing products to find one with less sodium is recommended.

Other Recommendations   Weight control is also important for decreasing your risk for CVD or even for managing your heart disease or blood pressure (8). Anyone who is overweight or obese (to check your body mass index [BMI], see p. 352-353) should focus on reducing total calorie intake and burning more calories through exercise. Studies have reported that weight loss can lower blood pressure, as well as improve overall cardiovascular health (for more details on weight management, see chapter 18). A critical review of your own diet and the decision to consume fruits, vegetables, and whole grains in preference to high-fat, highly processed options are very conducive to weight loss.

Finally, there has been speculation about the benefits of alcohol in relation to heart health. The AHA recommends moderation when it comes to alcohol consumption. This corresponds to one to two drinks per day for men and one drink per day for

---

■ Q&A

What about red wine and heart disease?

Some researchers have suggested that red wine may be associated with the reduced mortality seen with heart disease in some populations. Unfortunately, it is not clear if it is truly the wine or the grapes themselves or other components in red wine that may contribute to the reduced mortality. Further, it is difficult to separate out other lifestyle factors that may play a role. There has been evidence to suggest that drinking wine or alcohol in some populations can increase HDL cholesterol. However, regular exercise can do the same and has many more benefits.

women (8). Drinking too much alcohol can increase some fats in the blood (i.e., triglycerides). In addition, alcohol intake can influence blood pressure. For those who consume alcohol on a regular basis, reducing alcohol intake has been shown to lower resting blood pressure.

Heart-Healthy Diet Plans

There are many heart-healthy diets that are recommended for people who have heart disease or high blood pressure. One diet called Therapeutic Lifestyle Change, or TLC, may be recommended to you by your health care provider if you have high blood cholesterol or known CVD (16). This diet emphasizes reduced saturated fat and cholesterol intake with consumption of plant stanols/sterols and increased soluble fiber (see table 12.2). This diet was designed to lower LDL-cholesterol levels in the body. Consumption of plant stanols/sterols in the amount of 2 to 3 grams per day has been shown to lower LDL cholesterol by 6 to 15 percent (12). Further, fiber is important to consider, particularly soluble fiber. Research has shown that an increase in soluble fiber of 5 to 10 grams per day is associated with a 5 percent reduction in LDL cholesterol (26). Finally, total calorie (energy) intake should be adjusted to maintain a healthy body weight, and physical activity should be included to expend at least 200 kilocalories per day.

If you have elevated blood pressure, your health care provider may talk to you about the DASH diet or Dietary Approaches to Stop Hypertension diet (17). This diet evolved from several research studies conducted in the 1990s that showed the effect of this diet on blood pressure (9, 20). These dietary trials emphasized a low-sodium diet with consumption of foods rich in potassium, calcium, and magnesium. A 2,000-calorie DASH diet provides 4,700 milligrams of potassium, 1,240 milligrams of calcium, 500 milligrams of magnesium, 90 grams of protein, 30 grams of fiber, and 2,400 milligrams of sodium. Potassium, in particular, has been shown to have blood pressure–lowering properties (1). Food sources of potassium include milk, meat, fish, fruits (e.g., bananas, oranges, and other citrus fruit), and vegetables (e.g., potatoes, broccoli, carrots) (24).

Information on the DASH diet, including sample menus, can be found on the AHA website or the National Heart, Lung, and Blood Institute (of the National Institutes of Health) website (go to www.nhlbi.nih.gov and enter DASH into the search window). This site includes specific examples of healthful eating habits. In general, the recommendation is to eat several servings of fruit, several servings of vegetables, several servings of grains (with an emphasis on whole grains), and fat-free or low-fat milk products daily. You should limit fat, oils, and sweets and incorporate lean meats, poultry, and

TABLE 12.2   Therapeutic Lifestyle Change Diet Recommendations

Food group	Recommended intake
Saturated fat	<7% of total daily calories
Trans fat	As little as possible
Cholesterol	<200 mg
Total fat	25 to 35% of total daily calories
Carbohydrate	50 to 60% of total daily calories
Protein	15% of total daily calories
Fiber	25 to 30 g/day

Source: U.S. Department of Health and Human Services, National Heart, Lung, and Blood Institute, 2005.

fish into your diet. The overall recommendation for hypertensive adults is to adopt the DASH eating plan; the number of servings for each of the food group categories depends on your overall caloric intake (see table 12.3 for some general guidelines for the number of servings from various food groups). DASH is organized by servings for most food groups. The following are examples of DASH servings:

- *Grains*—1 ounce or equivalent; 1 slice bread
- *Fruits*—1/2 cup cut-up fruit or equivalent; 1 medium fruit
- *Vegetables*—1/2 cup cooked vegetables or equivalent; 1 cup raw leafy vegetables
- *Meats, poultry, and fish*—1 ounce cooked meats, poultry, or fish or one egg
- *Nuts, seeds, and legumes*—2 tablespoons peanut butter, 1/3 cup or 1 1/2 ounces of nuts, 1/2 cup cooked beans, or 1 cup bean soup
- *Fats and oils*—1 teaspoon soft margarine or vegetable oil, 1 tablespoon mayonnaise, 1 tablespoon regular salad dressing or 2 tablespoons low-fat dressing
- *Sugars*—1 tablespoon jam or jelly, 1/2 cup regular gelatin, or 1 cup regular lemonade

There are a few additional considerations related to diet if you are on medication. For instance, individuals who are on warfarin (i.e., Coumadin) should keep their vitamin K intake consistent to maintain stable levels of the drug in their body. Vitamin K is found in green leafy vegetables such as kale, spinach, Swiss chard, romaine lettuce, green leaf lettuce, mustard greens, and collards, as well as broccoli and asparagus. People taking diuretics may experience increased frequency of urination and as result may excrete more minerals, such as potassium, calcium, phosphorus, and magnesium, in their urine. Consult with your health care provider if you have any concerns before making any changes to your diet.

TABLE 12.3   DASH Eating Plan for Various Calorie Levels

Food group	Number of food servings by calorie level per day (unless noted as on a weekly basis)			
	1,600 calories	2,000 calories	2,600 calories	3,100 calories
Grains	6	6 to 8	10 to 11	12 to 13
Vegetables	3 to 4	4 to 5	5 to 6	6
Fruits	4	4 to 5	5 to 6	6
Fat-free or low-fat dairy products	2 to 3	2 to 3	3	3 to 4
Lean meats, poultry, and fish	3 to 4 or less	6 or less	6 or less	6 to 9
Nuts, seeds, and legumes	3 to 4 per week	4 to 5 per week	1	1
Fats and oils	2	2 to 3	3	4
Sweets and added sugars	3 or less per week	5 or less per week	≤ 2	≤ 2
Maximum sodium limit	2,300 mg/day	2,300 mg/day	2,300 mg/day	2,300 mg/day

Source: U.S. Department of Health and Human Services, National Heart, Lung, and Blood Institute.

Focusing on Physical Activity

High levels of habitual physical activity and structured exercise improve functional capacity and can help forestall the inevitable age-related declines in physiological function. Habitual physical activity and exercise also favorably influence many of the risk factors for CVD. This section focuses on exercise considerations for individuals with CVD.

Precautions for Exercise

Many individuals with heart disease, or risk factors for heart disease, have concerns related to cardiovascular events, such as a heart attack, when engaging in physical activity. An increased risk is seen particularly when people who are sedentary or who have CVD do vigorous-intensity exercise. This risk decreases, however, with regular physical activity (2). Thus, starting with low to moderate exercise and progressing gradually is key to promote safety along with improvements in health and fitness.

Proper screening is important for anyone about to begin an exercise program. To promote safety, individuals with a history of CVD should have medical clearance before beginning an exercise program. The medical clearance should include a medical exam by a health care professional, and very often an exercise test is also performed (2). If you have CVD, you may have started your exercise program in a cardiac rehabilitation facility. The principles that were used to design your exercise program in the cardiac rehabilitation program are likely similar to the principles discussed in this chapter.

Physical Activity Recommendations

Physical activity recommendations are similar in many ways to what has been presented in earlier chapters, although some special considerations for those with CVD are discussed in this section. A complete exercise program includes aerobic exercise, resistance training, and flexibility and neuromotor exercises.

Aerobic exercise should be performed at least three, but preferably most, days of the week. Exercising more frequently than three days per week can be helpful for people who want to lose weight because more frequent exercise causes expenditure of more calories. For those with high cholesterol, ACSM recommends at least five days per week to help maximize caloric expenditure. Also, each exercise bout can lower blood pressure for several hours, so exercising more frequently (five to seven days per week) can help persons with hypertension (2).

Aerobic exercise intensity will vary from person to person, but generally you should strive to perform moderate-intensity exercise, which corresponds to an exertion level of 5 or 6 on a 10-point scale (see chapter 5 for more information on intensity). Several points regarding intensity need to be emphasized (1). If you have been diagnosed with chronic angina by a health care provider and the provider is aware that you have some chest discomfort with exercise, the recommendation will likely be to keep your heart rate 10 beats below the chest discomfort threshold (2). Medications such as beta-blockers can lower your resting heart rate and lower your heart rate response to exercise. If you take these medications, you may not be able to achieve a high heart rate during exercise. Don't worry, though—you will still derive benefit from the exercise session and can focus on your perception of effort rather than heart rate (3). Medications such as diuretics (so-called water pills) can cause some individuals to become volume depleted, can alter electrolyte levels such as potassium, and can cause some to feel dizzy when they stand up or after an exercise bout. Your health care provider will regularly check your electrolyte levels, but you should let your doctor know if you get dizzy or light-headed after an exercise bout (2).

A general recommendation for exercise session duration is between 20 and 60 minutes, although you can begin with only 5 to 10 minutes per session and then gradually build up. If you are interested in weight loss, you probably want to get as close to 60 minutes per session as you can in order to maximize the calories that you burn. Also, you can strive for one continuous session or several sessions of at least 10 minutes each throughout the day (2).

Aerobic activities should form the backbone of your exercise routine. A reasonable goal for most adults is to expend about 1,000 calories (kcal) per week with the aerobic exercise program (or higher if your goal is to lose weight) (see chapter 5, p. 93, for steps to calculate the number of calories burned). This will vary depending on your weight, and it is important to emphasize that you will derive health benefits even if you are well below this value. No standard rate of progression is recommended for all individuals. The key is that the rate of progression for intensity and duration be should gradual to avoid injury (2).

Another way to reduce the risk of injury is to ease into and out of your exercise session. Warm-up should consist of low-intensity activities for approximately 5 to 10 minutes, typically doing the conditioning activity at a lower intensity than during the conditioning phase. An example is a period of slow walking prior to engaging in a more brisk pace for the conditioning phase. Following the conditioning activity, a cool-down should consist of low-intensity activity for approximately 5 to 10 minutes. Stretching and range of motion activities can also be incorporated into the warm-up or cool-down but should follow rather than precede the light activity.

The focus in this section thus far has been on aerobic exercise training, but it is important to highlight that resistance exercise training is also recommended on two to three days per week for individuals with CVD. Resistance exercise training should be included for improved muscle strength; however, isometric exercises (exercises in which a contraction is maintained or held in one position) should generally be avoided because they can lead to excessive increases in blood pressure. The intensity should generally be moderate. Remember to breathe normally while lifting (i.e., don't hold

▮ Q&A

Are there any special exercise considerations for those with high cholesterol or high blood pressure?

The general principles of the exercise prescription detailed in this chapter also apply to individuals with dyslipidemia (i.e., high cholesterol). However, typically, healthy weight maintenance is emphasized for individuals with high cholesterol. This means that caloric expenditure during the exercise session should be increased; in general, this is accomplished by exercising five or more days per week (rather than only three times) and exercising for 50 to 60 minutes per session (rather than 20 to 30 minutes).

Individuals with high blood pressure also benefit from regular exercise. Each exercise session can lead to a reduction in blood pressure; therefore near-daily or daily exercise is recommended (five to seven days per week). Moderate exercise intensity is also recommended; high-intensity exercise is not needed to derive the blood pressure–lowering effect of exercise. However, since blood pressure can decline immediately after exercise, an active cool-down is important to prevent blood pressure from declining too much.

your breath when lifting). For those with high cholesterol or high blood pressure, typically two to four sets of 8 to 12 repetitions for each of the major muscles groups are recommended (2). For additional information on resistance training and examples of exercises for the various muscle groups, see chapter 6.

Flexibility training is also beneficial for all adults, including those with CVD. In addition, although there are no recommendations unique to persons with CVD, inclusion of neuromotor exercise may be considered as part of a general exercise program. More information on flexibility and neuromotor exercises is presented in chapters 7 and 8 (2).

While the focus of this section is on the components of a structured exercise program, it is important to adopt a physically active lifestyle in general. Sedentary behaviors (i.e., a lot of sitting) can be detrimental, even in people who exercise regularly. Pedometers are one way to help promote regular physical activity, and most guidelines suggest a reasonable goal of 5,400 to 7,900 steps per day (2).

Influence of Medications

Sometimes lifestyle changes—the front line in cardiovascular risk reduction—are just not enough. You may need adjunctive drug therapy to better control certain risk factors. Of course, taking medication(s) does not take the place of the positive lifestyle modifications discussed in this chapter. Keep focused on heart-healthy nutrition choices and regular physical activity, understanding that medications may be needed in addition to those lifestyle behaviors to achieve goals.

Although a detailed description of cardioprotective drugs is outside the scope of this chapter, this section discusses medications used to address high cholesterol and high blood pressure. With any medication, additional considerations are the potential for interactions with food or other medications and for side effects or adverse reactions. Because of the complexity of this issue, ongoing consultation with your health care provider and pharmacist is recommended.

Lipid-Lowering Medications

Various types of drugs can be used to lower cholesterol, and they act on the body in differing ways. Many of the lipid-lowering drugs affect activity in the liver, so liver function should be routinely checked as a precaution against liver damage. One class of lipid-lowering medications is the statin drugs. Statins are powerful medications used to treat high blood cholesterol levels. These drugs block cholesterol production in the liver. Because the body needs a certain amount of cholesterol to function, it compensates by drawing on cholesterol present in the bloodstream. This reduces the amount of cholesterol that could damage arteries. Statins do have a downside. In rare cases, statins can cause elevations in some liver enzymes and ultimately result in liver damage. Thus, patients who use statin medications should have their liver enzymes evaluated once or twice yearly. In addition, statins are associated with muscle inflammation, a condition called rhabdomyolysis. The usual complaint is muscle soreness or pain. When someone who is exercising is taking a statin, muscle discomfort or pain may be a result of the medication and not the exercise. If you take a statin and notice any uncommon muscle discomfort or pain, report it to your health care provider.

Blood Pressure–Lowering Medications

Health care providers use several classes of medication to lower blood pressure, and most individuals with hypertension take more than one to control blood pressure.

Beta-blockers are one such medication. In addition, beta-blockers are used to relieve angina (chest discomfort) and to ward off heart rhythm disturbances. Beta-blockers decrease the work of the heart by inhibiting the activity of the sympathetic nervous system, which is responsible for increasing heart rate and blood pressure. Thus, both heart rate and blood pressure are suppressed in individuals taking beta-blockers. As a result, heart rate ranges are often not used to set intensity. An option to consider is the use of the relative scale (e.g., working at a level 5 on a 10-point scale) as discussed in chapter 5.

Other common medications used to help lower blood pressure include the following:

- Diuretics, commonly referred to as water pills, which increase urine output
- Angiotensin-converting enzyme (ACE) inhibitors, which block the production of a hormone that can elevate blood pressure
- Calcium channel blockers, which relax blood vessels

These medications lower blood pressure through different mechanisms of action. How each person responds to a given medication varies, so your health care provider will choose the most appropriate medication(s) for you. Your response will be monitored, and often dosage or type of medication will be adjusted to achieve blood pressure goals.

As reviewed in this chapter, a healthy diet and regular physical activity are both critical to achieve optimal cardiovascular health. Positive lifestyle choices are especially important for those with CVD, including heart disease and stroke. Proper diet and regular exercise favorably influence multiple risk factors and therefore lower your risk for disease. Adopting a healthy lifestyle will cause you to feel better, have more energy, and have an improved quality of life.

THIRTEEN

Diabetes

Diabetes is a common disease that is characterized by elevated blood glucose. More casually, this is often referred to as high blood sugar. Normally, after you eat, some of the food is broken down into glucose (a sugar) and is transported through the body in the bloodstream. This increase in blood glucose triggers the pancreas, a small organ in the abdomen, to release insulin. Insulin is a hormone needed to move the glucose into the body cells to either be used or be stored as energy for later use. In general, diabetes results from your body's inability to produce insulin (type 1) or to use the insulin properly to lower blood glucose levels to normal (type 2) (2).

Over 29 million Americans have some type of diabetes, and another estimated 86 million people have prediabetes, or slightly elevated blood glucose levels (44). Approximately 90 percent of people with diabetes have type 2. The remaining 10 percent have type 1 diabetes, which tends to occur in younger people, although it can develop at any age. Other categories of diabetes exist, including gestational diabetes, which occurs during pregnancy (2).

If you are reading this chapter, either you have diabetes or someone important to you does. After diagnosis, it's common to feel shocked, concerned, frustrated, sad, angry, or a combination of emotions. A diabetes diagnosis, however, can be an opportunity to examine how to take charge of your health. Although there is no magic wand to make diabetes disappear, exercise and attention to proper nutrition are two vital factors in managing diabetes and preventing its possible health complications. Exercise is the mainstay of treatment to improve insulin resistance and the effectiveness of any diabetes medications that you take (43). Diet, along with exercise, is also important in managing all types of diabetes and even potentially preventing type 2 diabetes (3). This chapter addresses how to safely include physical activity in your life and provides general nutrition guidelines for diabetes management. Insulin and various oral or other diabetes medications are discussed as well.

Causes of Diabetes

The origin of type 1 diabetes differs from that of type 2 diabetes. Type 1 diabetes is an autoimmune disease, which occurs when your body attacks its own cells (2). In type 1 diabetes, the cells in the pancreas that produce insulin are destroyed. Thus, insulin cannot be produced to lower your blood glucose after meals and snacks. As a result, blood glucose is not able to enter the cells, causing glucose levels in the blood to become elevated. A high level of glucose in the blood is called hyperglycemia. *Hyper-* means a high level, and *glycemia* refers to blood glucose concentrations. As a result of the deficiency in insulin production, type 1 diabetes must be treated with insulin, given as injections, delivered via an insulin pump, or sometimes inhaled.

Type 2 diabetes occurs when body cells cannot properly use the insulin produced by the pancreas (2). This is called insulin resistance (i.e., impaired insulin action in which body cells are resistant to the action of insulin). Insulin normally allows glucose to enter cells in the body to provide energy; but with insulin resistance, the glucose cannot enter the cells and thus remains in the blood. In type 2 diabetes, the body's ability to produce insulin usually decreases over time, which also contributes to hyperglycemia. As a result, some people with type 2 diabetes must also take supplemental insulin to control their blood glucose levels.

Obesity is associated with the development of type 2 diabetes, in particular upper body fat stores (i.e., an apple-shaped physique) (43). In the past, type 2 diabetes was called adult-onset diabetes because of the typically older age of onset. Unfortunately, the increased incidence of obesity and sedentary lifestyles has resulted in type 2 diabetes developing at earlier ages (6), thus exposing people to elevated blood glucose for longer periods of time and increasing their risk of health complications, such as kidney, eye, nerve, and heart disease. Other factors in addition to excessive body weight and inactivity increase the chances of developing diabetes (2):

- Prediabetes (see the sidebar How Do I Know If I Have Prediabetes or Diabetes?)
- Age (greater than 45 years old)
- Family history (parent or sibling)
- Other health concerns, including low high-density lipoprotein cholesterol, high triglycerides, high blood pressure

How Do I Know If I Have Prediabetes or Diabetes?

Blood glucose exists on a continuum from normal to elevated (diabetes). Prediabetes is diagnosed when the fasting blood glucose is above normal (greater than 100 mg/dL) but below the cutoff for diagnosing diabetes (126 mg/dL) (2). If your glucose level is in this range, you are at a higher risk for cardiovascular disease in addition to developing type 2 diabetes (33). Although a diagnosis of prediabetes increases your risk, it does not mean that type 2 diabetes is unavoidable or that prediabetes is not reversible. Losing weight and increasing your physical activity level will not only lower your risk for cardiovascular disease but also decrease your likelihood of progressing to fully developed type 2 diabetes (32). Losing at little as 5 percent of body weight (for example, 10 pounds [4.5 kg] for someone weighing 200 pounds [~90 kg]) has been found to decrease the risk of developing type 2 diabetes and other obesity-related complications in people who are overweight (35).

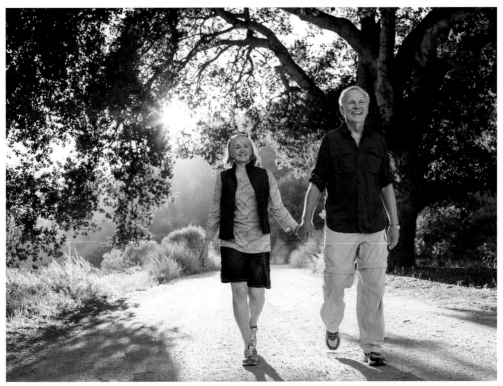

Exercise plays a pivotal role in preventing as well as managing diabetes.

- Certain racial and ethnic groups, including non-Hispanic blacks, Hispanic Americans, Asian Americans and Pacific Islanders, American Indians, and Alaska Natives
- Women who had gestational diabetes or have had a baby weighing 9 pounds (4 kg) or more at birth

Although a number of factors cannot be changed (e.g., your race or age), you can control your body weight and physical activity level. These factors are the focus of this chapter.

Healthy Approaches to Managing Diabetes

Physical activity and diet are two important lifestyle factors for anyone with type 1 or type 2 diabetes. This section discusses how both exercise and nutrition can help you manage your diabetes as well as improve your health and fitness.

Focusing on Nutrition

Weight loss may be a useful goal for people with type 2 diabetes who are overweight, and preventing excessive weight gain if you have type 1 diabetes can help keep your insulin action high and your insulin needs lower (9). Sustaining a weight loss of as little as 5 to 7 percent of body weight can lead to a decrease in insulin resistance and improvement in blood glucose control, therefore allowing for a reduction in the amount of medication taken (37). Weight management is discussed in detail in chapter

18; therefore the nutrition focus in this chapter is on the benefits of balancing carbohydrates, fats, and proteins in your diet to control blood glucose levels.

Dietary Macronutrients

The three macronutrients that provide energy for activity and routine body functioning are carbohydrates, fats, and proteins. Everyone, including persons with diabetes, benefits from an appropriate balance of these three nutrients. Obviously, because diabetes results from a break in the link between food eaten and the body cells receiving energy, diet is a major consideration in managing diabetes. Food choices do not need to be a frustrating mystery—just giving your diet some extra attention will allow for better control of the disease.

The macronutrients supply your body with energy or calories, although each of these nutrients has a different primary role. Protein helps to build muscle, while fat is important as a source of stored energy and contributes to the health of your brain, nerves, hair, skin, and nails. Carbohydrate is a major fuel source for your body, especially during physical activity, and is the primary supplier of energy for your brain, nerves, and muscles.

While each of these nutrients affects your blood glucose in different ways, carbohydrates in your diet have the greatest impact on the amount of glucose in your blood because they are turned into glucose quickly. You should check your blood glucose before and after meals to learn how foods affect your blood levels, particularly those containing a lot of carbohydrate (such as potatoes, bread, rice, and pasta). Focus on keeping portion sizes in check, which is helpful if weight loss is a goal and also helps manage your blood glucose levels by providing a good balance of carbohydrate, fat, and protein.

Fiber Intake

Dietary fiber, found in plant-based foods, is also a critical component of the meal plan for anyone with diabetes. Fiber cannot be digested completely because it resists acids and other digestive enzymes in the stomach and thus does not add extra calories to your diet. Fiber is found in foods such as oats, oat bran, ground flaxseed, beans and fruits, wheat bran, apple peel, and most vegetables.

Dietary fiber has many health and metabolic benefits (39). Fiber adds bulk and helps move food waste out of the body more quickly. Fiber also helps you feel full and can support your weight loss efforts. From a diabetes and health standpoint, dietary fiber may reduce blood glucose and cholesterol, all while slowing the digestion of carbohydrates to glucose, thereby keeping your blood glucose more stable. A high intake of dietary fiber, specifically cereal and fruit fiber, has been shown to lower the risk of heart disease by trapping fat and cholesterol during the digestive process and eliminating cholesterol through the stools. A good target intake is at least 20 to 35 grams of fiber per day.

Carbohydrate Intake

Your first reaction might be to avoid carbohydrates as a way to keep your blood glucose levels in check, but your body needs the fiber that is found in carbohydrate-based plant foods. Carbohydrates are also your body's first choice of fuels during many physical activities, and not having enough in your diet may limit your ability to exercise optimally. Many people with diabetes count the grams of carbohydrate in foods to help

How can I know how much carbohydrate is in a food item?

To determine the grams of carbohydrate in a given product, consult the package label. Be sure to check the serving size because serving sizes can be quite small—you may actually consume more than just one serving in a meal. For more details on reading food labels, see chapter 3.

---

them control their blood glucose levels, and others choose carbohydrates based on the glycemic index (how rapidly the food item raises blood glucose levels) (8). The exact amount of carbohydrate you should consume varies based on how active you are, the medications you take, and your overall insulin action. Typically, starches and sugars are factored into your daily total, whereas fiber and nonstarchy vegetables are not. Examples of nonstarchy vegetables are salad greens, peppers, tomatoes, beans, carrots, cauliflower, and onions.

As you review food labels for the number of carbohydrates in a given product, you may run across "sugar-free" products that contain sugar alcohols, which are reduced-calorie sweeteners (usually about half the number of calories of sugar). Your blood glucose response to different products may vary; but in general, sugar alcohols (like sorbitol) have less of an impact on your blood glucose level than other carbohydrates. Although helpful in reducing calories and the effect on your blood glucose, sugar alcohols are not completely calorie-free and may cause a laxative effect or other intestinal symptoms in some people.

Along with carbohydrates, do not forget to include proteins as well as fats to balance your meals, manage your body weight, and control your blood glucose levels most effectively. If your goal is to lose weight, the calories you consume must be less than the calories your body uses for basic functions, daily activities, and exercise. If some of your diabetes medications are causing you to gain weight (or keeping you from losing weight), talk to your health care provider about which medications may help you lose weight while controlling your blood glucose.

Focusing on Physical Activity

Exercise plays a pivotal role in preventing as well as managing diabetes. Potentially of even greater importance is the role that exercise can play in preventing the complications often associated with diabetes; the benefits of exercise for those who have diabetes are well documented (12, 45). Health care providers often prescribe exercise for type 1 and type 2 diabetes in conjunction with medication, or exercise alone for type 2 diabetes (16). Exercise can not only improve blood glucose levels and glycated hemoglobin or HbA1c levels (see Blood Glucose Control and A1c), but also reduce blood pressure and cholesterol levels, decrease the risk of heart disease, promote weight loss, improve brain function, and enhance self-image. Exercise may also reduce the amount of oral diabetic medications or the amount of insulin you require (3). Exercise needs to be continued to be effective; once it is suspended, the physiological benefits related to the control of blood glucose are lost within days (25).

Type 1 diabetes requires that blood glucose levels be fairly well controlled before exercise (46). When glucose levels are poorly controlled, the liver's production of glucose

Blood Glucose Control and A1c

Hemoglobin is a protein found inside red blood cells that carries oxygen around the body. When blood glucose levels are high (as with diabetes), hemoglobin links with glucose that enters the red blood cells. This is referred to as glycated hemoglobin or HbA1c (or commonly just A1c) (2). The higher the glucose levels in the blood are, the greater the A1c percentage is. Since red blood cells have a limited lifespan, looking at A1c levels can give a picture of the average glucose control over two to three months. A1c cannot be used to check short-term glucose levels (you need to use your blood glucose meter for those checks) but rather gives more of an overall picture. The A1c for someone without diabetes is 4 to 6 percent, but in those with diabetes it can be elevated to 10 percent or higher if glucose levels are out of control. Your health care provider will help you establish a target value; generally, well-controlled glucose is evident by an A1c less than 7 percent. Exercise is particularly important in improving A1c levels. In general, for every 1 percentage point drop in A1c, you can reduce the microvascular complications that affect the eyes, kidneys, and nerves by 40 percent (4).

increases, which can result in higher blood glucose levels during exercise. Higher blood glucose levels can also occur transiently after very intense exercise, such as sprinting or heavy resistance training (47). When blood glucose levels are controlled, moderate-intensity exercise can reduce blood glucose by increasing blood flow to the muscles, which increases the rate of glucose absorption into the cells (20).

Type 2 diabetes involves dual defects in insulin action (i.e., manner in which insulin helps cells take up glucose from the blood) and insulin secretion (i.e., body's ability to secrete insulin) (2). Exercise plays a major role in the control of type 2 diabetes (15). Being active significantly improves insulin action, and it decreases the amount of insulin needed for your body to lower blood glucose levels. Even in insulin users, improved insulin action can lead to decreases in the amount of insulin needed (46). Weight loss can also decrease abdominal fat, which can further improve insulin action and overall blood glucose levels.

Exercise is also well known to help prevent the onset of diabetes. People who have prediabetes and a family history of diabetes should focus on both diet and exercise to promote weight loss as a way to prevent type 2 diabetes. In one well-known study, the Diabetes Prevention Program, people who had a high probability of developing diabetes reduced their risk by 58 percent as a result of lifestyle interventions that included daily exercise, changes in diet, and average weight loss of about 12 pounds (5.4 kg) (32).

Precautions for Exercise

Do you need to see your doctor before you start to exercise? To determine this, follow preparticipation screening recommendations (see figures 2.1 and 2.2). In general, medical clearance is recommended if you have any signs or symptoms of disease, if you haven't been regularly active (even if you have no signs or symptoms of disease), or if you are desiring to increase your current exercise program from moderate to vigorous intensity (36). Whether you need medical clearance before beginning or whether the screening in chapter 2 indicates that this is not necessary, recognize the value of regular moderate to vigorous activity in actually reducing your risk of a heart attack (even if you have already had one) while realizing and respecting your limitations (15, 40).

If you have preexisting microvascular disease complications (eye, kidney, or nerve disease) or macrovascular disease (disease of the large blood vessels, such as those of the heart), you should not start a vigorous exercise program without being evaluated by a health care professional first. Your doctor may want you to have a cardiac stress test (i.e., treadmill test during which your heart rhythm is monitored) before exercising, particularly if you (15)

- are planning on participating in vigorous activities, not just easy or moderate ones;
- are over 40 years old (or over 30 if any of the following apply to you);
- have had diabetes for more than 10 years;
- have heart disease, a strong family history of heart disease, or high cholesterol;
- have poor circulation in your feet or legs (or lower leg pain while walking);
- have diabetic eye disease; kidney disease; numbness, burning, tingling, or loss of sensation in your feet; or dizziness when going from sitting to standing;
- have not consistently controlled your blood glucose levels well; or
- have any other concerns about exercising, including joint pain, arthritis, or other chronic health problems.

Some medical conditions related to diabetes may also influence exercise choices, including diabetic retinopathy, peripheral neuropathy, and nephropathy. Annual dilated eye exams done by an ophthalmologist can determine if you have any eye problems and should be considered before the start of a vigorous exercise program (5). Diabetic retinopathy is a disease affecting the retina of the eye. If this disease is present, certain activities should be avoided to prevent further damage (15). Mild background retinopathy will not affect your exercise choices, but if you have moderate nonproliferative diabetic retinopathy you will need to avoid exercises that unduly affect blood

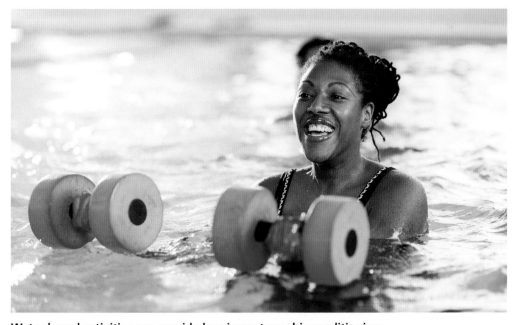

Water-based activities can provide low-impact aerobic conditioning.

pressure (e.g., heavy resistance training) (16). Avoid contact sports and heavy lifting if you have severe nonproliferative retinopathy. Anyone with unstable proliferative diabetic retinopathy should focus on low-impact cardiorespiratory exercises like walking, swimming, and stationary cycling, and people should never do any exercise if they have a retinal hemorrhage.

Another potential concern is peripheral neuropathy, which is nerve damage that can alter the sensation of the hands and feet as well as your balance (17). Falls are more common with this condition, as are joint and soft tissue injuries. Proper footwear is a must to prevent blisters or ulcers. Inspect your feet both before and after exercise for blisters or ulcers, using a mirror placed on the floor under your foot if that makes it easier for you to see. If you have had foot ulcers or foot deformities, schedule an

Precautions for Exercising With Diabetes

Having diabetes and engaging in physical activity requires some precautions to make sure that exercise is safe and effective. Follow these guidelines to get the most out of being active with diabetes:

- Have a blood glucose meter accessible to check your glucose level before, possibly during, and after exercise, or if you have any symptoms of low blood glucose.
- Immediately treat any hypoglycemia during or following exercise with quickly absorbed carbohydrates like glucose tablets, dextrose-based candy, or regular soft drinks.
- Inform your exercise partners about your diabetes, and show them how to give you glucose or another carbohydrate should you need assistance.
- Stay properly hydrated with frequent intake of small amounts of cool water, and take in adequate fluids before exercising, particularly if your blood glucose levels are elevated.
- Consult with your physician before exercising with any of the following conditions:
  - Proliferative retinopathy or active retinal hemorrhage (eye disease)
  - Neuropathy (nerve damage), either peripheral or autonomic
  - Foot injuries (including ulcers)
  - High blood pressure
  - Serious illness or infection
- Seek immediate medical attention for chest pain or any pain that radiates down your arm, jaw, or neck and for serious indigestion, any of which may indicate a lack of blood to your heart and a possible heart attack.
- If you have high blood pressure, avoid activities that cause blood pressure to go up dramatically, such as heavy weight training, head-down exercises, and anything requiring breath holding.
- Wear proper footwear and check your feet daily for signs of trauma, such as blisters, redness, or other irritation.
- Immediately stop exercising if you experience bleeding into your eyes caused by active, unstable proliferative retinopathy.
- Wear a diabetes medic alert bracelet or necklace with your physician's name and contact information on it.
- Carry a cell phone with you so that you can call someone for assistance if needed.

appointment with a podiatrist to be measured for shoes that fit well. Lower-impact activities, such as swimming and stationary biking, are preferred in these cases to limit complications, although aquatic activities are not an option with unhealed ulcers (17).

Since diabetes may also result in nephropathy (kidney damage), a kidney evaluation before starting an exercise program is suggested. One sign of kidney damage is the presence of proteins in the urine. Kidney damage can be exacerbated by strenuous activity because of the sudden increases in blood pressure, leading to further damage to kidney function (29). Blood pressure medications called angiotensin-converting enzyme (ACE) inhibitors or angiotensin receptor blockers protect kidney function and may be considered when one is faced with these conditions (24).

Although avoiding hypoglycemia is the goal, at times your blood glucose levels may drop. Always have some easily absorbed sources of glucose with you. When glucose levels are low (less than 70 mg/dL), consume a glucose-containing product that will rapidly become available in your blood (e.g., glucose tablets, hard candies, regular soda, or juice). Since fat and protein slow down the movement of glucose from the intestine into the blood, other snacks such as peanut butter and crackers or granola bars are better to use once glucose levels have risen or to prevent a later drop. To avoid overshooting and becoming hyperglycemic, a general recommendation is to consume 15 to 20 grams of carbohydrate and then wait 15 minutes to see how much your blood glucose level rises (13). If your glucose is still low, repeat the process. Letting those with whom you exercise know about your diabetes is important just in case your glucose levels drop so low that you become unconscious. If this happens, they can call for emergency assistance.

To avoid hypoglycemia, be consistent with your carbohydrate intake with regard to meal timing and exercise. Maintaining a regular time of day for your exercise routine is also helpful, and monitoring your blood glucose before and after exercise is a good idea especially if you take insulin or other oral medications that stimulate insulin release. If your exercise bout is prolonged, you may also want to check your blood glucose level during exercise if possible. Keeping blood glucose between 100 and 250 mg/dL (and no higher) optimizes safety by helping you avoid both hypoglycemia and hyperglycemia (14).

In individuals taking insulin or oral medications that increase the body's insulin secretion, physical activity can cause hypoglycemia if medication dose or carbohydrate consumption is not altered. Individuals on these therapies may need to ingest some added carbohydrate if preexercise glucose levels are <100 mg/dL (5.6 mmol/L), depending on whether they can lower insulin levels during the workout (e.g., with an insulin pump or reduced preexercise insulin dosage), the time of day exercise is done, and the intensity and duration of the activity. Hypoglycemia is less common in diabetic patients who are not treated with insulin or medications that cause insulin release, and no preventive measures for hypoglycemia are usually advised in these cases. Intense activities may actually raise blood glucose levels instead of lowering them (2).

You should also take special care if you exercise later in the day due to the potential for hypoglycemia to occur following the exercise session after you have gone to bed for the night, especially if you use insulin. Delayed-onset hypoglycemia is a phenomenon that typically occurs 6 to 15 hours after exercise (36). It appears to be a result of the liver and muscles replenishing their glucose stores after exercise. This underscores the need to monitor your blood glucose during that time and to eat an extra snack if necessary. If you need a snack, it should contain both carbohydrate (about 15 grams)

Effects of Blood Glucose on Exercise: Hypoglycemia

What you eat and when you eat are especially important for managing your glucose levels during exercise. Exercise itself helps to move glucose from the blood into the working muscles, but this also opens the possibility of blood glucose dropping too low. This is referred to as hypoglycemia (*hypo-* means low, and *glycemia* refers to blood glucose). Symptoms of hypoglycemia are as follows:

Shakiness	Hunger
Weakness	Headache
Abnormal sweating	Visual disturbances
Heart palpitations (fast heart rate)	Mental dullness
Nervousness	Confusion
Anxiety	Seizures
Tingling of the mouth and fingers	Coma

Checking your blood glucose on a regular basis is key to managing your diabetes and ensuring safety when exercising. Handheld glucose meters require only a small drop of blood and provide an immediate digital reading of your blood glucose level (see figure 13.1 for an example of a glucose monitor). Make a habit of checking your glucose before and after exercise.

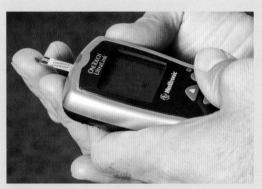

FIGURE 13.1 Glucose monitors provide quick feedback on blood glucose levels.

and protein (7 to 8 grams) to have a more lasting effect (30). Consult with your health care provider to solidify your plan of action based on your type of diabetes as well as the medications you are taking.

If you take insulin or are on a medication that stimulates insulin release (e.g., sulfonylureas or meglitinides; see table 13.4 later in this chapter for more information), be sure to check your glucose level before exercise. If your blood glucose level is low before an exercise bout (less than 100 mg/dL), you may need to consume some carbohydrate to avoid hypoglycemia during exercise, especially if you use insulin; but this really depends on how you manage your insulin doses and timing and the type of activity you do (47). Depending on the duration and intensity of your exercise session, you may need to take in additional carbohydrate and other food before, during, and after exercise to prevent hypoglycemia (14, 31).

On the opposite end of the spectrum from hypoglycemia is hyperglycemia, or high blood glucose. With type 1 diabetes, if your blood glucose is elevated (greater than 250 to 300 mg/dL), you may need to postpone or at least decrease the intensity of the exercise session (see figure 13.2 for a decision-making flowchart). You can base your decision on how you are feeling as well as whether you have ketones in your urine. Ketones make your blood more acidic, potentially causing ketoacidosis, a condition

■ Q&A

What is diabetic ketoacidosis, and how can I avoid it?

When your blood glucose levels remain elevated, the glucose needed for energy cannot enter your cells. As a result, fat is used for energy, resulting in the production of ketones (acids), which first build up in the blood and eventually also appear in the urine. You can check for ketones with a simple at-home urine test.

Situations that may result in ketones include insufficient insulin or inadequate calorie intake. Usually, ketoacidosis develops slowly, but if you become sick and are vomiting, it could develop within a few hours. Early signs include thirst or a dry mouth, frequent urination, high glucose levels, and high ketones in the urine. Over time other symptoms may appear, including constant feelings of tiredness, dry or flushed skin, nausea or vomiting, fruity-smelling breath, and confusion. Diabetic ketoacidosis is a serious medical condition, and if you have these signs or symptoms, drink plenty of water and contact your health care provider immediately (10).

---

that, if ignored, can cause coma and death (see What Is Diabetic Ketoacidosis, and How Can I Avoid It? for more information). Ketoacidosis is more commonly found with type 1 diabetes than with type 2 diabetes.

The American Diabetes Association suggests the following general guidelines to help keep your glucose levels in check (3):

- Avoid physical activity if your blood glucose is greater than 250 mg/dL and you have ketones in your blood or urine.

- Use caution if your glucose is above 300 mg/dL even if ketones are not present.

If your blood glucose level is elevated but you find no ketones in your urine and you feel well, then moderate-intensity exercise is appropriate and may actually be helpful in lowering your blood glucose level. However, if you have ketones in your urine, you should postpone exercise and contact your health care provider if you have not already

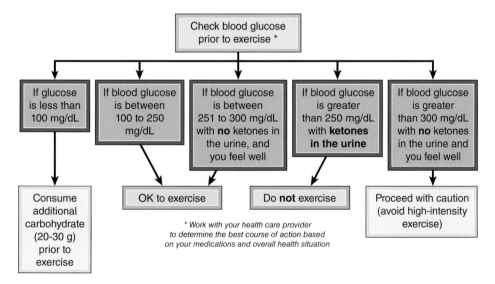

FIGURE 13.2 Decision-making flowchart for exercise for people with type 1 diabetes.

established a response plan for such situations. Often, treatment includes the administration of insulin to regain normal glucose levels, along with adequate hydration (10).

For type 2 diabetes, additional carbohydrate is not typically needed before exercise because hypoglycemia is not common unless one is being treated with insulin or insulin-stimulating medications (see the previous recommendations on carbohydrate consumption if these medications are included in your treatment plan). Other medications (e.g., metformin, thiazolidinediones, and alpha-glucosidase inhibitors) do not tend to cause hypoglycemia and thus do not require that you take in additional carbohydrate. With regard to hyperglycemia and type 2 diabetes, when ketones are present, vigorous exercise should be avoided. However, light to moderate exercise may actually help lower your blood glucose levels, especially if the high glucose level occurs after a meal (18). The American Diabetes Association suggests that as long as you feel well, are adequately hydrated, and have no ketones in your urine, it is not necessary to postpone exercise based on hyperglycemia alone. To optimize your safety when exercising, discuss your medical situation, including the medications you are taking, with your health care provider so you will know what steps are most appropriate for you.

Physical Activity Recommendations

All physical activity you do during the day counts toward your daily total. Until recently, it was believed that vigorous exercise was required for optimal health and fitness. While you may stand to gain more health benefits from harder workouts, almost any activity (including golfing, gardening, mowing the lawn, moderate walking) done for 30 to 45 minutes per day is also beneficial to your health. Furthermore, lower-intensity exercises are beneficial even if you do them for only 10 minutes at a time. The latest research shows benefits from simply breaking up sedentary time with any activity, even standing, once in a while (19). Start by standing up or walking around for 5 minutes after each hour that you spend doing something sedentary.

Exercise comes in many forms, and your structured exercise program should be tailored to your situation. Although your age and type of diabetes may call for different exercise programs, the goal is the same—to improve health outcomes. Following appropriate screening and armed with blood glucose monitoring skills, you are ready to get started. A complete exercise program should include aerobic activities, resistance training, and flexibility exercise, and even some balance training if you are over 40 years old.

Aerobic Exercise   Aerobic activities, which help improve the efficiency of the cardiovascular system, can be beneficial for regulating blood glucose levels. Examples include walking, jogging, swimming, and biking. If you cannot do weight-bearing or high-impact activities, chair exercises, water aerobics, and recumbent biking can be beneficial. Table 13.1 presents recommendations for type 1 and type 2 diabetes based on the FITT principle discussed in chapter 5, which addresses frequency, intensity, time, and type of activities (11, 15).

Working up to daily aerobic activity has benefits for both type 1 and type 2 diabetes (7, 27). For people with type 1, daily physical activity helps maintain the balance between insulin doses and food consumed. For those with type 2 diabetes, the focus is on burning calories and weight management, but improving overall fitness levels is also important for long-term health. Keep in mind that the recommendations in table 13.1 are targets, not initial levels. If you are just starting out, begin gradually because your body needs to adapt to the exercise, and you also have to monitor how your

TABLE 13.1 Aerobic Training Recommendations for People With Diabetes

	Type 1	Type 2
Frequency	Three to seven days per week	Three to seven days per week
Intensity	Moderate to vigorous	Moderate to vigorous (but may be low intensity to start)
Time	At least 150 min per week of moderate-intensity activity, 75 min of vigorous-intensity activity, or a combination of both intensities	At least 150 min per week of moderate- to vigorous-intensity activity
Type	Large-muscle group activities such as walking, biking, jogging, and water aerobics	Large-muscle group activities such as walking, biking, dancing, and water aerobics

Adapted by permission from American College of Sports Medicine, 2018.

blood glucose levels are affected. Consult chapter 5 for suggestions on beginning or advancing in your aerobic training program.

Resistance Training   Resistance training can lower A1c levels and confer other health benefits as well (see chapter 6 for more details on resistance training) (28). Including both aerobic exercise and resistance training can optimize the benefits related to managing your glucose levels (15, 21). A few precautions do need to be mentioned. If you have microvascular disease, be aware of the potential concerns about damage to the eyes, kidneys, and joints. Straining while lifting weights can lead to an increased risk of bleeding and retinal detachment for those with proliferative and severe nonproliferative eye disease. Resistance training may not be appropriate if you have unstable diabetic retinopathy. Also, be careful if you have nerve involvement; you are more susceptible to foot ulcers and bone damage because of the lack of sensation and weakening of the muscles and ligaments in the foot. If you have nephropathy (kidney damage) related to diabetes, strenuous activity can increase protein excretion. With these precautions in mind, you can implement a safe and effective resistance training program. Increasing your muscle mass while reducing fat tissue can decrease insulin resistance and improve blood glucose control. Having stronger muscles can also improve your balance, posture, ability to move, and daily functions.

The goal of resistance training is to focus on exercises involving the major muscle groups including the legs, back, chest, arms, shoulders, thighs, and abdominal area. Table 13.2 provides resistance training recommendations for type 1 and type 2 diabetes based on the FITT principle (15). Details regarding the many exercise options for resistance training are in chapter 6.

Flexibility   Flexibility is also an integral part of an exercise program for people with diabetes (26). Typically, static stretching is recommended. This involves placing the body into a position that creates tension in the muscles and holding that position for 15 to 30 seconds. Dynamic stretching done during movement can also work. Table 13.3 provides flexibility recommendations for persons with any type of diabetes based on the FITT principle (15). Details regarding stretching are found in chapter 7.

Balance Training   Particularly if you are middle-age or older, you will want to add one more activity to your weekly routine: functional fitness training that includes elements

TABLE 13.2   **Resistance Training Recommendations for People With Diabetes**

	Type 1	Type 2
Frequency	Two to three nonconsecutive days per week	Two to three nonconsecutive days per week
Intensity	Moderate to vigorous	Low to moderate to start, working up to moderate to vigorous
Time	8 to 15 repetitions per exercise 8 to 10 different exercises One to three sets per exercise	8 to 15 repetitions per exercise 8 to 10 different exercises One to three sets per exercise
Type	Resistance machines and free weights	Resistance machines and free weights

Adapted by permission from American College of Sports Medicine, 2018.

TABLE 13.3   **Flexibility Recommendations for People With Diabetes**

	Type 1 and type 2
Frequency	Two to three days per week
Intensity	Stretch to the point of tightness (not pain)
Time	10 to 30 sec per stretch (or dynamic stretching for that amount of time) Two to four repetitions per stretch
Type	Four or five exercises for both the upper and lower body (can be static or dynamic)

Adapted by permission from American College of Sports Medicine, 2018.

of balance training (23). Everyone starts to lose some natural balance with aging, but having diabetes can accelerate the loss and increase your risk of falling and losing your ability to live independently well into your later years (38). If you lose any of the feeling in your feet, this can alter the way you walk (your gait) and increase your risk, and having autonomic neuropathy that makes you dizzy when you stand up also raises your risk. Balance training can be as simple as practicing standing on one leg at a time. Resistance training that works the lower body or the core muscles improves your ability to balance while standing and walking. In addition, flexibility exercises that work the full range of motion around your joints can improve balance, as well as some alternative activities like tai chi and yoga. Even taking up dancing can help you stay on your feet at any age.

Influence of Medications

Diabetes can be controlled with the appropriate use of medications, including oral and injected medications (for type 2) as well as insulin injections (for type 1 mainly but also for some with type 2). A general understanding of how these medications work will help you see how they can fit into your total treatment plan.

Oral and Injected Medications for Type 2 Diabetes

Oral medications are the most common treatment for type 2 diabetes, but a few newer ones are taken by injection. In some situations, insulin, or a combination of insulin and other diabetes medications, is used to better control blood glucose levels (34, 42).

Several classes of medications are used to treat type 2 diabetes. Table 13.4 includes general information on how the medications work as well as some special considerations.

TABLE 13.4 Oral and Injected Medications for Type 2 Diabetes

Drug class	Primary mechanism	Possible side effects	Contraindications*	Comments
Biguanides	Decrease liver production of glucose and decrease insulin resistance	Diarrhea, stomach upset, lactic acidosis	Kidney disease as determined by creatinine in the urine greater than 1.5 mg/dL in males or greater than 1.4 mg/dL in females; liver disease and severe congestive heart failure	May cause weight loss; typically do not cause hypoglycemia
Sulfonylureas	Stimulate insulin release	Hypoglycemia	Caution warranted with sulfa allergies	Older adults may need lower doses; can cause exercise-related hypoglycemia
Meglitinides	Stimulate insulin release after a meal	Hypoglycemia	Use with caution in patients with hepatic or renal impairments	Take before meals; can be used by pregnant women; can cause hypoglycemia if exercise occurs soon after meals
DPP-4 inhibitors	Decrease liver production of glucose and stimulate insulin release	Usually well tolerated, but can cause upper respiratory tract infections and headaches	Reduce dose in anyone with kidney disease	Should not cause weight gain
Thiazolidinediones	Improve insulin sensitivity	Edema (swelling); weight gain; bone fractures with long-term use	Should not be used by people with congestive heart failure or liver abnormalities	Use lowest dose with insulin
Alpha-glucosidase inhibitors	Slow glucose absorption at the intestinal level	Diarrhea, abdominal pain, and flatulence	Avoid use in liver disease	Rarely used
GLP-1 agonists	Stimulate insulin release; inhibit the liver's release of glucose; delay stomach emptying	Mild to moderate nausea is common; diarrhea; headaches; dizziness	Stop use if gastrointestinal side effects are severe	When given as injection into the skin (subcutaneous), may aid in weight loss; may require dosage changes if combined with other medications that increase insulin levels
SGLT-2 inhibitors	Prevent kidneys from reabsorbing glucose, causing removal in the urine when above normal	Increased risk of urinary tract and yeast infections; dehydration; may lead to undetected ketoacidosis	Should never be used when blood or urinary ketones are elevated (ketoacidosis)	May aid in weight loss

*Consult with your doctor for other contraindications or considerations unique to your health situation.

Note: DPP-4 inhibitors = dipeptidyl peptidase-4 inhibitors, GLP-1 agonists = glucagon-like peptide-1 receptor agonists, SGLT-2 inhibitors = sodium-glucose transporter-2 inhibitors

As with all medications, there are side effects as well as situations in which certain medications may not be appropriate. Some of these issues are outlined in table 13.4.

For optimal outcomes, becoming more physically active and making other healthy lifestyle changes should be in conjunction with medication use. Exercise can contribute to weight loss, which can decrease insulin resistance and improve glucose tolerance. Exercise also increases insulin sensitivity and makes the body work more efficiently. In most people with well-controlled type 2 diabetes, most medications do not need to be adjusted for exercise. However, two classes of diabetes medications to watch closely are the sulfonylureas and the meglitinides, both of which can cause hypoglycemia (41). Insulin use also increases the risk of hypoglycemia. Discuss your exercise program with your health care provider to see if any of these medications need to be reduced on the days you exercise.

Frequent monitoring of blood glucose levels before, during, and after exercising is important to avoid potential problems (22). When you are exercising and losing weight, your overall medication doses may need to be decreased or discontinued. Work with your health care provider to adjust your medications (especially insulin if that is part of your treatment plan), instead of snacking and taking in more calories to prevent or treat hypoglycemia. When you are trying to lose weight, having to eat more to balance your glucose level will sabotage your efforts. Instead, enjoy the benefit of exercise for your body and be pleased that you have taken positive steps to decrease your reliance on medications.

Insulin Options for Diabetes

A number of types of insulin are used to treat type 1 and type 2 diabetes. Insulin must be injected; it cannot be consumed orally, although a new inhaled insulin (Afrezza) has been approved for use in people with type 2 diabetes. Insulin taken to provide background levels is called basal insulin, and what you use to cover meals or snacks is bolus insulin. One other option for delivering insulin is to use an insulin pump programmed to deliver basal and bolus doses.

The types of insulin are grouped based on their onset of action, time of peak activity, and duration of activity in the body. Details on these characteristics and common brands are listed in table 13.5. In general, rapid-acting and short-acting insulins have a relatively quick onset and time of peak action. These types of insulin are taken before meals and often need to be adjusted before exercise. The extent to which insulin

■ Q&A

What is an insulin pump, and how does it work?

Insulin pumps are small devices that are attached either directly to the body or indirectly via a tube (figure 13.3) to deliver insulin continuously throughout the day in a way intended to mimic the natural activity of the pancreas. Insulin levels can be adjusted up (when one is eating) or down (when one is being active) with a couple of button pushes. This gives users more flexibility with respect to timing meals as well as engaging in activity. For physically active people, the ability to more precisely administer insulin and reduce levels during and following exercise can make it easier to avoid hypoglycemia (13). In addition, the pump takes the place of separate insulin vials and syringes so it is much simpler to handle, especially for active, on-the-go people and youth.

should be decreased depends on the intensity of exercise. If activity occurs within 2 hours of eating, premeal insulin should be decreased 5 to 30 percent (5 percent for low-intensity exercise and 30 percent for high-intensity and long-duration exercise) (13). Intermediate-acting insulin has a longer onset of action as well as longer duration. Unless you are engaging in prolonged exercise, intermediate-acting insulin often does not need to be adjusted. Long-acting basal insulin does not have much of a peak; rather, it provides a low but constant level of insulin for 24 hours or longer (depending on the type). Like intermediate-acting insulin, long-acting insulin may or may not need to be adjusted for exercise (before or afterward).

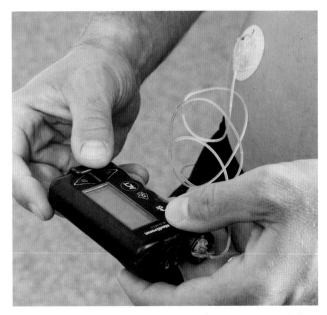

FIGURE 13.3   Insulin pumps are an alternate way to deliver insulin throughout the day.

Exercise is not recommended during peak insulin times unless doses are lowered before exercise or you eat extra carbohydrates to compensate (13, 14). The combination of the high levels of insulin and the glucose-lowering effect of exercise can lead to hypoglycemia unless you make adjustments. By monitoring your blood glucose levels (before, during, and after exercise), you can make additional adjustments to your food intake and insulin.

TABLE 13.5   Characteristics of Various Types of Insulin

Insulin type	Brand names	Onset	Peak	Duration
Rapid acting: Insulin aspart analog Insulin glulisine analog Insulin lispro analog	NovoLog Apidra Humalog	10 to 30 min	0.5 to 3 h	3 to 5 h
Short acting: Regular insulin	Humulin R Novolin R	30 min	1 to 5 h	8 h
Intermediate acting: Neutral Protamine Hagedorn (NPH) insulin	Humulin N Novolin R	1 to 4 h	4 to 12 h	14 to 26 h
Long acting (basal): Insulin detemir Insulin glargine	Levemir Lantus Toujeo (3× strength)	1 to 2 h	Minimal peak	Up to 24 h
Ultralong acting (basal): Insulin degludec	Tresiba	30 to 90 min	None	Over 24 h

Regular exercise and a sound nutritional plan are the two cornerstones of managing and thriving with diabetes. Your individualized exercise program should include aerobic activity as well as resistance training, stretching, and possibly balance training. Your exercise program should improve your health and blood glucose control without worsening or causing health-related complications. A health care provider or diabetes educator can be helpful with regard to making adjustments in medications and insulin when you are starting or expanding your exercise program. In addition, diet is a key part of managing blood glucose levels effectively. With type 1, balancing your intake of carbohydrate, fat, and protein will help you with sustained blood glucose control. With type 2 diabetes, attention to calories consumed is an asset for weight loss. A better diet is an essential complement to your exercise program to achieve the greatest possible control over your diabetes and your overall health.

FOURTEEN

Cancer

The cancer journey can begin many ways. For some, it begins with an abnormal screening test. For others, it begins with a symptom. Yet, for others, the journey begins with the diagnosis of a family member, followed by genetic testing. It was estimated that 1,658,370 Americans would be diagnosed with cancer in 2015 (2). Of these, it was estimated that 66.5 percent would live five or more years after their cancer diagnosis. For diagnoses of breast and prostate cancers, approximately 89 and 99 percent, respectively, of all incident cases are expected to live at least five years beyond their diagnosis. Five-year survival after endometrial, colon, and lung cancers is 82, 65, and 17 percent, respectively. These widely differing survival rates are a reflection of two realities. First, "cancer" should really be "cancers," plural. There are over 200 types of cancer. Further, progress in early detection and treatment success has varied greatly across these many different types of cancer. As a result, the population of 14.5 million cancer survivors alive in the United States today is tremendously diverse (7).

Causes of Cancer

Cancer occurs when a small number of cells in a particular body system begins to replicate more quickly than expected and without normal and expected planned cell death. All cells in the body replicate themselves, and all cells in the body should undergo planned cell death. When genetic changes occur, cells may begin to grow out of control. If the cells are replicating quickly and have no ability to spread to another part of the body, the growth (also called a tumor) is considered *benign*. If the cells have the characteristics that would allow them to grow beyond the tissue where they start, spreading through the blood or lymphatic vessels, the tumor is considered *malignant*. There are many reasons cells start to grow more quickly and fail to die as expected. People may have a gene mutation that was present at birth, passed on by a parent. An example is the BRCA1 and BRCA2 gene mutations. Both substantially increase the lifetime risk for breast and ovarian cancer among those who test positive for these mutations. Another reason for genetic changes that might contribute to the development of cancer is environmental. An example is exposure to asbestos and the development of mesothelioma.

Finally, there are lifestyle factors that explain the development of cancers as well. Cigarette smoking is the number one preventable cause of cancer. If you smoke and your goal with lifestyle change is to reduce your risk of cancer, quitting smoking should be your highest priority. In addition, it is estimated that one-third of all cancers in the United States are preventable with exercise, healthy eating, and weight control (9). Therefore, the exercise and nutrition information in this book is relevant for cancer prevention. It is also important to recognize that the reason any given person develops cancer is complex. People should not feel that they "caused" their cancer through their actions or inactions. This chapter focuses on how to recover the best possible function you can after a diagnosis of cancer.

Healthy Approaches to Managing Cancer

A diagnosis of cancer has been called a "teachable moment" with regard to developing and maintaining a healthy lifestyle. Published peer-reviewed evidence supports the benefits of healthful nutrition, weight control, and regular exercise for those who have had a diagnosis of cancer (10, 12, 16). This section outlines the benefits and provides guidelines on these lifestyle interventions. In addition, it provides guidance regarding preexercise precautions and evaluations, exercise prescription advice, and program suggestions for people currently undergoing treatment and those who have completed treatment. Two categories of concerns for cancer survivors are (1) persistent adverse treatment effects and (2) recurrence and survival; both of these are discussed.

Focusing on Nutrition

Every few years, the American Cancer Society (ACS) gathers a group of experts to discuss guidelines for nutrition (and physical activity) for people who have been diagnosed with cancer. The most recent publication from this process is from 2012 (12). The experts divide the nutrition guidance into sections: active treatment and recovery, living free of cancer or with stable disease, and living with advanced cancer. The most recent version of these guidelines from ACS is summarized in table 14.1 (12) and discussed in the following section.

If you are currently undergoing active treatment, your dietary focus should be on making sure you meet your nutrient and calorie needs, maintain a healthy body weight, avoid losing muscle mass, manage side effects related to nutrition, and improve quality of life. If you are struggling with any of these issues, ask for help. You can request that your doctor make a referral to a Registered Dietitian or another type of nutrition professional to help you as part of your cancer care team.

Many patients consider using nutritional supplements during cancer treatment. There are two things to know about nutritional supplements and cancer treatment outcomes. First, your doctor needs to know what you are using, given that some supplements may decrease the effectiveness of conventional treatments. Second, there is no evidence that nutritional supplements improve cancer treatment outcomes. In general, focus on getting your nutrients from food-based sources rather than supplements. During

TABLE 14.1   Guidelines for Nutrition After Cancer From the American Cancer Society

Time point during the cancer journey	Nutrition goals	Nutrition advice
During treatment and recovery	Focus on ensuring that all nutrient and calorie needs are met Maintain healthy weight Avoid losing muscle mass Prevent or manage nutrition-related side effects Improve quality of life	Consult with a Registered Dietitian or other qualified nutrition professional. Tell your doctor about any vitamin and mineral supplements you take (they may interfere with treatment).
Disease-free or living with stable disease	Set and achieve goals for weight management Be physically active Maintain healthy dietary patterns	Get to and stay at a healthy weight. Be active. Eat a variety of healthful foods from plant sources; limit the amount of processed meat and red meat you eat; eat 2½ cups or more of vegetables and fruits each day; choose whole grains rather than refined grain products.
Living with advanced cancer	Maintain well-being Improve quality of life Meet nutritional needs Change diet to address symptoms or side effects Maintain body weight	Consult with a Registered Dietitian or other qualified nutrition professional. Medicines are available to increase appetite if needed. Nutritional supplements can help maintain body weight.

recovery from treatment, there may still be symptoms and side effects of treatment that could be helped by specific nutritional interventions. Achieving and maintaining a healthy body weight remains important, whether this means losing or gaining weight. Nutrition counseling can assist with both of these issues.

When you are at the point of living disease-free or with stable disease, the ACS recommendations for achieving and maintaining a healthy body weight remain in place. There is increasing evidence that being overweight or obese is associated with a worse prognosis for people who have had a diagnosis of cancer. The nutrition guidance for cancer survivors is to eat a variety of healthy foods from plant sources, limit the amount of processed meat and red meat, consume 2.5 cups or more of vegetables and fruits each day, and choose whole grains rather than refined grain products.

For persons living with advanced cancer, the focus of nutrition guidance is on controlling symptoms and ensuring adequate calorie and nutrient intake. Medicines that can increase appetite might be used. The use of nutritional supplements and intravenous feeding can also be helpful in some patients with advanced cancer. The ACS website (www.cancer.org) has much more detailed information about the role of nutrition across the cancer journey, from diagnosis to prevention of cancer recurrence and for those living with advanced cancer (1).

Role of Exercise During the Cancer Journey

During the time period just before and after cancer diagnosis, exercise may be most useful for reducing the anxiety associated with waiting for test results. The journey continues with the active treatment period. For many people, the first type of cancer treatment is surgery, which sometimes occurs within weeks of diagnosis. Exercise can often continue right up until the day of surgery. The specific benefits of presurgical exercise are just beginning to be explored. The hypothesis is that exercise for even a few weeks before surgery may improve immediate surgical outcomes and decrease recovery time, including less time in the hospital.

During the time period immediately following surgery, the body needs to spend all of its energy healing. The rule of thumb for returning to exercise is anywhere from four to eight weeks after surgery, depending on your condition and the extent of the surgery. If adjuvant treatments such as radiation and chemotherapy are recommended, exercise can and should continue during this period. Exercise tolerance varies throughout the cycles of treatment. For example, if chemotherapy is received every three weeks, there may be a few days immediately after the infusion when exercise needs to be curtailed or even stopped. However, the recommendation from multiple leading organizations is that cancer patients continue to exercise throughout their treatment (10, 12, 16). At the end of chemotherapy or radiation treatment, some oral therapies may still be used. From this point and to the end of life, exercise is recommended and may be undertaken in a manner specifically designed to minimize adverse effects of treatment and maximize survival.

Focusing on Physical Activity

The benefits of exercise for persons who have had a diagnosis of cancer have been broadly documented and include both physical and psychosocial benefits (4, 5, 17). Hundreds of randomized controlled trials have been completed that document benefits of specific exercise regimens for specific outcomes (17). Exercise is like medicine in that it must be prescribed and dosed specifically for the outcome of interest. For example, low-intensity aerobic activity has been shown to improve fatigue and quality of life. However, to improve function and bone health may require strength training. To improve balance may require yet another type of activity (e.g., yoga). There is research to support the benefit of exercise on reducing risk for recurrence of breast and colon cancer as well (6).

ACSM, ACS, and National Comprehensive Cancer Network provide guidance for exercise after a diagnosis of cancer (10, 12, 17):

- Avoid inactivity, and return to activity as soon as possible after surgery.
- Build to 150 minutes per week of aerobic activity (e.g., walking, biking, swimming, dancing).
- Perform progressive strength training two to three times per week.
- Do flexibility activities on most days of the week.

The overall recommendations after therapeutic interventions (e.g., surgery) are to avoid inactivity and return to regular activity as soon as possible, including aerobic activities, resistance training, and flexibility exercises. With regard to aerobic exercise, low intensity is typically recommended. The ACSM guidelines are the only ones that specify an intensity of moderate to vigorous intensity, and this is based on the documentation of benefits from aerobic exercise at higher intensity levels.

▮ Q&A ▮

Where can I find a fitness professional to help guide me in my exercise program?

The ACSM, along with the ACS, has developed a certification that recognizes fitness professionals with expertise in working with cancer patients. Certified Cancer Exercise Trainers (CETs) can design and administer fitness assessments and exercise programs based on an individual's cancer diagnosis, treatment, and status. To find a CET near you, see the ACSM's Profinder webpage: http://certification.acsm.org/pro-finder.

Precautions for Exercise

As discussed earlier, many cancer survivors experience one or more persistent adverse effects of their cancer treatments. Some of these may alter the safety of certain types of exercise, which would suggest that survivors with these issues undergo a preexercise evaluation before getting started to avoid the potential that exercise might do more harm than good. In addition, most cancer survivors are older adults who enter their cancer journey with one or more chronic disease diagnoses, which also may alter the safety profile of exercise. This section discusses whether survivors should seek a preexercise evaluation by a well-trained exercise professional or physical therapist before starting exercise and then whether supervised or home-based activities are recommended.

How do you know whether you can proceed with exercise in a community or home-based, unsupervised setting versus needing a more structured, supervised exercise program after cancer? First, if you would like a supervised, structured program, go find that supervised program! Second, if you are going to do low-intensity activity such as walking, you can likely proceed without supervision or evaluation. However, if you intend to progress beyond low intensity, to include strength training or to do sports and higher-intensity outdoor activities (e.g., hiking mountains, skiing), it would be useful to understand your risk level. The ACSM and the National Comprehensive Cancer Network both have published guidelines on this topic (see table 14.2 for a summary)

TABLE 14.2   **Guidelines on Indications for the Need for Preexercise Evaluation**

Condition	Type of preexercise evaluation recommended	Supervised exercise recommended?
Survivors of early-stage cancer who have no comorbid health conditions (e.g., heart disease, diabetes, obesity) and who had a high level of activity before diagnosis	None	No
Persons with peripheral neuropathy, musculoskeletal issues, cancer in the bones, poor bone health, possible heart disease	Evaluation by an outpatient rehabilitation clinician (physical or occupational therapist) or physician	Determined by outcome of evaluation
Persons who have had lung or abdominal surgery or ostomy; those with cardiopulmonary disease, lymphedema, extreme fatigue, known cardiac disease	Physician clearance before exercise *and* evaluation by an outpatient rehabilitation clinician (physical or occupational therapist) or physician	Yes

(10, 16). There are three categories in both sets of guidelines: low-risk individuals who can exercise unsupervised without prior evaluation, moderate-risk individuals who are advised to undertake an evaluation to determine whether they need supervision, and high-risk individuals who are advised to find a supervised exercise program for their own safety.

The majority of individuals diagnosed with cancer are over age 65 and have at least one other chronic disease diagnosis at the time of cancer diagnosis (e.g., hypertension, obesity, asthma, arthritis). Therefore, the beginning exercise program draws heavily from the advice in chapters that focus on those specific conditions and the chapter on exercise for older adults. Ideally, starting an exercise program in a supervised setting helps to ensure that the exercises are being done properly before one continues the program in a community or home setting.

Physical Activity Recommendations

There are six elements common to all of the exercise components, toward the goal of ensuring that exercise is both safe and beneficial: frequency, intensity, time, type, volume, and progression (FITT-VP) (3, 19). Frequency refers to the number of times the activity occurs per week. Intensity refers to the degree of difficulty. This can be stated in absolute terms (e.g., lifting a given weight such as a 5-pound [2.3 kg] dumbbell) or in relative terms (50 percent of maximum effort). Time refers to the duration of a given exercise or session of exercise. Type refers to the mode of exercise, such as stationary bicycling, walking, or jogging. Volume is defined as the total amount of exercise done, which is a combination of intensity and time. Finally, progression refers to the need for exercise to progress with regard to volume in order for benefits to continue to accrue. One can increase the volume by increasing intensity or time.

Aerobic Exercise   To start an aerobic exercise program as a beginning exerciser, the frequency should be two to three times per week. Once you are comfortable with this frequency (e.g., no increase in fatigue or other adverse effects), another session can be added per week up to six sessions per week. There should always be at least one day of rest from aerobic exercise.

As to intensity, one easy way to determine this is to use the "talk but not sing" rule. If you can sing (hold a note) while doing your aerobic exercise, you are not working hard enough. By contrast, if you cannot talk while doing aerobic exercise, you are working too hard. Intensity needs to progress, however, for benefits to continue to accrue. Thus, it would be advisable to take note of your pace on a track or pathway or of your workload on any gym equipment you are using. For example, you could note how many blocks you can walk in your daily walking sessions and increase the number of blocks walked within a given time period as you continue. Tracking this information is helpful for ensuring that you get the most out of your workouts.

Regarding time per aerobic exercise session, a beginning exerciser who is starting after a cancer diagnosis might want to begin with as little as 5 to 10 minutes per session to be sure that the activity is tolerated. This is increased by 10 percent per week. For example, if you choose to do three 10-minute sessions in your first week of a walking program, the next week you would do 33 minutes, or 11 minutes per session. Within several months, you would be up to 30 minutes per session.

Typically with respect to the volume and progression of aerobic exercise for beginning exercisers after cancer, 30 minutes per week is a starting point, and then the time or intensity can be increased. The intensity can be increased by 10 percent per week, as can the time. However, it might be advisable to increase one of these per week, not both. That could mean increasing time one week and intensity another week.

Various types of aerobic exercise can be included in your exercise program. One common approach is a walking program. For those with balance or peripheral neuropathy, however, a stationary bicycle might be the best first step to aerobic fitness. The most important aspects of choosing a type of aerobic exercise are safety and enjoyment. If you get hurt or don't enjoy the activity, you won't keep doing it regularly.

Resistance Training   Resistance (strength) training is not just for young people and isn't just about lifting heavy weights in order to create bigger muscles and look better on the beach. Strength training can help cancer survivors regain strength that is lost during active treatment and is also helpful for promoting bone health (13, 15, 18). Strength training can help older adults by ensuring that they continue to have the strength to get on and off the toilet, climb stairs, carry groceries, and do other common functional tasks. Older adults lose muscle mass as they age, and cancer treatment can exacerbate that process. Strength training may be more important than aerobic exercise for some survivors.

The recommended frequency of strength training is two to three times per week. The time it takes per session may vary, but 20 to 30 minutes is adequate. The type could include dumbbells, variable-resistance machines, or strength training activities performed in a class.

Even if you have done strength training in the past, it would be advisable to start with very low levels of resistance during and after your cancer treatment. There is often a period of inactivity during active cancer treatment. This can result in loss of muscle mass and strength. Adjuvant treatments (e.g., chemotherapy and radiation) may also result in loss of muscle mass and strength. Thus, to avoid injury, it is recommended that those living with and beyond cancer start with low resistance. If you are using dumbbells, this would translate to 1 to 5 pounds (0.45 to 2.3 kg) per exercise. If you are using variable-resistance exercise machines at a fitness facility, start with one or two plates on each machine.

The type of strength training you do is not as important as doing it regularly. If you prefer to exercise at home, you might want to get a set of dumbbells or adjustable-weight dumbbells. If you enjoy exercising with others, you might like using variable-resistance machines in a circuit or in a class led by an instructor.

Progression of resistance should be slow after a cancer diagnosis for several reasons. First, many survivors experience a period of inactivity between the time of diagnosis and the time when the surgeon indicates it is safe to begin normal daily activities again. Deconditioning occurs when exercise is stopped. The extent of the deconditioning is determined by the length of time spent not exercising. When one is starting or returning to exercise after a period of deconditioning, there is a higher likelihood of muscle injury from overdoing. There is also an inflammatory response that occurs when one progresses resistance too much (e.g., a 50 percent increase, such as going from 5 to 10 pounds [2.3 to 4.5 kg] from one session to the next). This is pertinent because cancer-related fatigue is thought to be related to inflammation. Further, an inflammation-related adverse effect of cancer treatment called lymphedema can cause swelling of the area of the body affected by cancer. Lymphedema results from an increase in protein-rich fluid, which can happen with increased inflammation and

Effects of Cancer Relevant to Exercise

Developing exercise programming for such a diverse population requires consideration of physical and medical conditions before cancer diagnosis. Other important considerations include where the cancer is in the body, the body systems affected by the cancer and its treatments, and where survivors are with regard to their cancer journey.

Prediagnosis Physical and Medical Condition

The effect of a cancer diagnosis on the ability to exercise, as well as the ways in which exercise benefits a cancer survivor, varies according to how well one is at the point of diagnosis. As an extreme example, consider an 18-year-old testicular cancer survivor who was quite physically fit at the point of diagnosis compared to an 80-year-old man with prostate cancer who was obese, diabetic, and hypertensive when diagnosed. Clearly, any exercise advice needs to account for prediagnosis fitness, health, and other medical conditions such as obesity, high blood pressure, high cholesterol, diabetes, and other common chronic diseases.

Location of Cancer in the Body

The effects of cancer on the ability to exercise or on the benefits of exercise will vary according to where the cancer occurs. For example, a woman who had breast cancer treatment likely had surgery on her chest wall. She may also have elected to have reconstructive surgery. Both of these surgeries result in changes in the way she moves her shoulders and upper body. By contrast, a colon cancer patient may have had abdominal surgery and have a temporary or permanent alteration in the manner of waste elimination, including a bag to receive feces that is worn under the clothes (called an ostomy bag). This creates a higher level of risk with regard to infection since a hole in the abdomen exposes the inside of the body. There is also a higher level of risk for a hernia. As a result, the colon cancer survivor may now relate to abdominal exercises differently and wear different exercise clothing. A prostate cancer survivor may have issues with urinary incontinence, in part due to curative surgical procedures. Urine leakage could be embarrassing. An exercise plan minimizing activities that would increase leakage (e.g., jumping activities) might be desirable. Finally, a sarcoma survivor with a missing foot (and likely a prosthesis) would appreciate an exercise plan that accounts for the changes in balance and stability that have occurred due to limb amputation. In each case, these changes should not be taken as grounds not to exercise. Instead, the changes are reasons an exercise program needs to be individualized.

Body Systems Affected by Cancer and Treatment

Many of the changes that occur are a result of the surgeries undertaken to remove cancer. Adjuvant cancer treatments, such as radiation and chemotherapy, can also have adverse effects. These effects influence the ability to exercise as well as the benefits.

Adverse Effects of Radiation

Ionizing radiation continues to damage the specific area of the body that was treated for the remainder of life. Radiation techniques are changing and improving the "scatter" radiation can occur in the arms, breasts, and torso of breast cancer survivors and in the lower body after bladder, testicular, and gynecologic cancers, as well as after melanoma.

Although cancer survivors can safely do resistance training, in order to avoid increasing inflammation or muscle injury after deconditioning, they are advised to start with

that affects healthy tissue, but adverse effects continue to be documented. The effects are localized to the part of the body that received radiation. If radiation was received on the chest wall, it may cause damage to the heart and lungs. Development of arrhythmias (changes in heart rhythm) is the most common radiation-associated adverse effect with regard to the heart. Pulmonary fibrosis can also occur due to radiation to the chest wall. Radiation lower on the torso may result in gastrointestinal changes, including irritable bowel syndrome. Damage to soft tissue continues as well, which can result in stiffness and altered range of motion in the area that received radiation. For example, breast cancer survivors may find that they become tight (less flexible) on the side of the upper body that received radiation. The encouraging news is that exercise can be helpful for this issue.

Adverse Effects of Chemotherapy

Unlike what occurs with radiation, the effects of chemotherapy are systemic and thus the adverse effects may affect multiple body systems. The specifics of body systems affected and the nature of the changes vary according to the class of chemotherapy drugs. For example, anthracyclines are a class of drugs commonly used for breast cancer that can damage the heart, increasing risk for cardiomyopathies and heart failure. By contrast, all of the chemotherapy drugs that are platinum based (with names that end with "-platin") cause peripheral neuropathy (i.e., damage to nerves that can cause weakness, numbness, and pain) that may be permanent. Knowing what chemotherapy drugs were used in your treatment is important so that you can be aware of the adverse effects that might be associated with those drugs. Knowledge is power: Knowing what the possible adverse effects are allows you to know when to speak up with your doctor to ask for screening or treatment. Table 14.3 provides more details on these effects and whether there is evidence that exercise can help with the issue (8, 11, 14, 15, 16).

TABLE 14.3 Adverse Effects of Cancer Treatments and Benefits of Exercise

Adverse effects	Mode of exercise that may help
Cancer-related fatigue, quality of life, anxiety, depression, decreased lung function or heart function, immune suppression	Aerobic exercise
Peripheral neuropathy	Unknown—note the need to be careful regarding balance issues and fall risk during exercise
Bone loss, physical function decline	Aerobic exercise and strength training
Lymphedema (risk of onset or worsening)	Strength training
Sleep problems	Yoga

low weights (below 5 pounds [2.3 kg] for dumbbells, one or two plates on variable-resistance machines) and progress resistance in the smallest possible increments. As always, allow changes in symptoms to be your guide. Finally, if you find that you need to take an "exercise holiday" (e.g., because of caring for an ill relative, vacation), be sure to back off on the resistance used in your strength training exercises. If you take three weeks off, start over with the lowest weight and rebuild. To avoid injury and any excessive inflammatory responses, maintain a regular strength training routine performed at least twice weekly. But make sure you have at least one day between each session to allow the muscles to recover.

The exercises you perform should work the major muscle groups: chest, back, shoulders, arms (biceps and triceps), front of thighs, back of thighs, buttocks, and calves. You should also do exercises for the muscles commonly referred to as the core: the abdominal muscles and lower back. The exercises shown in chapter 6 of this book would form an excellent program for cancer survivors. The only change would be to start at a low weight and to progress more slowly than indicated in chapter 6.

Flexibility and Neuromotor Exercises   With age, range of motion generally decreases, which can make it difficult to perform common activities that require reaching or twisting. The deconditioning that commonly surrounds diagnosis and surgery for cancer patients can also increase stiffness. To maintain a healthy range of motion and optimal function of all muscle groups, it is useful to do flexibility exercises. In addition, although specific benefits related to cancer have not been studied, inclusion of neuromotor exercise involving balance, agility, coordination, and gait may be considered as part of a general exercise program, especially for older adults (3). The flexibility program outlined in chapter 7 would be an outstanding program for cancer survivors, and options for neuromotor exercises are provided in chapter 8. No adaptations are needed unless symptoms indicate otherwise.

Influence of Medications

A broad variety of medications are prescribed to cancer patients and survivors that may affect both the ability to exercise and the potential benefits of exercise. Since reviewing all possible options is beyond the scope of this chapter, consider this general advice

■ Q&A

Are there benefits of yoga for cancer survivors?

There is evidence that yoga can help cancer survivors sleep better (11). Further, many cancer survivors enjoy yoga for the benefits of relaxation and quality of life improvements. The challenge in recommending yoga to cancer survivors is that there are many types of yoga, and not all of them would be suitable for cancer survivors. Vinyasa, Bikram, Hot, Ashtanga, Power, Jivamukti, and Kundalini yoga might be more advisable for cancer survivors who had been practicing these types of yoga for a long time before diagnosis.

The forms of yoga that might be more advisable for cancer survivors include Yin, Hatha, Iyengar, and Restorative yoga. Ultimately, there is no hard and fast rule to determine what is safe for a specific person. Thus, use caution when approaching yoga in all forms by starting slowly, progressing slowly, and letting symptoms be your guide. This is good advice for all other forms of exercise as well. There is value to moving more. If you are attracted to a form of exercise that isn't discussed in this chapter and wonder whether it would be advisable for you as a cancer survivor, there is a simple way to proceed: with caution. Do a small amount of the activity and see how it feels. Progress the time and intensity gradually. And, as always, allow your symptoms to be your guide.

■ Q&A

Can exercise really help following chemotherapy?

Problems sleeping and persistent tiredness are common. Although it seems counterintuitive, a program of aerobic activity helps with fatigue. In addition, yoga has benefits for sleep outcomes in cancer patients, as well as the expected benefits for balance and muscular fitness. Consult with your health care provider for recommendations on local programs specifically designed for cancer survivors (e.g., YMCA or hospital-based fitness centers).

that applies to all cancer survivors: Ask your doctor and pharmacist what effects your medications have on the body beyond the purpose for which they were prescribed. Ask whether the medication will alter your ability to exercise safely or the likelihood that exercise would be beneficial. If there are body systems affected by your medications, be aware of any changes you experience in your ability to exercise or in how your body adapts to the exercise. And as always, start slowly, progress slowly, and let your symptoms guide you.

There is compelling scientific evidence that exercise is safe and beneficial for those on a cancer journey, from the point of diagnosis through to the balance of life. There was a time when cancer doctors would tell their patients to rest, take it easy, and not push themselves. More recently, that advice has changed. Three major national organizations have issued guidance that cancer survivors should avoid inactivity and exercise regularly, both during and after treatment. Survivors who do so can experience improved physical function and quality of life, among other benefits.

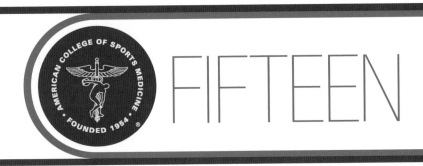

Alzheimer's Disease

Having a family member diagnosed with Alzheimer's disease is a daunting experience as you face the reality that you or your loved one has a serious, progressive, and ultimately fatal neurodegenerative condition. As the cognitive and physical abilities of people with Alzheimer's progressively decline, family members face challenging emotional and financial decisions regarding long-term care. Thus early diagnosis, support group participation, appropriate nutrition, and regular physical activity are important for both the person with Alzheimer's and the health of those providing care.

Once considered a relatively rare disorder, Alzheimer's disease is listed as the sixth leading cause of death in the United States and considered a major public health challenge affecting more than 5 million Americans, the majority of whom are over the age of 65 years. The prevalence of dementia, with Alzheimer's disease accounting for two-thirds of the cases, increases with age, affecting nearly 14 percent of the population over the age of 70 years. This creates a challenging public health issue, as the prevalence of neurodegenerative conditions like Alzheimer's doubles every five years beyond age 65 (38). At the dawn of the 21st century, approximately 35 million Americans (12.4 percent of the total population) were 65 years or older. By 2015, nearly 46 million Americans (15 percent) had reached the age of 65; and by 2030, when the last of the baby boom generation hits this milestone, one in five Americans will be over age 65 (14).

Alzheimer's disease is named after Dr. Alois Alzheimer, the German neurologist and psychiatrist who first described the condition, in 1906, when he reported on changes in the brain tissue in a woman who had died of an unusual mental illness. Her cluster of symptoms included memory loss, language challenges, disorientation, behavioral problems, and hallucinations. Following her death, Dr. Alzheimer studied her brain tissue and described two of the primary hallmarks of Alzheimer's disease—numerous abnormal clumps or globs of sticky proteins (now referred to as amyloid plaques) and tangled bundles of fibers within the neurons (now called neurofibrillary or tau tangles) (38).

How does the brain work to regulate daily activities?

The brain is a phenomenal organ that allows each person to carry out every aspect of daily living, from internal body functions such as breathing and digestion to conscious functions such as speaking, moving, and making decisions. The brain is made up of more than 100 billion nerve cells or neurons and is served by over 400 billion tiny blood vessels called capillaries. The vast majority of the brain consists of the left and right cerebral hemispheres, which are connected by a large bundle of nerve fibers. Each of these cerebral hemispheres has an outer layer (cerebral cortex) where the brain regulates cognitive functions such as learning, remembering, and decision making; controlling voluntary movements; and processing sensory information.

Despite intensive and ongoing research efforts, currently there is no medication or other medical intervention that can "cure" Alzheimer's. Thus medical treatment focuses on managing symptoms and prolonging, for as long as possible, the person's ability to carry out activities of daily living.

Effect of Alzheimer's on the Brain

Alzheimer's disease is present years before symptoms of memory loss and other cognitive deficits appear. This is referred to as the preclinical stage of Alzheimer's disease, in which people appear to function normally but a number of toxic changes within the brain are progressing. Among the abnormal changes, two primary features have been identified (38):

- *Amyloid plaques*—These consist of insoluble deposits of beta-amyloid, a toxic protein fragment. Generally found in the spaces between the brain's nerve cells, they are more abundant in people with Alzheimer's disease.

- *Neurofibrillary or tau tangles*—Found inside the nerve cell, these consist of abnormally shaped or twisted protein collections that stick together and build up, eventually disrupting cell communication and even causing cell death.

These toxic changes can cause healthy neurons to shrink, lose connections with other brain cells, stop functioning, and even die. As more and more neurons are affected, the given brain areas lose volume and shrink (see figure 15.1). This appears to initially occur in the hippocampus (a critical area for learning, short-term memory, and conver-

Healthy brain

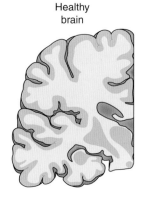

Severe Alzheimer's

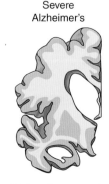

FIGURE 15.1 Cross sections of the brain comparing healthy brain to brain affected by Alzheimer's disease.

Source: National Institutes of Health and Human Services, National Institute on Aging.

sion of short-term memories to long-term storage in other areas of the brain) but then spreads to other areas of the brain, eventually affecting one's cognitive abilities. By the final stage of Alzheimer's, the damage is pervasive and brain volume significantly declines.

While Alzheimer's can occur early in life, 95 percent of the cases are late onset and occur after the age of 60 years. Early-onset Alzheimer's is thought to be caused by gene changes inherited from a parent, but a small number of cases currently have no specifically identified cause. The more prevalent late-onset form results from a variety of factors that occur and progress over decades. These include possible genetic mutations (such as the apolipoprotein E gene, or APOE), environmental and social factors, and poor lifestyle choices.

Since Alzheimer's disease develops over a period of many years, the condition can go unrecognized until outward symptoms are displayed. Early in the Alzheimer's disease process, symptomatic changes are very subtle. You or your loved one may experience memory problems that are fairly mild but slightly greater than expected based on age, but they generally do not interfere with everyday activities. As Alzheimer's progresses, memory challenges increase and other cognitive difficulties are manifested, such as personality and behavior changes, difficulty handling money and paying bills, challenges with multistep tasks such as dressing and cooking, and wandering. At the severe stage of Alzheimer's, people lose their ability to communicate, often becoming completely dependent on others for their daily care and perhaps requiring admittance to a care facility.

Healthy Approaches to Managing Alzheimer's

What can you do to stay healthy and independent as you grow older? Similar to the risk factors for heart disease and other chronic health conditions, eating poorly, not exercising, smoking, being overweight, or having high blood pressure or type 2 diabetes increases your susceptibility to Alzheimer's disease. The good news is that research suggests that modifying these lifestyle factors and conditions may help optimize brain health with age. While the importance of these risk factors differs from person to person, it appears that what you choose to eat and how much you move each day are critical factors in maintaining good health and thinking power. Being physically active also provides opportunities to interact with others, thus maintaining important social connections.

Focusing on Nutrition

A nutritious diet with appropriate portion sizes is critical for overall health and well-being, regardless of one's current age and health status. Consuming appropriate nutrients and calories is especially important if you are an older adult striving to maintain your physical and mental functions, independence, and associated quality of life.

Although healthy eating patterns have been associated with a lower risk of cognitive decline, there is no definitive answer yet about the role lifestyle factors may play in reducing Alzheimer's disease risk (29, 42, 44, 51). However, healthy food choices and regular physical activity can help manage your waistline, lower the risk of chronic diseases, and improve overall health and well-being.

The strongest evidence so far suggests that what's good for the heart also benefits brain health. Memory loss in Alzheimer's disease is linked to the abnormal clumping of protein in the nerve cells, causing them to malfunction and die. The presence or absence of vascular disease may explain why some people develop characteristic Alzheimer's plaques and tangles but do not develop cognitive decline. The role of atherosclerosis in the development of cognitive impairment and dementia may be related to the degree of atherosclerotic calcification in the brain (9). Eating a heart-healthy diet, one rich in fruits and vegetables and lower in saturated fat, appears to help keep the mind and body healthy.

Healthy Fat Recommendations

A growing body of evidence indicates that while total fat intake is not a key factor in brain health, eating healthy fats and less saturated fat may help protect your brain. Most of the fat you eat should come from unsaturated food sources (fish, nuts, vegetable oil). Omega-3 fatty acids, monounsaturated fat, and polyunsaturated fat are considered heart-healthy fats. Saturated fats are primarily found in food from animals, such as meat and whole-fat dairy products, as well as many processed foods. All types of fat are high in calories, so healthy fats should be substituted for saturated fats rather than adding more fat to your diet. Table 15.1 provides examples of healthy fat choices (1).

Diet Plans

Both the Dietary Approaches to Stop Hypertension (DASH) eating plan and the Mediterranean diet have been found to help reduce heart disease and may also lower dementia risk (45). The longevity of people living in the Mediterranean region has led to research on the role their traditional diet may play. While there is no one "Mediterranean" diet, the typical meal plan consists of plant-based foods (fruits, vegetables, whole grains, nuts, legumes), seafood, and olive oil while limiting intake of red meat, sweets, and eggs. Most of the fat in a Mediterranean diet comes from unsaturated sources (fish, nuts, and olive oil) (27, 32). Consider these tips on adopting a Mediterranean-inspired diet:

- Include fruits and vegetables at every meal and choose them for snacks as well.
- Switch from refined to whole-grain bread, cereal, rice, and pasta products.
- Nuts and seeds supply protein, healthy fat, and fiber. Limit your portion to no more than a 1-ounce serving (approximately 1/3 cup), as they are high in calories.

TABLE 15.1 Choose Healthy Fats

Monounsaturated and polyunsaturated fat sources	• Avocado • Nuts and seeds: almonds, cashews, peanuts, pecans, pine nuts, pumpkin, sesame or sunflower seeds • Olives and olive oil • Peanut butter • Vegetable oils: corn, cottonseed, safflower, sunflower
Omega-3 fat sources	• Canola oil • Eggs (check label for those high in omega-3s) • Fish: albacore tuna, herring, mackerel, rainbow trout, salmon, sardines • Flaxseed and flaxseed oil • Walnuts

- Eat fish at least twice per week. Limit red meat to no more than a few times per month.
- Use spices and herbs to flavor foods instead of salt.

Wine is commonly consumed in the Mediterranean diet. Moderate intake is defined as no more than 5 ounces (148 mL) of wine daily in women and men older than age 65, and in younger men no more than 10 ounces (296 mL) daily. Although some research indicates that light to moderate alcohol intake may have a positive impact on dementia risk, the U.S. Dietary Guidelines make it clear that no one should begin drinking or drink more often on the basis of potential health benefits (44).

The DASH eating plan is lower in sodium than the typical American diet (less than 2,300 milligrams daily). It limits intake of saturated fat and emphasizes foods rich in potassium, calcium, magnesium, and fiber. The plan is based on research studies sponsored by the National Heart, Lung, and Blood Institute (NHLBI), which showed that DASH lowers high blood pressure, improves levels of fats in the bloodstream, and reduces the risk of developing heart disease. The DASH eating plan emphasizes daily intake of vegetables, fruits, fat-free or low-fat dairy products, more whole grains, lean protein (fish, poultry, legumes, nuts, seeds) and vegetable oils and less sodium, sweets, sugary beverages, and red meats. The DASH plan recommendations are summarized in chapter 12 (37).

Researchers from Rush University in Chicago combined elements from the heart-healthy Mediterranean diet and the DASH diet to create the MIND diet (Mediterranean–DASH Intervention for Neurodegenerative Delay). The Rush Memory and Aging Project found that people whose diet most closely conformed to the MIND diet had a 53 percent lower risk of developing Alzheimer's. Participants who had moderate adherence demonstrated a 35 percent reduced disease risk. High adherence to the DASH and the Mediterranean diets also conferred protective benefits (30).

The MIND diet focuses on 10 brain-healthy foods and five foods you should limit to avoid "brain drain" (see table 15.2). The diet was specifically designed to include

TABLE 15.2 MIND Diet Characteristics

Brain power foods	
Berries (blueberries, strawberries)—two or more servings per week	**P**oultry (chicken or turkey)—two times a week
Relax with a glass of wine daily	**O**live oil—use as your main cooking oil
A serving of leafy green vegetables (spinach, salad greens)—at least 6 days per week and one other vegetable at least once a day	**W**hole grains—three or more servings daily
Include dried peas, beans, and legumes every other day	**E**at fish at least once a week
Nuts—five servings a week	**R**eplace saturated fat with healthy fat

Reduce your intake of foods high in saturated fat:
- Butter and stick margarine—less than 1 Tbsp daily
- Cheese—less than one serving per week
- Fried or fast food—less than one serving per week
- Red meat—less than four servings per week
- Sweets and pastries—less than five servings per week

Adapted from M.C. Morris, C.C. Tangney, Y. Wang, et al., 2015.

■ Q&A

Does type 2 diabetes impact the risk of developing Alzheimer's?

Type 2 diabetes and Alzheimer's disease have been thought to be independent disorders whose incidence increases with aging. Evidence now suggests that having diabetes increases the risk of developing Alzheimer's disease and that insulin resistance may contribute to amyloid deposition in the brain (2, 4, 49). Even among people who do not have diabetes, higher blood glucose levels have been associated with a greater risk of dementia (16). The results of these studies reinforce the importance of achieving and maintaining optimum levels of blood sugar.

---

the foods and nutrients that evidence has shown to be good for the brain. Researchers believe that people who follow the diet for long periods of time acquire the greatest protection from Alzheimer's. The MIND diet includes the following components:

- Plant-based foods (berries, vegetables, nuts, legumes, and whole grains)
- Olive oil as a healthy fat source
- Eating fish at least once a week and poultry twice per week
- Drinking wine in moderation

Nutritional Supplements

The National Center for Complementary and Integrative Health reports that there is no convincing evidence from a large body of research that any dietary supplement can prevent the worsening of cognitive impairment. This includes research on the use of ginkgo biloba, omega-3 fatty acids, vitamins B and E, Asian ginseng, grape seed extract, and curcumin (derived from turmeric root) (31). Research on the use of Huperzine A, a moss extract that has been used in traditional Chinese medicine, also demonstrated no effect in delaying or preventing Alzheimer's disease (5, 33, 34).

The Role of Antioxidants   As you age, damaging molecules called free radicals can build up in nerve cells and may play a role in the development of Alzheimer's. Research results on the use of antioxidants (natural substances such as vitamins E and C, beta-carotene, flavonoids) that are thought to help protect the body from the damaging effects of free radicals have been mixed (18, 23, 48).

A recent research review found no convincing evidence that vitamin E is of benefit in the treatment of Alzheimer's disease or mild cognitive impairment (20), although some studies suggest that consuming a diet rich in vitamin E and vitamin C may be associated with a reduced risk of Alzheimer's (29). Vegetable oils, almonds, and sunflower seeds are among the richest sources of vitamin E, and significant amounts are found in green leafy vegetables and fortified cereals (35). Sources of vitamin C include citrus fruits, broccoli, peppers, and fortified foods and beverages.

Vitamin D   Studies have demonstrated an association between vitamin D deficiency and increased risk of Alzheimer's disease (2, 7). Vitamin D deficiency is common among older adults due to reduced sun exposure and their skin's decreased ability to synthesize vitamin D. Fish liver oil and fatty fish such as salmon, tuna, and mackerel are natural sources of vitamin D. Small amounts are also found in beef liver, cheese, and egg yolks. Foods fortified with vitamin D such as milk, orange juice, and breakfast cereal provide the majority of vitamin D in the American diet. While it appears there is a link between vitamin D and the development of Alzheimer's, more research is needed to determine cause and effect.

Omega-3 Fatty Acids   Increased intake of omega-3 fatty acids, such as docosahexaenoic acid (DHA) found in fish, may also have beneficial effects on brain function (50, 53). Docosahexaenoic acid is one of the most abundant fatty acids in the brain and is critical for healthy development and function. Its anti-inflammatory effects promote cardiovascular health and may also be beneficial to the brain (17, 26). Thus far, research in relation to dementia risk has yielded mixed results, so there is not yet sufficient evidence to recommend DHA or other fatty acid supplements to treat or prevent Alzheimer's disease (5, 6, 12, 40).

Homocysteine and B Vitamins   An elevated level of the blood protein homocysteine is an established cardiovascular risk factor and also appears to increase the risk of Alzheimer's disease. Certain B vitamins (folate, B_6, B_{12}) have been shown to lower blood homocysteine levels, leading to hopes that supplementation may prevent or halt the progression of Alzheimer's. However, while supplementation can lower homocysteine levels, studies generally have not reported improvements in cognitive performance, and additional research is needed (13).

Resveratrol   Resveratrol, a compound found in red grapes that has both anti-inflammatory and antioxidant properties, has been correlated with a lower risk of dementia in a small number of studies (47). Researchers continue to explore whether resveratrol therapy can delay or alter memory deterioration and functional decline in Alzheimer's disease.

Impact of Combining Supplements

Most studies of individual vitamins and supplements have shown limited to no benefit. More recent findings suggest that improved cognitive function may occur with formulations containing a combination of nutrients (41). Future research studies are needed to examine various combinations and the potential for benefits related to cognitive function.

Practical Aspects of Diet for Someone With Alzheimer's

While good nutrition is generally not a concern in the early stages of Alzheimer's disease, help with cooking and grocery shopping may be needed. Behaviors related to disease progression include refusal to eat or to sit long enough for meals, problems with chewing and swallowing, and changes in physical activity level. These changes may result in issues with weight loss, poor nutrition, and dehydration. The National Institute on Aging suggests these Alzheimer's caregiving tips (36):

- Avoid new routines. Serve meals at consistent times in a familiar place and way whenever possible.
- Be patient. Extra time may be required to finish meals.
- Serve well-liked foods and respect cultural and religious food preferences.

Because there is no known cause or cure for Alzheimer's disease, people are often tempted to try dietary supplements or "medical foods" that are touted to boost brain health. Supplements are not regulated by the Food and Drug Administration as stringently as medications, and there may be concerns regarding their effectiveness and safety as well as potential reactions with other medications. Always check with your physician before using supplements or alternative therapies.

Focusing on Physical Activity

As discussed in chapter 1, physical activity is an essential component of a healthy lifestyle that reduces the risk of developing cardiovascular disease, diabetes, and other chronic health conditions; burns additional daily calories to promote maintenance of normal weight; and keeps muscles and joints strong and mobile to allow life to be lived to the fullest. Being physically active is also important for maintaining the health of your brain as you move through life.

Regular physical activity improves attention, focus, and academic performance in children; enhances attention, working memory, and the ability to multitask in young adults; and can delay the process of cognitive decline and neurodegenerative diseases such as Alzheimer's in older adults (39). Numerous scientific research studies have analyzed the relationship between physical activity and the risk of developing Alzheimer's disease with aging. The findings have consistently shown that people who regularly exercised (three or more days per week) had slower rates of cognitive decline and were less likely to develop full-blown Alzheimer's disease than those who exercised less.

However, while these studies have highlighted a strong association between physical activity and Alzheimer's disease, they do not definitively show that a true cause-and-effect relationship exists, nor do they reveal why certain benefits occur. Thus scientists continue to conduct a variety of animal and human research studies to confirm these associations, better understand their underlying mechanisms, and hopefully, at some point, uncover specific causation and curative treatments.

Being physically active is one of the most important steps you can take to maintain and even improve your overall health profile. And while scientists continue to dig deeper in their efforts to identify effective prevention strategies for Alzheimer's, exercise is recommended to promote health for those at risk for as well as those with Alzheimer's.

Physical Activity and Cognitive Decline Prevention

Many research studies have noted that regular physical activity has positive benefits on cognitive function. Benefits identified include delaying the onset of dementia, decreasing the chance of developing Alzheimer's, and slowing progression in those diagnosed with the disease (3, 15, 25, 28, 52). Studies have shown a significantly higher risk of developing Alzheimer's, and significantly greater dementia, in people who did minimal physical activity versus their more active counterparts (22). For example, in a recent study in which daily physical activity was tracked (including cleaning, gardening, cooking), those with the highest activity had a twofold decreased risk for developing Alzheimer's compared with the most inactive individuals (10). Thus, there is evidence that maintaining a physically active lifestyle supports your brain health and may lower your risk of developing Alzheimer's disease.

However, while these and other research studies highlight the association between aerobic fitness, improved cognitive function, and decreased manifestation of dementia and Alzheimer's disease, the specific physiological mechanisms are not yet clearly defined (11). Development of Alzheimer's is a progressive and complex disease process; thus the positive physiological mechanisms induced by physical activity are most likely multifactorial and interlinked. This section describes a few possibilities.

Maintenance of Cerebral Blood Flow   Similar to the effect that cardiovascular disease has on blood flow to the heart and vasculature, atherosclerotic cerebrovascular disease affects blood flow to the brain. Many of the same risk factors that affect your heart, such as hypertension, hyperlipidemia, obesity, glucose intolerance, diabetes, smoking, and inflammatory processes also increase your risk for stroke and cognitive decline (11, 24). Physical activity is an important intervention for each of these risk factors. By keeping your heart effectively pumping and the arteries serving your brain functioning appropriately, blood flow to your brain is maintained. Physical activity may also stimulate the development of additional cerebral blood vessels or capillaries. These vessels provide the key chemicals and nutrients that help maintain the brain's network connections and can also induce the growth of new connections that are vital to our cognitive abilities.

Brain-Derived Neurotrophic Factor   Perhaps the most extensively studied brain chemical is brain-derived neurotrophic factor (BDNF), one of the chemicals (neurotrophins) that stimulate neurogenesis, which simply means the brain's ability to grow new neurons (brain cells) and synapses (connections). Brain-derived neurotrophic factor also increases the release of neurotransmitters that enhance communication connections within the brain, and may provide a protective factor for existing brain cells against the toxicity resulting from the development of amyloid plaques. Low levels of BDNF have been documented in the brain tissue of people who died from Alzheimer's disease. Numerous animal and human studies have documented increased levels of BDNF following both long-term aerobic and short-term vigorous exercise training (3). This exercise-stimulated increase in BDNF has been correlated with improved cognitive function and increased hippocampal volume.

Brain Volume and Cognitive Reserve   In middle age, the hippocampus decreases in size by approximately 1 to 2 percent per year, and over time this shrinkage can affect memory and other cognitive functions. Regular aerobic exercise can slow this atrophy process and even promote the growth (neurogenesis) of new brain cells. This new growth is important for preserving the size of the hippocampus and other brain areas that are essential for memory and other mental processes.

Brain imaging studies have noted Alzheimer's disease pathology in the brains of older adults who never displayed the cognitive deficits and symptoms typical of Alzheimer's (19). Why this occurs is not well understood, but researchers have proposed the concept of "cognitive reserve" as one possible explanation (8). In research studies, the primary difference between the brains of people with and without manifestation of symptomatic Alzheimer's disease was their brain size, particularly that of the hippocampus area. Preservation of brain size, or cognitive reserve, might allow the brain to maintain its function by recruiting alternate brain networks or connections that have developed over time (8, 43). Exercise appears to be one mechanism that stimulates this preservation process by stimulating brain chemicals such as BDNF, blood flow enhancements, and other factors that preserve hippocampus volume (21).

What is important to note is that a growing body of scientific evidence suggests that regular physical activity is beneficial for long-term brain health and maintenance of cognitive capabilities. While additional research will help to refine recommendations

Key Physical Activity Tips for Alzheimer's

Physical activity is encouraged for all adults and older adults. Specific exercise programs may need to be individualized as Alzheimer's disease progresses; general tips on promoting physical activity are included here.

Start Now

It is never too early or too late in life to get started; the benefits are substantial and too important not to take advantage of. Remember, most chronic health conditions like Alzheimer's develop over long periods of time and ultimately impair your quality of life.

Exercise Regularly

The key to gaining fitness and preventing Alzheimer's and other chronic health conditions is consistency over time. You should be physically active on most if not all days of the week.

Move More

Look for ways throughout the day to move and try to avoid extended periods of sitting when at home or at work. See Sit Less, Move More in chapter 1.

Set Goals

Strive to meet or even exceed the recommended guidelines for your age group as discussed in chapters 10 and 11. At a minimum you should build up to and maintain at least 150 minutes or more of moderate-intensity exercise each week (e.g., five 30-minute sessions of walking, cycling, swimming, or some other form of aerobic activity you enjoy). As your fitness improves, including short bouts of higher-intensity exercise can stimulate further fitness gains.

Mix It Up

Incorporate a number of different exercise activities into your routine; mix it up and don't do the exact same thing day after day.

Add Resistance Training

Some form of resistance training at least two times per week is important. This can consist of lifting weights, using dumbbells and resistance bands, or performing functional exercises that use your body weight for resistance. Maintenance of muscle strength is an important component of maintaining independence with aging and prevention of falls.

Be Social

Maintaining social links and interacting with others may be an important component in preventing Alzheimer's. Consider participating in a group exercise class. Most fitness centers and many community centers offer group classes that range from chair exercises for older adults to more intense aerobic activities such as spinning, functional training, and step aerobics. Dancing can be fun and is an excellent aerobic activity that connects you with others.

Consult a Professional

Degreed and certified professionals such as Personal Trainers, Exercise Physiologists, and Clinical Exercise Physiologists can assist you with developing your exercise program and provide guidance as you progress along your health and fitness journey. Ask your health care provider if this might be beneficial for you.

on the amount, intensity, and type of physical activities that promote optimal brain health, considering all the health benefits of being active, there is no reason to wait to get started. Since cognitive decline and the development of Alzheimer's disease occur over a period of many years, the sooner you can incorporate physical activity into your daily routine, the greater the benefits may be. Now is the time to get moving!

Role of Physical Activity in Treating Alzheimer's Disease

People diagnosed with Alzheimer's disease should remain physically active for as long as possible. A consistent routine of physical activity promotes better sleep, improves mood, reduces anxiety, slows the rate of cognitive and physical decline, and allows you or your loved one to remain independent for a longer period of time.

One of the pivotal challenges in Alzheimer's disease is a progressive decline in physical function and mobility. This process can be accelerated when people with Alzheimer's stop exercising and become sedentary. The resulting loss of physical fitness places them in a progressive downward spiral that negatively affects their muscles, bones, and physical capabilities. Joints lose their mobility and become stiff, and when this is combined with weakened muscles, gait changes make walking more challenging. The loss of strength and mobility affects balance, predisposing the person to falls, potential fractures, and other medical complications.

As cognition and physical fitness progressively worsen, depression, inadequate sleep, and mood changes become more apparent; daily living functions such as getting dressed and undressed, bathing, preparing meals, and transferring from one place to another become challenging. This results in a loss of autonomy and increases the need for care assistance.

Exercising and staying physically active is critical to slowing this downward slide and maintaining independence and quality of life for as long as possible. The type of physical activity that is best for the person with Alzheimer's depends on age, abilities, current fitness level, stage of Alzheimer's disease, symptoms, and other health-limiting conditions. Younger people with Alzheimer's and those at earlier stages of the disease process may be able to undertake a greater amount and intensity of activity than those who are older, are at later stages of the disease, or have not previously maintained a physically active lifestyle.

In the early stages of Alzheimer's disease it is important to establish a regular exercise routine that can be maintained for as long as possible. The primary objective is to maintain and even improve the physical functions that allow independent living. As the disease progresses, activities need to be modified and simplified. Many community centers and fitness facilities, such as medical fitness centers and YMCAs, offer specific programming for people with dementia and Alzheimer's. These centers have trained health and fitness professionals who can assist with developing an appropriate program, provide instruction regarding technique, and make modifications as necessary. These are a few things to consider:

- Check all workout areas and your home environment for potential safety hazards such as inadequate lighting, rugs, cords, and other trip-and-fall obstacles.
- Keep it simple, especially as Alzheimer's progresses and memory becomes more impaired. Remembering how to do complicated movements may be challenging, and safety could become an issue.
- If balance is an issue, installing and exercising within reach of a grab bar or with assistance should be considered.

Maximize Safety: Steps to Take Before Starting an Exercise Program

Before initiation of an exercise program, consultation with one's physician is warranted. This is especially important in the presence of any coexisting health factors such as high blood pressure, heart or vascular conditions, or history of falls, or symptoms like shortness of breath, chest discomfort, dizziness, and fainting. Ask the doctor for advice related to these questions:

- What type(s) of physical activities will be best?
- What physical activities should be avoided?
- How frequent should the activity sessions be and for what duration?
- What is the recommended intensity?
- Is referral to a health professional, such as a physical or occupational therapist or ACSM Clinical Exercise Physiologist, who can help create and monitor an appropriate physical activity program recommended?

- Choose activities that are enjoyable; the key is remaining physically active for as long as possible.
- Walking is an excellent activity and does not require complicated equipment. Activities such as gardening, cleaning, cooking, and dancing are also beneficial.
- Some form of resistance training should be incorporated. If a fitness facility is accessible, this could include weight machines and other available equipment. Resistance bands and cords can easily be incorporated at home, as can a variety of body weight exercises.
- Start slow; even 10-minute sessions spaced throughout the day are beneficial.
- As ambulation becomes limited, seated exercise activities can be incorporated.
- Establish a calm and soothing environment that is devoid of loud noises and distractions; familiar, calming music can be helpful.

Over the past century, numerous medical and public health advances have served to significantly increase lifespans, allowing more and more people to live into their 90s and beyond. Parallel to enhanced longevity is a substantial increase in the risk of developing Alzheimer's disease and other forms of dementia. While additional research is required to carve out the definitive underlying causes, it is apparent that a number of lifestyle factors play a significant role. The health benefits derived from being physically active and consuming a nutritious diet are far-reaching and include the health of your brain. Nutritional and physical activity habits are important components for preventing the development of Alzheimer's disease in some people and delaying manifestation of symptoms in others, and are important treatment interventions in those who have symptomatic Alzheimer's.

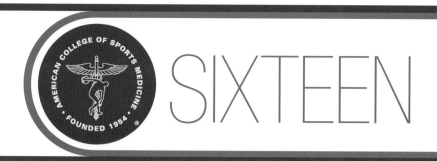
Osteoporosis and Bone Health

Imagine the internal structure of bone as being like the wood foundation of a house. The process of osteoporosis is similar to what happens during a termite infestation in a home's foundation. At some point, so much wood is consumed that the strength of the foundation is compromised and it begins to fail. This is not unlike the progression of osteoporosis; over time, the internal architecture of bone is eroded as a result of a number of factors that eventually increase your risk for fracture. The term *osteopenia,* or *low bone mass,* refers to a condition of reduced bone density that has not yet progressed to osteoporosis. Those diagnosed with this condition should still be monitored to ensure that the condition does not get worse. Figure 16.1 shows a comparison of healthy bone and bone affected by osteoporosis.

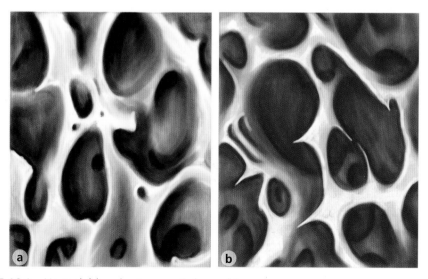

FIGURE 16.1 Normal *(a)* and osteoporotic bone *(b).*

Osteoporosis is the most common disease affecting the skeleton and is one of the most important public health issues facing America. More than 50 percent of women and 25 percent of men over the age of 50 will suffer an osteoporotic fracture at some time in their lives (12). Sadly, one in six women will experience a hip fracture, the most devastating type of osteoporotic fracture (3). This risk is equal to a woman's chance of developing breast, uterine, and ovarian cancer combined (17). Newest estimates of hip fracture show that while the number of hip fractures among women will decrease slightly over the next 20 years, the number of hip fractures among men will rise more than 50 percent (21). While education, new medications, and improvement in healthy behaviors may explain the reduction of fractures in women, the fact that men are now living longer explains the staggering projections for osteoporosis and subsequent fracture.

Fracturing a bone is a serious complication of osteoporosis. Fractures can cause severe pain, affect posture and appearance, and even be deadly. Fractures of the spine can cause a person to lose height and become permanently hunched over. An estimated 20 percent of people who fracture a hip die within one year due to complications of the broken bone or the surgery to repair it. Most who survive a hip fracture never regain their previous level of independence. Although an osteoporotic fracture can be devastating, the good news is that because osteoporosis progresses slowly, you can take a number of steps throughout your life to reduce your risk of developing it.

Causes of Osteoporosis

During growth and young adulthood, the skeleton is busy changing in size, shape, and density to ultimately support the physical needs of an adult. In adulthood, the skeleton remains relatively stable but is still constantly undergoing a process called bone remodeling, in which bone repairs and replaces itself in roughly the same amount. Many processes, however, can "uncouple" bone balance. With normal aging, bone breakdown outpaces replacement, causing up to 1 percent of bone to be lost per year after around age 30. Certain conditions—such as estrogen loss from menopause or reduced testosterone in men, an overactive thyroid gland, diabetes, certain autoimmune diseases and cancers, and gastrointestinal disorders like celiac disease or irritable bowel syndrome—may increase bone breakdown and slow down bone replacement, causing further overall loss of bone. On the other hand, pharmaceutical agents that stop the breakdown of bone, as well as physical activity, which causes bone to be built, can cause a net bone gain.

Because bone is a dynamic tissue throughout life, strategies to slow bone breakdown and to build new, stronger bone are useful at any life stage. Some of the factors you can control, and others you cannot (see Risk Factors for Osteoporosis). Take a look at figure 16.2. On the left side of the scale are factors that have a positive influence on bone; the right side of the scale includes factors that have a negative influence. Positive factors may contribute to bone gain while negative factors may cause bone loss. If you're interested in learning more about your risk for osteoporosis, the World Health Organization has adopted a scientifically validated tool that predicts 10-year probability of sustaining an osteoporosis-related fracture called the WHO Fracture Risk Assessment Tool, or FRAX. This tool enhances patient assessment by integrating clinical risk factors alone or in combination with your bone mineral density (if you know it): www.shef.ac.uk/FRAX/.

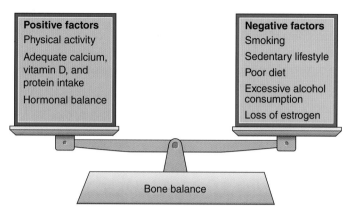

FIGURE 16.2 Factors that influence bone balance.

Risk Factors for Osteoporosis

Your risk of osteoporosis is influenced by many factors, some of which you can control or modify, and others that are outside of your control.

Risk Factors You Cannot Control

- Being female
- Having a thin or small frame
- Being of advanced age
- Having a family history of osteoporosis
- Being postmenopausal, including early or surgically induced menopause
- Being male with low testosterone levels
- Being Caucasian or Asian (although African Americans and Hispanic Americans can be at risk as well)

Risk Factors You Can Control

- Having a diet low in calcium, vitamin D, and protein
- Being inactive
- Smoking, including exposure to secondhand smoke
- Excessive use of alcohol (more than three drinks per day)

Risk Factors You May Be Able to Control

- Loss of menstrual periods not related to menopause (amenorrhea)
- Anorexia nervosa (eating disorder characterized by low body weight) or bulimia nervosa (purging food, which reduces absorption of vital nutrients)
- Prolonged use of certain medications, such as corticosteroids and anticonvulsants
- The presence of other chronic diseases such as heart disease, high blood pressure, or high cholesterol related to poor lifestyle choices or obesity.

Smoking and alcohol consumption are two lifestyle factors you can manage. Avoid smoking, being in contact with secondhand smoke, and excessive alcohol consumption, as these influence the absorption of key nutrients. Other controllable factors that affect the health of your bones include reproductive hormone levels, dietary adequacy (namely, of calcium and vitamin D), and physical activity. Near or at the onset of menopause, typically around age 50, women's bodies produce less estrogen. This loss of estrogen can cause bone to be lost two to five times more quickly than bone loss as a result of age alone. Although estrogen and hormone therapy have been shown to effectively stop menopause-related bone loss (2), many women choose not to take hormones because of a history of breast cancer or other concerns, such as a potential increased risk of heart attack or stroke (6). For men, age-related reductions in testosterone and estrogen may also contribute to fracture risk. Although some men with osteoporosis also have low testosterone levels, low testosterone does not inevitably lead to osteoporosis.

Most of the options for maintaining normal hormone levels are drug related and are discussed later in this chapter, but some behaviors can also influence hormone levels.

Assessment and Diagnosis of Osteoporosis

The gold standard technique for osteoporosis evaluation is called dual-energy X-ray absorptiometry, or DXA, also called a bone density test. Dual-energy X-ray absorptiometry measures the density of the mineral in your bones using a low-dose digital X-ray. Bone density is a very accurate index of bone strength and risk for fracture. Bone density is typically measured at the bones that are most often fractured—the hip, spine, and forearm. The test is very simple: You lie on a large, flat table while the measurement device passes over your body and takes the necessary readings.

Your risk of fracture is evaluated through the comparison of your bone density values to that of a young adult (20 to 29 years old). If your bone density is significantly less, then you are diagnosed with osteoporosis.

You may be asking yourself whether you should have a DXA test. The National Osteoporosis Foundation (17) suggests that people in the following categories be tested for bone density:

- Women age 65 and older
- Men age 70 and older
- Anyone who breaks a bone after 50 years of age
- Younger postmenopausal women with risk factors
- Postmenopausal women under age 65 with risk factors
- Men age 50 to 69 with risk factors
- Estrogen-deficient women at clinical risk for osteoporosis
- Individuals with vertebral abnormalities
- Individuals receiving, or planning to receive, long-term glucocorticoid (steroid) therapy
- Individuals with primary hyperparathyroidism
- Individuals being monitored to assess the response or efficacy of an approved osteoporosis drug therapy

As with all medical procedures, discuss your situation with your health care provider to determine whether an assessment would be beneficial.

In particular, you should avoid excessive exercise training coupled with strict dieting. Women who exercise excessively and restrict their eating are prone to disturbances in their menstrual cycle as a result of low estrogen levels caused by low energy availability. In other words, you must consume enough calories each day to support the amount of exercise you do. The amount and type of exercise recommended in this book would not put someone at risk for such a problem. This chapter explains which types of exercise are best for your bones to keep them healthy while helping you better understand all the factors that influence your risk of osteoporosis so you can make the best choices.

Healthy Approaches to Managing Osteoporosis

Although many factors can influence bone health, this chapter focuses on the impact of diet and physical activity. These two lifestyle factors are under your control and can have a major impact on the strength of your bones.

Focusing on Nutrition

The quality of your diet can influence the health of your bones. A healthy, well-balanced diet as outlined in chapter 3 should provide the necessary building blocks for healthy bones. Even with the best efforts, however, your diet may fall short of meeting recommended levels. In this case, dietary supplements may help you meet the recommended dietary intake. In particular, calcium and vitamin D are two nutrients of importance for healthy bones, as is adequate protein, which supports muscle and improves absorption of calcium from the diet.

Calcium

Calcium is a critical mineral for bone health, and the body strongly defends its blood levels of calcium. Humans are not very good at moving calcium from the food eaten into the bloodstream, and this gets worse with age. Therefore, dietary calcium recommendations also increase with age (see table 16.1 for age-related calcium intake recommendations) (10).

TABLE 16.1   **Recommended Dietary Intake of Calcium**

Age	Calcium (mg)
Birth to 6 months	200
Infants 7 to 12 months	260
1 to 3 years	700
4 to 8 years	1,000
9 to 18 years	1,300
19 to 50 years	1,000
51+ years (men)	1,000
51+ years or postmenopausal (women)	1,200
Pregnant or lactating adult	1,000

Adapted from Institute of Medicine, 2011, p. 349.

■ Q&A

What are common food and beverage sources of calcium?

As with all nutrients, calcium is most usable by the body when it is ingested in the form of food. Dairy products such as milk, yogurt, and cheese are high in calcium; other foods such as nuts, fish, beans, and some vegetables are less calcium dense but can help you achieve your calcium requirement (see table 16.2 for examples of calcium-rich foods) (17). Many nondairy foods are now fortified with calcium, such as orange juice, bread, and cereals, but be sure to read the label because some foods contain more fortification than others.

It is vital that growing children get as much calcium in their diets as they can because it may make a large difference in their bone health when they are adults. For adults, studies show that calcium intake at or above recommended levels cannot increase bone density but is very important in preventing bone loss over time. Excessive calcium intake, on the other hand, could contribute to kidney stone formation in certain people, and taking more than 2,500 milligrams per day should be avoided.

When you cannot consume sufficient calcium in your diet, supplements in the form of calcium phosphate, calcium carbonate, and calcium citrate may be warranted. Supplements should be evaluated on the basis of their elemental calcium content (usually between 200 and 600 mg per tablet or chew), and not on the overall milligrams of calcium compounds. Because the stomach can absorb only about 500 milligrams of calcium at a time, it is best to spread supplements throughout the day.

Some supplements made from bone meal, dolomite, or unrefined oyster shells may contain substances such as lead or other toxic metals and should be avoided. One way to help ensure that the supplement you are taking is safe and effective is to

TABLE 16.2   Calcium Content of Selected Foods

Food	Amount	Calcium (mg)
Milk (skim, low fat, whole)	1 cup (240 mL)	300
Yogurt (low fat, plain)	6 oz (170 g)	310
Yogurt (Greek)	6 oz (170 g)	200
Hard cheese (cheddar)	1 oz (28 g)	205
Cottage cheese (2%)	4 oz (113 g)	105
Ice cream, vanilla	8 oz (227 g)	85
Tofu (prepared with calcium)	4 oz (113 g)	205
Sardines with bones	3 oz (85 g) canned	325
Salmon, canned, with bones	3 oz (85 g)	180
Broccoli	8 oz (227 g)	60
Kale	8 oz (227 g)	180
Collard greens	8 oz (227 g)	360
Orange	1 medium	55

Source: National Osteoporosis Foundation.

look for products that have a USP symbol on the label, which stands for United States Pharmacopeia. This is a nongovernmental, official public standards-setting authority. Unfortunately, testing of supplements is voluntary, so not all suitable products have this notation.

Vitamin D

Vitamin D is another nutrient important to bone health because it helps the body absorb and store calcium. Low vitamin D levels are related to low bone density and increased risk of fractures (23). The recommended daily intake of vitamin D is 600 international units (IU) for adults and pregnant and lactating women (800 IU for those over the age of 70), which can be obtained from food and sunlight. Vitamin D–rich foods include eggs, fatty fish, and cereal and milk fortified with vitamin D (see table 16.3 for examples of foods rich in vitamin D) (17). Based on recent research studies linking vitamin D supplementation to reduced risk of fractures and some chronic diseases, the Institute of Medicine is considering increasing the recommended intakes. Studies suggest that intakes in the range of 800 to 1,000 IU per day of vitamin D are associated with better health outcomes (1, 17) and are well below the 2,000 IU daily limit that would avoid any harmful effects of excess vitamin D.

Vitamin D is sometimes referred to as the sunshine vitamin because when UV rays from the sun make contact with the skin, vitamin D is formed. Minimal sun exposure (to feet, hands, and face) of about 15 to 20 minutes per day is usually enough to get most of the needed daily vitamin D, although this ability does decline with age. Sunscreen can reduce vitamin D synthesis by the skin, and deficiencies may also occur in those who are housebound, reside in extreme northern latitudes, do not consume vitamin D–fortified foods, or have kidney or liver disorders that interfere with normal vitamin D metabolism.

Protein

Protein makes up about half of the volume of the bone and about one-third of its mass. Though it may seem confusing, research has shown both pros and cons about protein in the diet and the impact on bone health—but really, it's the amount of protein that matters. Protein helps balance hormones and improves absorption of calcium from food. Very high protein diets can cause too much calcium to be lost in the urine, but very low protein diets hamper the body's ability to grow and repair bone. Most older adults do not consume enough protein and should increase their intake to recommended levels in order to support muscle and bone health. Research has shown that

TABLE 16.3   **Vitamin D Levels in Selected Foods**

Food	Amount	Vitamin D (IU)
Egg	1 large	41
Salmon	3.5 oz (99 g) cooked	447
Tuna, canned in water	3 oz (85 g)	154
Ready-to-eat fortified cereal	3/4 to 1 cup (180 to 240 mL)	40
Yogurt, fortified	6 oz (170 g)	80
Milk (nonfat, low fat, or whole)	1 cup (240 mL)	120

Data from National Institutes of Health Office of Dietary Supplement.

TABLE 16.4   **Protein Requirements Across the Lifespan**

Age	RDA (grams protein per kilogram body weight)*
Infants 0 to 6 months	1.52 g/kg per day
Infants 7 to 12 months	1.20 g/kg per day
Children 1 to 3 years	1.05 g/kg per day
Children 4 to 13 years	0.95 g/kg per day
Children 14 to 18 years	0.85 g/kg per day
Adults 19+	0.80 g/kg per day

*Kilograms body weight = weight in pounds ÷ 2.2.

To calculate RDA (Recommended Dietary Allowance), multiply kilograms body weight by the factor shown in the table.

Adapted from Institute of Medicine, 2005.

increasing protein along with fruits and vegetables in the diet is the best approach for keeping calcium loss at a minimum (9).

Protein intake requirements are based on a person's body weight because of the wide variation in lean mass based on body size. Table 16.4 lists protein requirements based on nitrogen balance studies across the lifespan (11).

Focusing on Physical Activity

Exercise can improve bone health by increasing bone mass or by slowing or preventing age-related bone loss. Researchers continue to examine what type and how much exercise is necessary for bone health. Though leisurely levels of physical activity are a good starting point for beginning an exercise program, more moderate to vigorous levels of activity are necessary to challenge the skeleton. Exercise is also important for fall prevention, and certain types of exercise have been shown to lower fall risk. To realize the potential benefits of exercise, some precautions should be considered.

Precautions Before Exercise for Those With Osteopenia or Osteoporosis

Specific exercise recommendations tend to be difficult for those diagnosed with osteopenia or osteoporosis because of the limited number of research studies. If you have been diagnosed with osteoporosis, even if you have not yet experienced a fracture, you should avoid activities that put high stresses on the bone, such as jumping or deep forward-trunk flexion exercises (e.g., rowing, toe touches, and full sit-ups). A regular brisk walking program with hills as tolerated, combined with resistance training to improve balance and muscle strength, may reduce your fall risk. Exercise options may be limited for those with osteoporosis who are restricted by severe pain. It may be a good idea to begin exercise with a warm pool–based program, which, although not weight bearing, can improve flexibility and provide some muscle strengthening.

Exercise training after hip fracture and surgery has been found to significantly increase strength, functional ability, and balance as well as to reduce fall-related behavioral and emotional problems in elderly people (8). Recommendations for specific exercises should come from a physical therapist because the activity program needs to be individualized. Generally, these programs begin with safe range of motion activities and muscle-strengthening exercises for the muscles surrounding the hips, trunk, pelvis, and lower body. Typically, exercise recommendations include avoiding high-impact activities such as basketball, volleyball, soccer, jogging, and tennis. These activities can damage the new hip or loosen its parts. Resistance exercises that cause hip abduction or adduction (swinging the leg from side to side) should generally be avoided initially to prevent dislocation of the new hip. Recommended exercises often include walking, stationary bicycling, and swimming.

Rehabilitation after vertebral fracture should include exercises to maintain proper posture while moving and exercises specifically aimed at strengthening the back extensor muscles (the muscles that help you stand up straight). Gentle yoga and tai chi are excellent activities to increase postural awareness and muscle strength and to improve balance. The goals of this type of program should be to reduce pain, improve mobility, and contribute to a better quality of life.

Physical Activity Recommendations

You have probably heard that exercise must be weight bearing to benefit your bones. Some of the first evidence that weight bearing was important to the skeleton came from observations of bone loss in astronauts while in space, when the invisible force of gravity on the skeleton is removed. Examples of this include immobilization (as when a limb is in a cast), long periods of bed rest (from prolonged illness), or being physically inactive. Unfortunately, the body quickly adapts to the reduced loads placed on it. Similarly, non–weight-bearing exercise, such as swimming and cycling, may not be an ideal exercise for bones because the body weight is supported by the water or the bike.

Studies of athletes have provided the basis for the design and testing of exercise interventions aimed to improve bone health. These interventions can better answer the question of what type and how much exercise strengthens bones. The Position Stand on Physical Activity and Bone Health from ACSM (13) and the U.S. Surgeon General's National Report on Bone Health (22) recommend important lifestyle modifications, including exercise, to improve bone health. This information forms the basis for the exercise recommendations and sample programs outlined in this chapter.

■ Q&A

Is walking enough?

Walking is often advocated as a weight-bearing exercise that is good for bones. True, walking is weight bearing, but unfortunately, most research studies of inactive women who begin a moderate walking program fail to find any effect of walking on bone mass. Survey studies show that women who walk fracture less often than women who are inactive. However, it is possible that walkers also engage in other healthy behaviors that could lower their fracture risk, such as better calcium intake or less smoking.

Only two walking studies out of many showed a positive effect of walking on spine bone mass (but not the hip). In these studies, however, women walked at a very fast race-walking pace of around 5 to 6 miles per hour (8 to 9.6 km/h), which is much faster than the usual 2 to 3 miles per hour (3.2 to 4.8 km/h) pace of most women. Because walking confers so many other benefits to the body, if you love walking, don't stop! Increasing the intensity of your walking program to include bursts of very fast walking or walking briskly up hills, however, will burn some extra calories and keep your heart healthy as well as help your bones.

The best program is one that incorporates multiple types of activity and applies the principles of training with bone health in mind. Table 16.5 outlines the basic guidelines for exercise to promote bone health and overall fitness, and each exercise type is covered in more detail in the following sections. With respect to bone, exercise is site specific. In other words, a particular bone must be directly stressed to receive benefits. A multimodal program can provide multiple benefits for musculoskeletal, cardiorespiratory, and metabolic health plus reduce the risk of injury.

Aerobic Exercise   Moderate to vigorous aerobic exercise can improve or maintain bone mass of the hip and spine and has additional benefits to the cardiovascular, muscular, and nervous systems. To challenge the skeleton, the aerobic exercise should be weight bearing, although rowing may have particular benefit to the spine. Examples of weight-bearing aerobic exercises that have been shown to build or preserve bone density when done at moderate to vigorous intensity include aerobic dance, fast walking (5 miles per hour or faster, or 8 km/h), jogging (may begin with walking and intermittent jogging), stair climbing or bench stepping, tennis, and rowing.

The general recommendation for aerobic exercise aimed to improve bone health is to reach a minimum target of 30 minutes of continuous moderate-intensity exercise five days each week for a total of 150 minutes. Another option is 75 minutes of vigorous-intensity exercise per week (about 20 to 25 minutes three days each week), similar to the general public health recommendations for physical activity described in chapter 2.

To see more improvement, you can increase the amount of exercise by increasing the intensity, duration, or frequency. Generally, the upper range for effective aerobic exercise is 60 minutes of vigorous-intensity exercise five to seven days per week. Any more than this and your risk of injury or burnout increases.

TABLE 16.5   **General Exercise Recommendations for Those With Osteoporosis**

	Aerobic	Resistance	Flexibility
Frequency	4 to 5 days/week	Start with 1 to 2 nonconsecutive days/week. May progress to 2 to 3 days/week	5 to 7 days/week
Intensity	Moderate intensity (rating of 3 to 4 on a scale of 0 to 10, with 0 being resting and 10 being maximal effort)	Adjust resistance so that the last two reps are challenging to perform High-intensity training is beneficial in those who can tolerate it	Stretch to the point of tightness or slight discomfort
Time	Begin with 20 min Gradually progress to a minimum of 30 min (with a maximum of 45 to 60 min)	Begin with one set of 8 to 12 reps; increase to two sets after ~2 weeks No more than 8 to 10 exercises per session	Hold static stretch for 10 to 30 sec; two to four reps of each exercise
Type	Walking, cycling, or other individually appropriate aerobic activity (weight bearing preferred)	Standard equipment can be used with adequate instruction and safety considerations	Static stretching of all major joints

Adapted by permission from American College of Sports Medicine, 2018.

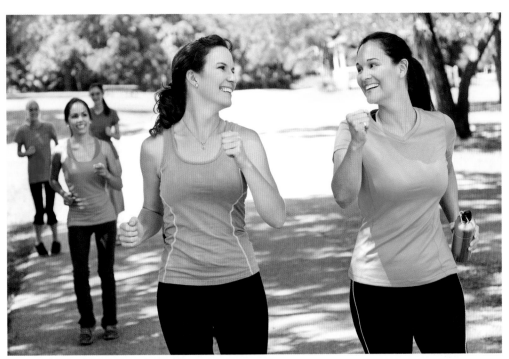

Weight-bearing aerobic activities can benefit your bones.

If you already have been diagnosed with osteopenia or mild osteoporosis, a low- to moderate-intensity exercise program is recommended to improve bone mass or prevent or slow further bone loss. If you have advanced osteoporosis or have had a recent fracture, this type of program may be too rigorous. Consult your health care provider to determine the level of activity suitable for your circumstances.

Resistance Training   Resistance or strength training can have a positive effect on bone because the strong muscle contractions required to lift, push, or pull a heavy weight place stress on the bones. Resistance exercises can be done using weight machines, free weights such as dumbbells and barbells, weighted vests, elastic tubing, or elastic bands. In general, strength training using any means of applying sufficient resistance will maintain or slightly improve hip and spine bone mass (14, 15, 16).

Resistance training has an added benefit of strengthening muscles that are important for fall prevention and to perform strength-based tasks such as lifting groceries, rising from a chair, and climbing stairs. Strong leg muscles can also contribute to better balance and locomotion, which reduces the risk of falls. In addition, resistance exercise can help to lower blood pressure, improve cholesterol and triglyceride levels, and aid in weight reduction. There are many good reasons to include resistance training in your exercise plan.

Resistance exercise, like aerobic exercise, must be slightly rigorous to affect bone. Low-intensity resistance training like sculpting or toning exercises performed with light weights and for many repetitions generally does not help because this type of training doesn't place enough force on the bones. See the sample exercise program for a beginning progression. This level gives you an opportunity to become familiar with resistance training and start to build a base of strength. Try to do most of your

Exercise With Impact: Jumping!

Impact exercise, such as jumping, has been used for years by athletes to improve their muscular strength and power. Jump training may offer a quick and simple means to specifically improve bone mass at the hip, an area where fractures are especially debilitating. Jumping exercise works because it transmits forces up the skeleton and challenges bones in a way that they do not experience during normal daily activities. The skeleton responds by laying down more bone to make it stronger.

In general, studies have shown that women who perform jumping exercise, either alone or added to a program of other exercise such as walking or resistance training, maintain or improve their hip and spine bone mass (14). In one study, middle-age and older women who regularly engaged in resistance exercise plus 50 to 100 jumps, three times per week, were able to increase or maintain hip bone mass; this even included women with low bone density (20, 24). Unfortunately, jumping exercise alone does not appear to improve the bone health of the spine because the forces generated from landing are quite small by the time they reach the spine. Remember, to improve a bone, you must challenge it.

Jump training has not been studied extensively. In most studies, women have performed a variety of jumping routines, including simply jumping straight up and down (see figure 16.3). When the height of the jump

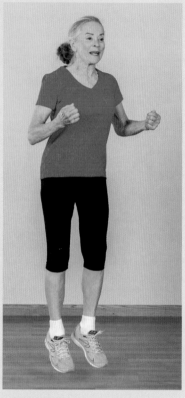

FIGURE 16.3   Jump training.

(jumping on and off small steps) or the weight of the person jumping is increased (jumping while wearing a weighted vest), the jump produces more force on the lower body. In general, doing 50 to 100 jumps in place three to five days per week in sets of 10 is recommended based on current research. Also keep in mind that bone responds slowly and is lost when you stop exercising (24), so a lifelong commitment is required for the best results.

People who have been diagnosed with orthopedic and joint limitations or are significantly overweight should discuss jump exercise with their health care provider before starting a program and may wish to consider other types of exercise first.

resistance training exercises while standing, which engages smaller muscles and is much more functional.

Resistance exercise is recommended for everyone, especially older adults who may have had some bone and muscle loss from age. Following proper guidelines, even 90-year-olds have safely performed resistance exercise. For complete details on resistance training, including specific exercises, see chapter 6. Resistance exercise may be new for you, but it could make a real difference in your life, so give it a try.

Flexibility and Neuromotor Training   Stretching at least two to three days per week should be part of your exercise program to maintain or improve your flexibility and joint mobility (see chapter 7 for details). In addition, neuromotor exercises are also

■ Q&A

What strategies can be used at home to avoid falls?

Use these simple strategies to avoid a fall in the first place.

- Wear supportive, low-heeled shoes rather than walking in socks or slippers.
- Ensure that rooms are well lit.
- Use a rubber mat in the shower or bathtub.
- Use the handrails when going up and down stairs.
- Avoid the use of area rugs, but if you do have them, use skid-proof backing and secure corners to the floor or carpet underneath.
- Keep floors and walkways clutter free.
- Keep phone and electrical cords out of the way.
- If needed, keep glasses handy rather than moving about with impaired vision.
- Realize the potential influence of medications on balance, and talk with your health care provider about any medications you are taking.
- Consider the fact that some hip fractures occur as a result of tripping over small pets.

valuable. People with weak legs, poor balance, and gait problems are much more likely to fall than those who are strong, are stable, and move easily. Because falls are a leading cause of fracture, along with weak bones, focusing on fall prevention is key. For a list of proactive steps you can take to prevent falls, see "What strategies can be used at home to avoid falls?"

For specific suggestions on functional (neuromotor) exercises, see chapter 8. Some nontraditional forms of exercise (such as tai chi) have also been shown to reduce the risk of falls, suggesting that both muscle strength and the ability to transfer weight while in motion can maintain stability. Many research studies underscore how important strong muscles are for fall prevention.

Sample Exercise Program for Bone Health

A sample program of bone health exercise that incorporates multiple types of activity is shown in figure 16.4. Note that rest is included to allow bone to be responsive to the next loading bout. This program would be appropriate for a beginner exerciser who is otherwise healthy and has no known orthopedic problems. If you have any concerns about your readiness to begin exercise, consult with your health care provider.

As you can see, the sample program includes activities focused on aerobic and muscular fitness as well as flexibility. In addition, balance training is another consideration for fall prevention for anyone with osteoporosis. Each of these components is important to include in your exercise plan.

Influence of Medications

If you have known osteoporosis, medical treatment that reduces your risk of fracture is important. New drugs continue to be developed, and new formulations of current drugs are being made to improve effectiveness while reducing side effects. It is important

FIGURE 16.4

Sample multimodal beginner exercise program*.

	Mon.	Tues.	Wed.	Thurs.	Fri.	Sat.	Sun.
Week 1	Bench step** at a slow, steady pace for 15 to 20 min	Three sets of four two-footed jumps from the ground; stretch	One set of 8 to 12 reps of upper and lower body strength training exercises*** at a weight you can't lift more than 12 times	Three sets of six two-footed jumps from the ground; stretch	Walk at a steady pace (with short bursts of faster walking) for 15 to 20 min	Day off or stretch	See Wednesday
Week 2	For week 2, note the increased time for aerobic activity and number of sets and repetitions for jumps and strength.						
	Bench step** at a slow, steady pace for 20 to 25 min	Four sets of six two-footed jumps from the ground; stretch	One set of 8 to 12 reps of upper and lower body strength training exercises using the same weight as week 1	Four sets of eight two-footed jumps from the ground; stretch	Walk at a steady pace (with short bursts of faster walking) for 20 to 25 min	Day off or stretch	See Wednesday
Week 3	For week 3, note the increased intensity for aerobic and strength training and number of repetitions for jumps.						
	Bench step** for 20 to 25 min at a faster pace than week 2	Four sets of eight two-footed jumps from the ground; stretch	Two sets of 8 to 12 reps of upper and lower body strength training exercises, increasing the weight from week 2	See Tuesday	Walk at a steady pace (with bursts of faster walking or jogging) for 20 to 25 min	Day off or stretch	See Wednesday
Week 4	For week 4, the time per session is increased.						
	Bench step** for 25 to 30 min at the same pace as week 3	Five sets of eight two-footed jumps from the ground; stretch	Two sets of 8 to 12 reps of upper and lower body strength training exercises, using the same weight as week 3	See Tuesday	Walk at a steady pace (with bursts of faster walking or jogging) for 25 to 30 min	Day off or stretch	See Wednesday

*Every exercise session should include a 5- to 10-minute warm-up before exercise and a 5- to 10-minute cool-down afterward. The cool-down period is a perfect time to include flexibility exercises for good mobility and function.

**The bench step exercise can be replaced by any aerobic activity listed in chapter 5, including aerobic dance, walking (try adding intermittent jogging), tennis, or rowing.

***Include exercises for the hips and legs, chest, back, shoulders, low back, and abdominal muscles. Examples of exercises to target these areas can be found in chapter 6.

to remember, however, that although many of these drugs can effectively reduce fracture rates by up to 50 percent, none are 100 percent effective. Thus, it is important to consider all of the factors that contribute to fracture risk (e.g., exercise, nutrition, falling) to ensure that you follow a comprehensive program that may include drug management.

Most of the drugs currently approved by the U.S. Food and Drug Administration (FDA) for the management of postmenopausal osteoporosis are called antiresorptives. They increase bone density by rendering the cells that break down bone inactive while leaving alone those cells that form bone. Drugs in this category include estrogens, calcitonin, bisphosphonates, denosumab, and selective estrogen receptor modulators. Two drugs have been shown to reduce fracture by actually stimulating bone-forming cells: parathyroid hormone (brand name, Forteo) and strontium ranelate (brand name, Protelos). The latter, however, has recently been restricted to use in those with severe osteoporosis due to an increased risk for heart attack.

The class of drugs called bisphosphonates is currently the most widely used to reduce osteoporotic fractures. Several forms of bisphosphonates are currently available: alendronate (brand name, Fosamax or Fosamax Plus D), risedronate (brand names, Actonel, Atelvia), ibandronate (brand name, Boniva), zoledronic acid (brand names, Reclast and Zometa), and calcitonin (brand names, Fortical and Miacalcin), just to name a few. On average, these drugs increase bone density by 4 to 8 percent at the spine and 1 to 3 percent at the hip over the first three to four years of treatment (2, 5). This small increase can actually reduce the risk of vertebral fractures by 40 to 50 percent and nonvertebral fractures (including hip fractures) by as much as 20 to 40 percent (7, 18).

Despite the impressive potential of bisphosphonates to reduce fractures, new studies are questioning their long-term safety. These drugs remain in the skeleton for decades, and bone turnover can be affected for up to five years after the drugs are discontinued. Recall that bone remodeling is a natural process that allows the body to repair microdamage due to everyday wear and tear. If bisphosphonates prevent breakdown and bone renewal, the concern is that bone could become brittle. Furthermore, the rare but serious disorder called osteonecrosis of the jaw (a condition characterized by pain, swelling, infection, and exposure of bone) has been associated with bisphosphonate use, mainly in patients receiving high doses in combination with cancer treatment. While experts have not come to a concrete consensus on how long bisphosphonate therapy should be continued, preliminary clinical recommendations state that 3 to 5 years of treatment is probably sufficient for someone with mild risk of fracture, 5 to 10 years of treatment for those with moderate risk of fracture followed by a drug "holiday" of 3 to 5 years, and 10 years of treatment for those with high risk of fracture followed by a 1- to 2-year drug holiday and reevaluation (4).

Hormone therapy (HT, combination of estrogen and progesterone) and estrogen therapy (ET) offset the estrogen-related bone loss associated with menopause and even cause a slight increase in hip and spine bone density that plateaus after three years of use. Studies show that HT and ET reduce the incidence of fractures of the hip and spine by 30 to 50 percent. Hormone therapies are currently approved to reduce postmenopausal bone loss as a means to prevent osteoporosis but are ineffective at preventing bone loss in men. To be most effective at preventing bone loss, therapy should begin close to, if not a few years before, the menopausal transition. After the publication of the Women's Health Initiative study in 2002, the role of long-term postmenopausal HT and ET for the prevention and management of osteoporosis became controversial because of a suspected increased risk of cardiovascular events.

You may be wondering whether HT or ET is appropriate for you. Consulting with your health care provider, who has an understanding of your complete health picture, is best. The FDA currently recommends that HT not be taken to prevent heart disease; and although it is effective for the prevention of osteoporosis, it should be used only by women with a significant risk of fracture who cannot take antiresorptive medication. For other women at risk for osteoporosis, the FDA favors the use of antiresorptive agents and only short-term use of HT around menopause in women with menopausal symptoms or those at risk for fracture (19).

Selective estrogen receptor modulators (SERMs) represent a class of agents that, although similar in structure to estrogen, exert their effects only on target tissues. The most widely studied is raloxifene (brand name, Evista). Its overall effect is more modest than that of bisphosphonates, and its effect on hip fractures has not been marked. For this reason, it is recommended for women with milder osteoporosis or for those with osteoporosis primarily in the spine.

Because each person's health history is unique, your choice of medication should be made with your health care provider in light of your total health situation. Table 16.6 lists the pros and cons of common osteoporosis medications.

TABLE 16.6   Pros and Cons of Common Osteoporosis Medications

Drug class (examples)	Approved for	Pros	Cons
Bisphosphonates (Actonel, Fosamax, Boniva, Reclast, Zometa)	Postmenopausal osteoporosis; post-menopausal bone loss; male bone loss; glucocorticoid-induced osteoporosis	Large increase in bone density at hip and spine; reduction of spine and hip fractures by up to 50%	Inconvenient dosing regimen; small risk of upper gastrointestinal side effects
ET, HT (Estrace, Prempro)	Postmenopausal bone loss	Modest increase in bone density; reduction of spine and hip fractures by up to 30%	Increased risk of cardiovascular events; slight increase in breast cancer risk
SERMs (Evista, Nolvadex)	Postmenopausal bone loss	Modest increase in spine bone density; preservation of hip bone density; reduction of spine fractures by up to 50%; reduction of breast cancer risk and "bad" cholesterol	No effect on hip fractures
RANKL inhibitor–human monoclonal antibody (Denosumab, Prolia)	Postmenopausal women and men at high risk for fracture	Reduced new spine fractures by 68%, hip fractures by 40%	Injectable; requires blood tests, may lower blood calcium
Synthetic hormone: calcitonin (Fortical, Miacalcin, Calcimar)	Postmenopausal osteoporosis	Modest increase in spine bone density; reduction of spine fractures by up to 36%	No effect on hip bone density or fractures
Synthetic hormone: parathyroid hormone (Forteo)	Men and women with osteoporosis and high risk of fracture	Potentially large increase in spine bone density (8 to 10%)	Little to no effect on hip bone density; ability to reduce hip or spine fractures not tested

Osteoporosis is a progressive weakening of the skeleton that makes bones more susceptible to a fracture. Osteoporosis is referred to as the silent disease because bone loss is not painful and produces no noticeable symptoms, but a bone density test can easily diagnose osteoporosis and also determine the risk of osteoporosis before it develops. Depending on the diagnosis, medication may be recommended. Many factors contribute to the health of the skeleton, and many of these are under your control, such as diet and physical activity. A bone-healthy diet includes sufficient calcium, vitamin D, and protein from dietary sources, brought up to recommended levels with supplements if necessary. Everyone should engage in bone-healthy exercise, but especially women and men who are concerned about their risk of fracture. Because the bone benefits from exercise are lost when you stop training, your commitment to exercise that targets the bones must be lifelong.

SEVENTEEN

Arthritis and Joint Health

Arthritis is a chronic disease affecting joints, muscles, and sometimes other body systems. Because of the resulting pain and disability, arthritis is the leading cause of impaired functioning in adults and affects more than 52.5 million Americans. There are more than 100 forms of arthritis, though the most common forms are osteoarthritis (OA), rheumatoid arthritis (RA), fibromyalgia, and the spondyloarthropathies (SA) (6). Osteoarthritis is primarily joint specific while the others are systemic and affect more than just the joints, although even OA has systemic inflammatory responses.

The most common symptoms of arthritis, regardless of the type, are stiffness, joint or muscle pain, and fatigue. Unfortunately, you may have stopped exercising when you started to have this joint or muscle pain, believing that the activity would make your pain worse or speed up the degenerative process. However, proper exercise actually decreases pain. Exercise does not speed up the joint degeneration; rather it helps you maintain normal function.

Causes of Arthritis

Trauma to a joint, abnormal biomechanics (movement), or repetitive joint stress can damage the articular cartilage (the special covering within the joint that absorbs stress and smooths motion) (9, 34). As the damage progresses, the joint space narrows and the bone underlying the cartilage experiences abnormal stresses and deforms. However, for some people, there is no identifiable cause for their arthritis; and with the systemic forms of arthritis, an abnormal immune system response is often the cause of the joint destruction.

There are several risk factors for arthritis. Although some, such as age and sex, cannot be altered, addressing some of the other risk factors may help to control the discomfort of arthritis. Risk factors include the following:

- *Age.* Your risk increases with advancing age.
- *Sex.* Females are at higher risk for most types of arthritis.

- *Overweight and obesity.* Increased body weight may result in increased stress on the joints and may alter biomechanics.
- *Previous joint injury.* Joint injuries usually cause long-term changes to the joint surface and lead to the development of arthritis. In addition, muscle strength may decrease after an injury, transmitting more force through the joint and altering biomechanics.
- *Occupation.* Jobs that require sustained positions or repetitive motions place increased stress on the involved joints (e.g., butchers must use sustained grips, with repeated impact, and thus have a higher incidence of hand arthritis).
- *Smoking.* Smoking is a risk factor for RA and can also lead to complications following joint replacement.

Arthritis is often self-diagnosed during the initial stages. Most people do not go to the doctor until the pain and perhaps loss of motion limit their activity. Diagnosis of arthritis is done by correlating a health history and a physical examination to X-ray and various laboratory test results (1, 4, 7). Some people have little joint damage but significant pain, whereas others have significant damage and little pain. Regular activity appears to diminish the presence of pain. Laboratory tests are most helpful in diagnosing the systemic arthritis diseases.

As noted previously, stiffness is the most common symptom of arthritis, and thus its presence is used to help diagnosis the disease. Generally, if morning stiffness lasts less than 30 minutes, the condition is OA; most of the systemic forms result in stiffness that lasts at least an hour. Osteoarthritis is initially limited to one or two distinct joints, whereas RA is diagnosed by the presence in multiple joints, and fibromyalgia has distinct muscle tenderness at points all over the body.

Types of Arthritis

The two most common forms of arthritis are OA and RA (1). Osteoarthritis is most common (85 percent of arthritis is in this form). It is a local degenerative joint disease and as such most commonly affects the hands, hips, knees, and spine. One or more joints may be affected. Damage to the joint may be due to trauma, infection, mechanical stress, or often an unidentified cause (27). For many with OA, initial symptoms include aching within a joint or stiffness after prolonged sitting. Cartilage damage within the joint is the main problem with OA, and over time the joint may become deformed and lose motion.

Rheumatoid arthritis is the second most common form (1 to 2 percent of the adult population, although it can occur at any age). The cause is unknown, but risk factors include age and being female. Unlike OA, which is more localized, RA is body-wide (systemic) and affects tissues throughout the body. Symptoms develop slowly and include fatigue, weight loss, weakness, and general joint pain. Similar to what occurs with OA, joints become deformed and motion becomes difficult.

Two other common systemic conditions are fibromyalgia and SA (a category). Fibromyalgia is an arthritis-related condition found more often in women than in men that causes widespread muscle tenderness. With fibromyalgia, numerous "tender points" occur in various places (e.g., neck, shoulders, back, hips, arms, legs) when pressure is put on the area. Several forms of SA exist; ankylosing spondylitis is the most common. This condition causes back pain and eventually complete immobility in joints of the spine.

Healthy Approaches to Managing Arthritis

Physical activity and diet are two important lifestyle factors over which you have control. This section explains how both improved nutrition and regular exercise can help you manage your arthritis while also improving your health and fitness.

Focusing on Nutrition

Maintaining an appropriate body weight decreases the risk of developing arthritis; it also helps lessen pain if you already have arthritis (27). Experts speculate that decreased weight results in less force to the joint. If you are overweight, you can use exercise and proper nutrition to control your weight. A loss of as little as 10 pounds (4.5 kg) has been shown to decrease the pain associated with arthritis (26). Because obesity is a risk factor for arthritis, you may want to consult chapter 18, which focuses on weight management. The nutritional guidelines outlined in chapter 3 provide a solid plan for ensuring optimal nutrition. Some nutritional supplements may be helpful and are discussed in "Influence of Supplements" later in this chapter.

Focusing on Physical Activity

In general, the benefits of exercise are similar across all types of arthritis. A proper exercise program can diminish the associated pain and disability. Some studies have shown an immediate decrease in joint pain after gentle exercise, whereas participation in a regular exercise program results in more significant reductions in pain (10, 28). In addition to reducing the pain associated with arthritis, you may also be able to reduce the amount of medication you take to control pain. As noted in the section on medications, many medications have some associated risks, so reductions in dosage are considered a very positive benefit.

Decreased muscle strength and joint motion often result in functional limitations and disability. Regular exercise improves strength and joint motion, thus improving function (21). Additionally, some studies have shown that even low-intensity exercise slows the progression of functional loss, although more intense exercise confers even more benefits (15, 17, 22, 29, 35). A common myth is that those with arthritis should participate only in low-intensity activities. In reality, more intense exercise does not speed the joint degeneration or worsen symptoms as long as you have progressed your program gradually and are protecting your joints appropriately.

If you have one of the systemic forms of arthritis, such as RA, you have a higher risk of heart disease and other systemic complications. Participating in a regular exercise program will help decrease these risks as well.

Precautions for Arthritic Conditions Before Exercise

To maintain a safe and effective training program, you may have to make some modifications. One problem you may have is flare-ups—periods in which the joint swells more than it does normally and the pain is worse. These are more common with the systemic forms of arthritis. During a flare-up you may need to alter your program, reducing the intensity or temporarily eliminating a specific activity if it makes your symptoms worse. Balancing activity and rest is important, especially with systemic arthritis, because of the involvement of the immune system. However, it is not good to stop all activity.

Another concern with arthritis is joint instability and laxity (32). As the joint becomes more degraded and the joint space narrows, the tissues that normally stabilize the joint become slack. When this happens, they are no longer able to properly control the joint movement. In addition, the joint often becomes slightly deformed and out of alignment. Instability is the sensation of the joint "giving way" when you are active and is not necessarily related to laxity, though it is related to a decrease in function.

You may need a brace to provide stability and alignment if you are engaging in activities that stress a joint prone to laxity or joint instability. If joint alignment is the primary problem, especially for the lower extremity, you may benefit from an orthotic, which is an insert placed in a shoe to correct the alignment of the foot (33). Correction of foot position has been shown to decrease knee pain.

If you are having any of these issues, consider consulting with a health professional with expertise in orthopedics or sports medicine. In particular, a professional evaluation is a good idea if you are experiencing your knee giving way with pain, clicking, or catching. Shoulders also are a joint at risk for being unstable.

If you have arthritis in the lower extremity, proper shoes are a must. Your shoes should provide support as well as cushioning. Good shoes can help with minor alignment problems, whereas worn shoes can turn minor problems into major discomfort.

Physical Activity Recommendations

Exercise comes in many forms, and you should tailor your program to your current health status. A complete exercise program includes aerobic activities, resistance training, flexibility, and neuromotor training.

For the primary components of aerobic and muscular fitness, you can safely set up a program following the Physical Activity Guidelines as endorsed by the ACSM and as described in chapters 5 and 6 (3). If walking is difficult, biking is an excellent alternative that can be very effective (24). You will require more flexibility activities than in a typical program (as described in chapter 7); depending on the severity of your arthritis, you should do range of motion activities on a daily basis, and perhaps several times a day.

■ Q&A

What type of shoes are recommended?

The right shoes can have a major impact on your enjoyment of exercise. A good shoe does not have to be the most expensive. These are some qualities to look for in a shoe:

- A sole that provides shock absorption and cushioning.
- Good arch support.
- A roomy toe box that accommodates toe deformities.
- A snug fit along the width of the shoe, especially in the heel counter. When purchasing, walk or jog around the store in the shoes—the heels should not slip.
- Secure closure. Lace-up is preferable, but Velcro may be necessary if you have trouble managing laces because of arthritis in your hands.
- A design appropriate for the activity.

Also, if you have orthotics, be sure to bring them along when you shop for shoes so you can try them in the shoes before making your purchase.

Aerobic Exercise   Aerobic fitness is often lower in people with arthritis than in those of the same age without arthritis. Much of this is likely due to decreased activity. Furthermore, some of the systemic forms of arthritis such as RA bring a higher risk of heart disease, implying that aerobic activity is important to help to reduce the cardiac disease risk. Not only does aerobic exercise improve circulation to the muscles and joints, but also the rhythmic nature of the activities helps lubricate joints and provides nutrition to the joints, thereby decreasing pain. Aerobic exercise is one of the easiest ways to reduce the stiffness associated with arthritis. You can safely follow the guidelines for aerobic activity outlined in chapter 5, though you may want to make a few modifications (3).

If you have not been doing much physical activity, you should start at a lower intensity (e.g., two to three 10-minute sessions a day) until your joints get used to the increased activity. This will also allow you to develop your lower extremity (thigh and leg) strength before engaging in higher-intensity or longer-duration sessions. Increased strength helps absorb forces around your joints, such as the knees, which should help decrease the stress through the joint and the pain.

Although walking is often the easiest and most functional aerobic activity, if you are a runner, there is no reason to give up running. Running does not increase the speed of joint breakdown; many regular runners report less pain with regular training. If you have severe joint instability (the sensation of the knee giving way or buckling), you might want to start with cycling or pool activities until you can decrease the instability. Some exercise ideas to address joint instability appear at the end of this chapter.

If your arthritis is more advanced and you have access to a pool, aquatic activities are an option to consider, although the cardiovascular benefits are not as good as with land exercises (11). The buoyancy helps to unload your weight-bearing joints and allows you to work on joint motion as well. Because the shoulder joint is less stable, if you have arthritis in your shoulders, you should start shoulder stability exercises before swimming. Water activities in general are great for arthritis, but not everyone with arthritis in the shoulders tolerates swimming laps.

If you prefer group activities, many facilities have special classes for people with arthritis. Such classes may not be rigorous enough to build aerobic fitness, but they may be good for alternate training days. Tai chi can help improve lower extremity strength, improve flexibility, and provide some aerobic benefits (18). Aquatic classes are another alternative, especially if you are looking for activities with reduced weight bearing. Other group aerobic classes can be good as long as you make sure to modify movements that seem to stress your involved joint(s) and start at an appropriate intensity based on your level of fitness.

Warm-up activities are particularly important for people with arthritis, especially those who are very stiff. Before your exercise session, loosen up the joints and muscles

■ **Q&A** ▬▬▬▬▬▬▬▬▬▬▬▬▬▬▬▬▬▬▬▬▬▬▬▬▬▬

Does running cause arthritis?

Although running affects joints more than walking does, scientists have not found evidence that links running, in itself, with arthritis. Actually, moderate levels of running may decrease the symptoms and loss of function associated with arthritis compared to being inactive.

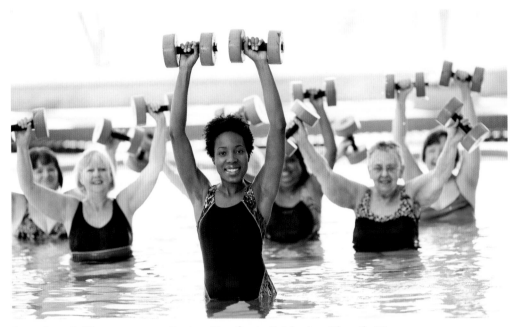

Aquatic activities are an excellent option for individuals with arthritis.

that are stiff. A good way to warm up is to do some gentle rhythmic activities, starting with small movements and increasing the range of the movements as you loosen up. The objective is controlled movement with a slowly increasing range of motion.

Resistance Training   Resistance training may be one of the most important fitness activities you can do to reduce symptoms and protect your joints (5, 13). When there is pain around a joint such as your knee, the nervous system can also inhibit muscle contraction. For many, this results in a knee buckling unexpectedly, usually secondary to pain. After starting a strengthening routine, people with this concern have less pain and fewer problems with their knees giving way. Some have found that strengthening alone does not decrease their joint instability. In such instances, combining strengthening with some balance and movement activities has proven effective (14, 32).

You can safely follow the guidelines for resistance training outlined in chapter 6. A program of two to three days per week that emphasizes the major muscle groups is appropriate (3). Start at a lower level of exertion and gradually work up to a moderate level in order to allow your body time to adapt. A resistance that allows you to do one set of 10 to 15 repetitions in a controlled manner is a good start and is adequate for obtaining some strength benefits.

If you prefer to exercise at home, you can start with a few dumbbells and cuff weights or use resistance bands. Many resistance bands have handgrips and cuffs so you can do upper or lower extremity exercises (see figure 17.1 for an example of a shoulder-strengthening exercise using a resistance band). Resistance bands allow you to progress the resistance with the use of different densities of tubing (see chapter 6 for more information).

You can also do resistance training without equipment by simply using your own body weight. For example, the wall sit, as shown in figure 17.2, is an easy way to strengthen the front of the thigh, or the quadriceps. This exercise decreases the amount of pressure on the knee while still working the muscle. Stronger quadriceps can help distribute forces that are being transmitted through the knee and also improve function, such as going up and down stairs. You can do the wall sit as a timed activity by holding the position for 15 seconds, returning to an upright stance, and then repeating three to five times (progressing the time as you get stronger). You can also do repetitions by using a towel (something that will allow your body to slide up and down against the wall) or a ball behind your back. Another way to increase the resistance is to use tubing with a partial squat.

Flexibility Joint motion is usually lost as arthritis progresses, but regular stretching and range of motion activities can help slow this loss. Furthermore, if you do not move

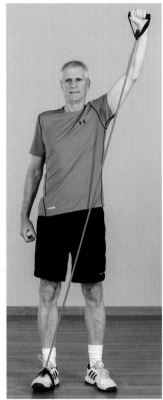 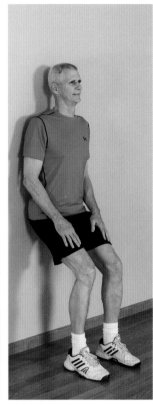

FIGURE 17.1 A shoulder-strengthening exercise using a resistance band.

FIGURE 17.2 Wall sit for strengthening the quadriceps (thighs).

an involved joint, you may lose joint motion more quickly, with an associated increase in pain. Flexibility and joint range of motion can be restored if the loss is temporary, but the longer the impairment lasts, the more difficult it will be to regain your motion. Regular motion of each joint decreases the stiffness and associated pain. Although the typical recommendation is to do flexibility exercises three days per week, you will benefit from daily stretching and range of motion activities (3, 27).

Stretching focuses on increasing the extensibility of tight muscles. Stretching techniques include static and dynamic, as well as those that use assistive devices. You can use any of these safely as long as you follow a few guidelines. You should never hold a stretch that is causing increased pain; rather, stretching should be gentle. Because arthritis can cause laxity in a joint, you should not stretch beyond what is considered normal for that joint. Several factors can affect your response to stretching. With age, muscles tend to lose elasticity, which means that the tissues do not respond as easily to stretching even though much of a stretching response is neural (i.e., nervous system control of the resting tension in the muscle).

You can improve the response to stretching by warming your muscles, which improves elasticity. You can do this by increasing the blood flow to a muscle with a repetitive activity or by using external heat. Some people find that an elastic support not only provides a sense of stability to an affected joint but also helps to keep the joint warm.

Staying hydrated is also important, because dehydration decreases the elasticity of your muscles. The use of a prolonged stretch (several minutes) may be helpful if you are extremely tight—just make sure to find a comfortable, supported position. For example, if you have tight hamstrings, you might lie on the floor with one foot on a wall (see figure 17.3). You should find a position that puts a gentle but tolerable stretch on the hamstring.

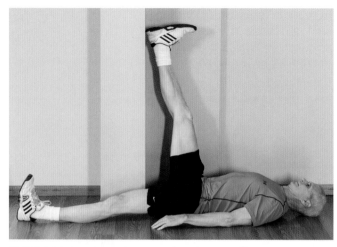

FIGURE 17.3 Hamstring stretch using a wall.

Range of motion is simply moving a joint through its entire range without holding it at any one position. This type of activity may be even more important than stretching because you can use it to prevent loss of motion and throughout the day to decrease stiffness. You should be moving every joint through its full range every day. If a joint stiffens with sitting or lack of activity, simply moving that joint through its range a few times helps to decrease the pain and stiffness. For example, if you work at a desk and have arthritis in your knees, you might slide your feet back and forth (moving the knees) in the middle of a long session of work. Five to 10 repetitions will help to lubricate the joint and prevent discomfort. Most aquatic classes emphasize joint motion in the comfort of the water; thus they are a nice way to work on flexibility. Yoga and tai chi are popular activities that are beneficial for improving flexibility and have the added benefit of improving balance (8, 18).

Neuromotor Training   A typical result of arthritis is the loss of proprioception, which is the feedback to the brain regarding joint position and motion. This loss also contributes to the instability noted earlier. You will need to do some specific activities to address the problem. Neuromotor training addresses joint proprioception and includes agility, balance, and other types of activities that stimulate feedback between the muscles and the brain (15).

Although general guidelines suggest two to three days per week, you will benefit from a more frequent program of five to seven days per week (3, 14). Tai chi is an excellent activity to train the connection between the nervous system and the muscles; it addresses all of the necessary components (18). Tai chi focuses on slow, controlled movements throughout the range of motion with limited impact on the lower extremities. Tai chi decreases pain, improves function, and has the side benefit of relaxation. If you don't want to take a class, you may elect to get a DVD and participate in the comfort of your home. Some people like starting their day with tai chi because it helps reduce morning stiffness. Yoga has also been shown to improve function and balance (8).

You can also design your own neuromuscular training program (14). Because this is the most distinctive component of the training program, a sample is provided in figure 17.4, which includes both land- and water-based activities. Note that if your knees give way frequently, you might want to start balance and agility activities in

FIGURE 17.4

Sample neuromotor training program.

Land-based activities		
Crossover walking	Bring your leg across the midline with each step for 10 ft (3 m), both forward and backward. Repeat three times in each direction.	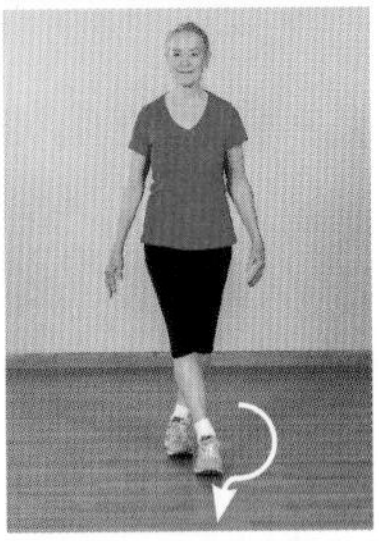
Braiding	Walk sideways, alternating placing one leg behind or in front of the other leg for 10 ft (3 m), both to the left and to the right. Repeat three times in each direction.	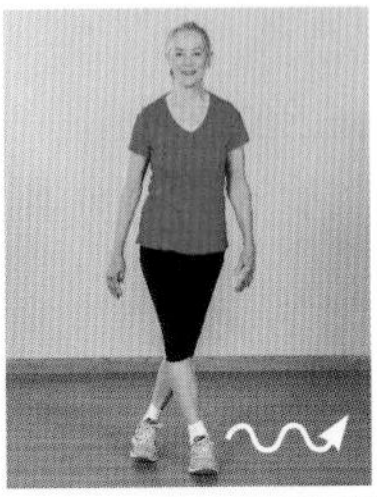
Double-leg stance on foam pad	Stand on a foam pad and shift from side to side, holding for 10 sec. Repeat 10 times on each side.	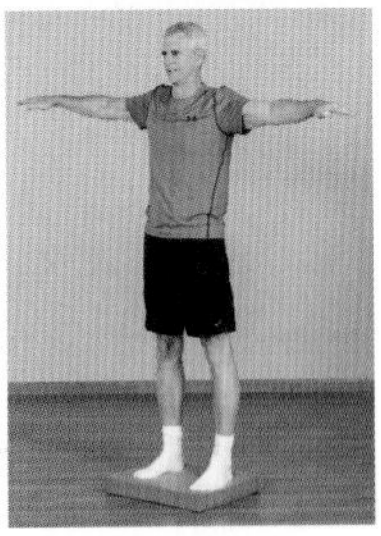
Single-leg stance	Shift to stand on just one leg (hold the other foot off the ground a couple of inches, or about 5 cm), holding for 10 sec. Repeat five times on each leg. Increase to 30 sec and repeat five times on each leg. Then, progress to a single-leg stance on a foam pad, holding for 10 sec, and repeat five times on each leg.	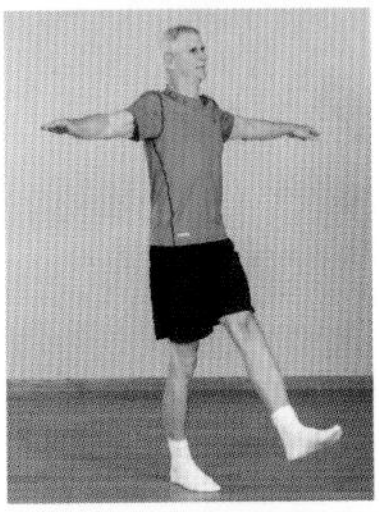
Water-based activities*		
Braiding	Walk sideways, alternating placing one leg behind or in front of the other for 10 ft (3 m), both to the left and to the right. Repeat three times in each direction.	
Crossover walking	Bring your leg across the midline with each step for 10 ft (3 m), both forward and backward. Repeat three times in each direction.	
Leg raises	Raise your leg forward and backward as well as right and left for each leg. Repeat five times in each direction.	

*Include water activities two to three times per week; start in chest-deep water and then progress to waist-deep water. Warm up by walking back and forth for 10 minutes.

the pool to remove the influence of gravity on the joint and decrease the chance of the knee buckling while doing the activity. Furthermore, if the knee does give way, you are protected by the water against falling. Once you are not having pain with the activities and can do them without your knees giving way, you can progress to land activities or alternate between water- and land-based activities.

Influence of Medications

Acetaminophen is recommended for people with mild to moderate pain due to arthritis. The most common, though still rare, side effects are upper gastrointestinal (GI) bleeding and liver damage. Nonsteroidal anti-inflammatories (NSAIDs) are the next type of medication taken to help control the pain of arthritis. The strength ranges from medications that are available over the counter (aspirin and ibuprofen) to stronger forms that require a prescription and have different modes of action within the body. As with acetaminophen, GI bleeding is a possible side effect. Naproxen sodium also has the potential of raising blood pressure and lower extremity swelling. Some of the prescription anti-inflammatories have a decreased risk of GI bleeding but may have some cardiovascular-related risks (20).

If you have a systemic form of arthritis, you are likely to be on a disease-modifying antirheumatic drug (DMARD), glucocorticoid (steroid), or biologic drug (2). Possible side effects include liver and kidney damage and, with the steroids, a risk for infections. On the positive side, these drugs are the most effective for pain relief and for slowing the associated joint deterioration. Because these drugs affect the immune system, you may need to slightly decrease the intensity of your program. A summary of the benefits and possible side effects of common arthritis medications is presented in table 17.1.

Influence of Supplements

A few nutritional supplements have been shown to decrease the pain associated with arthritis. A positive aspect of these supplements is that they do not have the health risks associated with some of the medications. For this reason, they could be worth

TABLE 17.1   Benefits and Possible Side Effects of Common Arthritis Medications

Category	Example	Benefits	Possible side effects
Pain relievers	Acetaminophen	Decrease pain	GI bleeding, ulcers, liver damage
NSAIDs (nonsteroidal anti-inflammatory drugs)	Aspirin, ibuprofen, ketoprofen, Naproxen	Decrease pain, decrease inflammation	GI bleeding, ulcers, leg swelling
DMARDs (disease-modifying antirheumatic drugs)	Gold, methotrexate	Decrease pain, decrease inflammation, slow progression of joint destruction	Liver damage, kidney damage, some cancers
Glucocorticoids	Prednisone, cortisone	Decrease pain, decrease inflammation	Increase risk of infection
Biologics	Etanercept	Decrease pain, decrease inflammation	Increase risk of infection

Potentially Risky Supplements to Watch Out For

Dietary supplements are not tested as rigorously as medicines are and thus may have harmful effects. They are not necessarily labeled properly, and they may interact with medications you take. Some have been linked to heart irregularities, increases in blood pressure, seizures, and even death. Steer clear of the following risky substances:

- Ephedrine or ephedra (used in weight loss or energy supplements)
- Kava (purported to produce relaxation and reduce sleeplessness)
- Prohormones or herbal anabolic supplements, such as androstenedione or yohimbine

Even vitamins and minerals can be toxic if taken in excessive quantities. Consider the following:

- Vitamins B_6 and B_{12} can cause liver damage.
- Vitamin C can cause stomach upset and interfere with copper and iron status.

Check with a knowledgeable person who is qualified to give you information about a supplement before you try it, such as a physician, pharmacist, or Registered Dietitian.

Also, the National Institute of Health's Office of Dietary Supplements provides summaries of many supplements at http://ods.od.nih.gov/HealthInformation/makingdecisions.sec.aspx.

trying. When considering use of various supplements, it is recommended that you check with your health care provider regarding your particular situation. This section discusses glucosamine and chondroitin, fish oil, flaxseed, and antioxidants. Although other supplements have been identified in the popular literature, the research is still lacking on many. See Potentially Risky Supplements to Watch Out For to read about supplements that you may want to avoid.

One of the most common nutritional supplement therapies is a combination of glucosamine and chondroitin. These compounds are normally found in body tissues, and it is thought that increased levels might protect and even improve the joint cartilage. Although the advertised promises are overwhelmingly positive, the research findings are varied. Some studies have shown decreased pain for those with OA, whereas others have not shown any benefit (25). Some of the studies reporting positive effects used supplements in addition to glucosamine and chondroitin, such as manganese ascorbate (a compound formed from ascorbic acid, or vitamin C, and the mineral magnesium) (19, 28). Typical daily dosage recommendations are 1,500 milligrams for glucosamine and 1,200 milligrams for chondroitin. Benefits are typically seen within a few weeks and may be related to the severity of the arthritis and your body's ability to respond to the supplement.

Fish oil, which contains omega-3 fatty acids, has been shown to reduce the pain associated with arthritis (19, 30). In several studies people were able to reduce the amount of NSAIDs or other medications they were taking when they consumed fish oil. Another positive side benefit of fish oil may be a reduced risk for heart disease and reductions in blood pressure that are associated with omega-3 fatty acids. The primary side effect is GI discomfort, which one can address by reducing the dosage and taking the supplement with foods. The recommended daily dosage varies between 3 and 8 grams per day, usually divided into two or three doses (2.6 grams two times per day for RA).

Flaxseed contains both omega-3 and omega-6 fatty acids, but research related to arthritis has been limited, and there are some side effects. Flaxseed can alter the absorption of some medications and thins the blood, so you should check with your physician if you are considering this supplement.

Newer research has looked at the use of other antioxidants that can be found in different types of foods (12). Cherry juice has been shown to decrease inflammatory markers in the blood for some individuals (23). Supplementation of vitamin C (ascorbate) or vitamin E (α-tocopherol) reduced the progression of OA and had anti-inflammatory effects (31).

Exercise is important for people with arthritis. A balanced exercise program that includes aerobic activities, resistance training, stretching, and neuromuscular training (i.e., balance and agility) can help you maintain normal function. Medications used for arthritis can have side effects in addition to the intended benefits. Exercising may allow you to reduce the amount of medication you take to control pain. Although supplements are widely advertised, few have proven to be beneficial. Some people benefit from a combination therapy of glucosamine and chondroitin or from fish oil (omega-3 fatty acids). In addition to physical activity, a healthy diet helps to maintain an appropriate body weight; overweight and obesity are concerns related to risk of developing arthritis as well as the pain associated with arthritis.

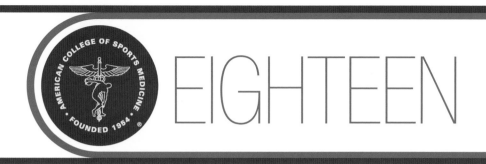

Weight Management

Weight management is a struggle for many people, but controlling body weight has many health benefits. The U.S. Centers for Disease Control and Prevention (CDC) has classified the American society as "obesogenic" due to the environmental factors that promote excessive intake of unhealthy, high-calorie foods coupled with physical inactivity. This combination has resulted in a culture primed to make its citizens gain body fat. This transformation toward overfatness has not occurred overnight. The number of overweight and obese Americans has gradually increased over the past 20 years. For adults 20 years of age and older, approximately 69 percent are overweight or obese; 35 percent of these adults are classified as obese (4).

Assessing Body Composition: Body Mass Index and Waist Circumference

The terms overweight and obesity are both used to refer to situations in which body weight is higher than recommended for optimal health (since being overweight or obese increases your risk of developing many diseases or health problems) (1). You are overweight if you weigh more than expected for someone of your stature (height), and you are obese if you weigh a lot more than expected. To be more specific, body mass index (BMI) is used to classify people into four subclasses: underweight, normal, overweight, and obese (3). To calculate your BMI, choose your unit of measurement and follow these instructions:

Pounds and Inches
Calculate BMI by dividing weight in pounds by height in inches squared and multiplying by a conversion factor of 703, as follows:

[weight in pounds ÷ (height in inches)^2] × 703

For example, if you weigh 150 pounds and are 5 feet 5 inches (65 inches), your BMI calculation would look like this:

$$[150 \div (65)^2] \times 703 = 25.0$$

Kilograms and Meters (or Centimeters)

With the metric system, the formula for BMI is weight in kilograms divided by height in meters squared. Because height is commonly measured in centimeters, divide height in centimeters by 100 to obtain height in meters, as follows:

$$\text{weight in kilograms} \div (\text{height in meters})^2$$

For example, if you weigh 68 kilograms and are 165 centimeters (1.65 m) in height, your BMI calculation would look like this:

$$68 \div (1.65)^2 = 25.0$$

You can also look up your BMI if you know your height in inches and your body weight in pounds using the calculator (see figure 18.1).

FIGURE 18.1

Body mass index (BMI) calculator.

	Normal						Overweight					Obese					
BMI	19	20	21	22	23	24	25	26	27	28	29	30	31	32	33	34	35
Height (inches)	Body weight (pounds)																
58	91	96	100	105	110	115	119	124	129	134	138	143	148	153	158	162	167
59	94	99	104	109	114	119	124	128	133	138	143	148	153	158	163	168	173
60	97	102	107	112	118	123	128	133	138	143	148	153	158	163	168	174	179
61	100	106	111	116	122	127	132	137	143	148	153	158	164	169	174	180	185
62	104	109	115	120	126	131	136	142	147	153	158	164	169	175	180	186	191
63	107	113	118	124	130	135	141	146	152	158	163	169	175	180	186	191	197
64	110	116	122	128	134	140	145	151	157	163	169	174	180	186	192	197	204
65	114	120	126	132	138	144	150	156	162	168	174	180	186	192	198	204	210
66	118	124	130	136	142	148	155	161	167	173	179	186	192	198	204	210	216
67	121	127	134	140	146	153	159	166	172	173	185	191	198	204	211	217	223
68	125	131	138	144	151	158	164	171	177	184	190	197	203	210	216	223	230
69	128	135	143	149	155	162	169	176	182	189	196	203	209	216	223	230	236
70	132	139	146	153	160	167	174	181	188	195	202	209	216	222	229	236	243
71	136	143	150	157	165	172	179	186	193	200	208	215	222	229	236	243	250
72	140	147	154	162	169	177	184	191	199	206	213	221	228	235	242	250	258
73	144	151	159	166	174	182	189	197	204	212	219	227	235	242	250	257	265
74	148	155	163	171	179	186	194	202	210	218	225	233	241	249	256	264	272
75	152	160	168	176	184	192	200	208	216	224	232	240	248	256	264	272	279
76	156	164	172	180	189	197	205	213	221	230	238	246	254	263	271	279	287

Adapted from U.S. Department of Health and Human Services, National Heart, Lung, and Blood Institute, 1998.

Body mass index is commonly used because it is very easy to measure and also correlates strongly with the percentage of body fat. Excess levels of body fat contribute to a number of health concerns including heart disease, hypertension, diabetes, stroke, and some cancers. Typically, body fat levels are higher as BMI increases. As shown in table 18.1, a BMI between 18.5 and 24.9 kg/m² is considered normal or healthy (1); this is because BMI within this range is associated with the lowest risk of developing a chronic disease or of dying. People classified as overweight have an increased risk of disease and death, and those who are obese have the highest risk of developing a number of diseases (4, 5).

Calculating your BMI is a useful starting point for determining whether you would benefit from losing weight. One thing to keep in mind is that BMI does not distinguish between simply having a higher weight than expected and having excess fat. For example, because muscle is much denser than fat, a very muscular male athlete with low body fat could have a BMI that classifies him as overweight or obese. His weight would be higher than expected for his height, but he would not be overfat and thus not at a higher risk for disease based on body composition. If your BMI is 25 kg/m² or

Extreme Obesity																		
36	37	38	39	40	41	42	43	44	45	46	47	48	49	50	51	52	53	54
172	177	181	186	191	196	201	205	210	215	220	224	229	234	239	244	248	253	258
178	183	188	193	198	203	208	212	217	222	227	232	237	242	247	252	257	262	267
184	189	194	199	204	209	215	220	225	230	235	240	245	250	255	261	266	271	276
190	195	201	206	211	217	222	227	232	238	243	248	254	259	264	269	275	280	285
196	202	207	213	218	224	229	235	240	146	251	256	268	267	279	278	284	289	295
203	208	216	220	225	231	237	242	248	254	259	265	270	278	282	287	293	299	304
209	215	221	227	232	238	244	250	256	262	267	273	279	285	291	296	302	308	314
216	222	228	234	240	246	252	258	264	270	276	282	288	294	300	306	312	218	324
223	229	235	241	247	253	260	266	272	278	284	291	297	303	309	315	322	328	334
230	236	242	249	255	261	268	274	280	287	293	299	306	312	319	325	331	338	344
236	243	249	256	262	269	276	282	289	295	302	308	315	322	328	335	341	348	354
243	250	257	263	270	277	285	291	297	304	311	318	324	331	338	345	351	358	365
250	259	264	271	278	285	292	299	306	313	320	327	334	341	348	355	362	369	376
257	265	272	279	286	293	301	308	315	322	329	338	343	351	358	365	372	379	386
265	272	279	287	294	302	309	316	324	331	338	346	353	361	368	375	383	390	397
273	280	288	295	302	310	318	325	333	340	348	355	363	371	378	386	393	401	408
280	287	295	303	311	319	326	334	342	350	358	365	373	381	389	396	404	412	420
287	295	303	311	319	327	335	343	351	359	367	375	383	391	399	407	415	423	431
295	304	312	320	328	336	344	353	361	369	377	385	394	402	410	418	426	435	443

TABLE 18.1   **Body Mass Index Classification**

BMI (kg/m²)	Classification
Below 18.5	Underweight
18.5 to 24.9	Normal or healthy
25.0 to 29.9	Overweight
30 or higher	Obese

greater, use your judgment to determine whether you should make weight loss your goal. If you are an athletic person with large muscles and defined musculature, then BMI may not be the best tool for determining your level of body fatness. In such situations, having body composition (percent body fat) measured may be of value, although these techniques require the assistance of a qualified fitness professional (5).

Body fat distribution is also a predictor of health risk associated with obesity. Accumulation of fat around the abdominal area, often referred to as an apple-shaped physique, carries a higher health risk than fat around the hips and thighs (pear-shaped physique). Taking a measurement of your waist circumference is one way to look more closely at abdominal obesity:

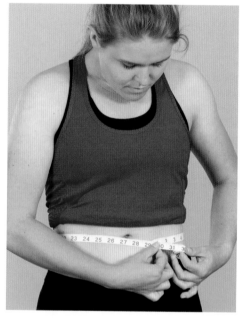

- In a standing position, place a tape measure horizontally near your belly button, just above your hip bones, as shown in figure 18.2.

- Make sure the tape is snug but not compressing the skin.

- Take the measurement once you have comfortably exhaled (1).

FIGURE 18.2   Site for measuring waist circumference.

Waist measures of more than 35 inches (89 cm) for women or more than 39 inches (99 cm) for men classify people as being at increased risk for developing chronic disease (1). Use of both BMI and waist circumference can be helpful in tracking your success at managing your weight (5).

Causes of Obesity

The shape and size of your body is due to a combination of genetic and environmental factors working in unison. Though our genes have not changed over the years, our environment has changed significantly. There is now an abundance of high-calorie, cheap foods and a decreased level of physical activity. In general, your genes create starting points and boundaries that shape how fat or muscular you are likely to become. Although these genetic limits are beyond your control, this does not mean that your body size is set. Environmental factors such as behaviors and lifestyle choices, including food selections and your level of physical activity, ultimately determine how close to your genetic potential you become (4).

Genetic Factors

Genetics play a role in determining a person's height, weight, body fat distribution, and metabolism. Research studies of twins reared apart having similar body weights and adopted children resembling their biological parents in body type support the genetic influence. Determining the impact of genetic factors is difficult, but genetics may contribute from 50 to 90 percent of a person's body weight. This means that somewhere between 10 and 50 percent of one's body weight is a result of environmental factors and lifestyle choices. In addition to body fat, people also tend to inherit specific body types, such as tall and thin or short and stout. This is important to remember because some people may not be able to achieve a desired body shape no matter how hard they train or how diligent they are about food choices. For example, a very tall and thin person may never be able to put on enough muscle mass to look like a bodybuilder; a very muscular, stocky person may never achieve extreme thinness. Another factor out of your control is where body fat is deposited. Some people naturally gain body fat around the abdominal area whereas others accumulate fat in their hips and thighs (10).

Other areas of genetic research include the concept of a thrifty gene and the set point theory. The thrifty gene notion proposes that humans slow their metabolism and store more body fat in times of food scarcity. This may have been an important survival mechanism many years ago in times of famine, but is not so desirable today when one is restricting food consumption voluntarily to lower body weight. Whether there is actually a specific gene associated with this phenomenon is a question scientists continue to examine. In any case, your body's attempt to protect you when you restrict calories can make it difficult to lose weight.

The set point theory proposes that the brain, hormones, and enzymes work in unison to regulate body weight at a genetically determined level. Any attempt to change your body weight from the set point initiates a series of body responses that ultimately result in a return to your genetically predetermined weight. These body responses may include becoming more efficient at storing fat or controlling metabolism, hunger, or feelings of fullness through the action of various hormones. As tempting as it may be, you should not use the set point theory as an excuse to conclude that weight control is impossible. You may not attain aesthetic perfection, but you can achieve and maintain a body weight and composition that are best for your health and well-being (10).

■ Q&A

What is a healthy body weight?

Sometimes the number is not the most important thing. People may have an unrealistic expectation about body weight (e.g., returning to their high school weight) that may not be achievable or desirable. A healthy body weight is one at which you are free of or are managing chronic disease, feel good, and can complete physical activities with ease. This may or may not be the number in a formula or a body weight maintained during early adulthood.

Environmental Factors

Your environment is another factor that determines your body weight. Although genetic factors limit what you can accomplish, healthy behaviors and choices, such as choosing the correct foods and portion sizes, getting sufficient quantity and quality of physical exercise, and learning behavioral modification techniques, certainly can help you reach your genetic potential. Overeating and underexercising are often learned behaviors that can become lifelong habits. Children who are not taught to eat a healthy diet and who are not encouraged to engage in voluntary physical activity begin their lives at a clear disadvantage when it comes to maintaining a healthy body weight. It is very difficult to break old habits when the new behaviors, although healthier, are perceived as comparatively unpleasant. Telling children who typically eat ice cream while watching television after school that they instead should eat an apple and then play outside may generate a less than enthusiastic response. Over time, new habits can be established by building on small positive changes. Behavior modification strategies are discussed later in the chapter.

Determining Energy Requirements

Establishing or maintaining a healthy body weight requires an understanding of how the body uses food to provide energy. In addition, when weight loss is desired, a plan of action is needed for long-term success.

Energy Balance

Understanding the concept of energy balance (EB) is critical if you want to understand how body weight is regulated in human beings. Energy balance in its simplest form is simply a comparison of the amount of energy consumed as food with the amount of energy expended through the combination of resting metabolism, activities of daily living, and voluntary physical exercise. The three possible states of EB are positive, negative, and neutral. Positive EB occurs when you consume more energy (calories) than you expend, resulting in weight gain. Negative EB occurs when you expend more calories than you consume, resulting in weight loss. Neutral EB occurs when the amount of calories you consume equals the amount that you expend as shown in figure 18.3 (10).

Energy balance is most meaningful when it is measured over a reasonably long period of time. Being out of EB for one day has no discernible impact on body weight, but being out of EB over several weeks or months can cause significant weight gain or loss. Whereas the small daily positive EB is not discernible to the naked eye, being in positive EB for long periods is definitely noticeable. Unfortunately, most people notice that they are in positive EB only after they have gained weight.

Although the concept of EB is relatively straightforward, actually implementing a weight loss program is not quite as simple. Seeking the advice of qualified nutrition and exercise professionals, such as a Registered Dietitian or an ACSM-certified exercise professional (see chapter 2 for information on finding a certified professional), is a wise approach if you are unsure how to most effectively balance dietary intake with regular physical activity.

Many external factors control your food intake and physical activity patterns. Factors that influence food intake include cultural rituals; childhood experiences; educational

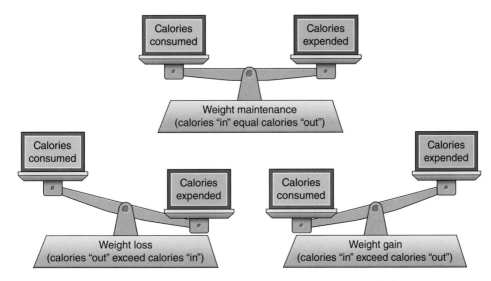

FIGURE 18.3 Energy balance: calories consumed versus calories expended.

and socioeconomic status; nutrition knowledge; convenience; and food flavor, texture, and appearance (10). Motivation, perceived lack of time, and lack of knowledge may contribute to the choice not to exercise. Qualified nutrition and exercise practitioners have the knowledge and skills to help you control the factors that determine whether you are in positive, negative, or neutral EB.

Components of Calorie Expenditure

The number of calories you burn on a daily basis is commonly referred to as total energy expenditure (TEE). Three major components contribute to TEE: the calories expended at rest; the calories expended during exercise; and the calories expended during the digestion, absorption, and storage of food after eating. The largest component, which accounts for about 60 to 70 percent of TEE, is the calories used while the body is resting comfortably, also known as resting metabolic rate (RMR) or basal metabolic rate (BMR).

Energy Balance and Weight Loss

There are approximately 3,500 calories in a pound of body fat. This means that for each pound of body fat, the body must achieve a negative EB of 3,500 calories. For example, to lose 1 pound (0.45 kg) in the upcoming week, an energy deficit of about 500 calories per day (3,500 calories divided by 7 days) is needed. (Note that this is a general estimate; many physiological factors influence the precise rate of weight loss.) One can reach this caloric deficit by reducing calorie intake, increasing energy expenditure, or, ideally, combining the two. To achieve this short-term goal one could consider walking 3 extra miles (4.8 km) and drinking one less nondiet soda per day than normal, or walking only 1 extra mile (1.6 km) and drinking two fewer sodas. The most effective approach over the long term is to combine moderate calorie restriction with moderate daily exercise.

The term resting metabolism is actually a misnomer because the body is never truly at rest. Inside your body a constant array of activity is occurring that must be fueled at all times. For example, your heart beats about 70 times per minute, your neurons fire at lightspeed 24 hours per day, and your white cells are constantly fighting invaders and replacing old or damaged tissue. All of these activities that keep you alive and allow you to look basically the same from one day to the next are exceedingly costly from an energy standpoint. So, your resting metabolism is essentially what makes you "you," and the more of "you" there is, the greater your RMR is. Thus, it is not surprising that RMR is highly related to body mass, particularly the amount of muscle you have. Skeletal muscle is a highly active tissue that contributes a great deal to resting metabolism. The quantity of skeletal muscle in your body is something that you can control to some extent through resistance training, which is discussed further in the section on physical activity.

A second component of TEE includes all energy burned off during physical exercise. This is also known as the thermic effect of activity. It represents any movement your body performs above the resting level and includes fidgeting, doing chores, and participating in formal exercise. This component makes up 15 to 30 percent of the TEE in most people; however, it is the most variable. For example, it may be lower than 15 percent in a very sedentary person and more than 50 percent in a marathoner. As long as you do not have a physical disability, this is the component over which you have the most control. You can choose how many calories you burn through various forms of physical activity (1, 10).

The third component of TEE encompasses all the activities that occur in the body after consumption of food, including digestion, absorption, and the transport and storage of nutrients throughout the body. This incremental energy cost of eating, also known as the thermic effect of food, is a relatively small (5-10 percent) component of TEE. The thermic effect of food is not something you can control to any significant extent for the purpose of weight management. Some diet books claim that you can increase the thermic effect of food by exploiting the fact that more energy is required to digest and metabolize carbohydrates and proteins than fats, but the total number of extra calories burned using these techniques is not very high and probably not worth the effort.

Estimating Energy (Calorie) Needs and Expenditure

Probably the first question that comes to mind when contemplating your own body weight is how many calories you need. There are sophisticated laboratory techniques to estimate this, but these tests are not practical for most people. One simple way to estimate how many calories you need to maintain current body weight is displayed in table 18.2 (13). Simply find the column that best fits your activity level and you can see the estimated calorie requirements based on age and sex.

This method provides just an estimate and a value for maintaining your current weight. If you want to lose weight you need to reduce your calorie intake. An alternative, more accurate method is available from the Choose MyPlate website, devised by the U.S. Department of Agriculture (USDA) (www.choosemyplate.gov and then select the SuperTracker from the list of online tools). This website is completely free and maintained by the USDA. You can create a profile and have a password-protected account that you can use to calculate your energy needs and then track your food intake and energy expenditure over the long term. You will be asked to create a profile that

TABLE 18.2 Estimated Calorie Needs per Day by Age, Sex, and Physical Activity Level

Age	Sedentary[a]	Moderately active[b]	Active[c]
Males			
18	2,400	2,800	3,200
19 to 20	2,600	2,800	3,000
21 to 25	2,400	2,800	3,000
26 to 30	2,400	2,600	3,000
31 to 35	2,400	2,600	3,000
36 to 40	2,400	2,600	2,800
41 to 45	2,200	2,600	2,800
46 to 50	2,200	2,400	2,800
51 to 55	2,200	2.400	2,800
56 to 60	2,200	2,400	2,600
61 to 65	2,000	2,400	2,600
66 to 70	2,000	2,200	2,600
71 to 75	2,000	2,200	2,600
76 and up	2,000	2,200	2,400
Females[d]			
18	1,800	2,000	2,400
19 to 20	2,000	2,200	2,400
21 to 25	2,000	2,200	2,400
26 to 30	1,800	2,000	2,400
31 to 35	1,800	2,000	2,200
36 to 40	1,800	2,000	2,200
41 to 45	1,800	2,000	2,200
46 to 50	1,800	2,000	2,200
51 to 55	1,600	1,800	2,200
56 to 60	1,600	1,800	2,200
61 to 65	1,600	1,800	2,000
66 to 70	1,600	1,800	2,000
71 to 75	1,600	1,800	2,000
76 and up	1,600	1,800	2,000

[a]Sedentary refers to a lifestyle that includes only the physical activity of independent living.

[b]Moderately active refers to a lifestyle that includes physical activity equivalent to walking around 1.5 to 3 miles (2.4 to 4.8 km) per day at 3 to 4 miles (4.8 to 6.4 km) per hour, in addition to the activities of independent living.

[c]Active refers to a lifestyle that includes physical activity equivalent to walking more than 3 miles per day at 3 to 4 miles per hour, in addition to the activities of independent living.

[d]Estimates for females do not include women who are pregnant or breastfeeding.

Source: U.S. Department of Health and Human Services and U.S. Department of Agriculture.

includes your age, sex, physical activity level, height, and weight. Once you complete this you will be given your energy expenditure estimate and be directed toward suggested meal plans to help achieve your goals. If you are trying to lose weight, you can set your profile based on a weight loss goal or a daily calorie reduction. Once your profile is complete, you can look up the nutrition information for food items; track your weight, daily food intake, and physical activity; set goals; and even keep track of your favorite recipes.

Please be aware that this site is designed for people who are free of disease or medical conditions that could affect nutrient requirements. It does not replace the advice of a Registered Dietitian who is trained to address the unique needs of people with various medical conditions. Rather, the MyPlate website is a tool to help you get started in managing your body weight.

It is important to understand that these methods provide only estimates that should not be accepted as absolute values. The estimates are designed to meet the average requirements, but there are interindividual differences that cannot be ignored. You should use these estimates as a starting point but be prepared to adjust your food consumption if you are not progressing as expected. If you consume the suggested amount of calories and your body weight changes unexpectedly, then you will need to adjust your calorie intake up or down depending on your desired outcome.

The MyPlate website can help you estimate energy expenditure during exercise. In addition, if you are using exercise equipment, many devices display the number of calories burned during an exercise session. If you plan to use such readings to help manage your body weight, be sure to enter your age, weight, and sex into the machine's console to achieve the most accurate estimate of calories burned; otherwise, the estimate you receive will be based on the average person and may not be accurate for you. Also, try to use the machines as they were designed to be used. For example, hanging on to the side bars while walking on a treadmill produces erroneous calorie expenditure results because not all of your body weight is being supported throughout the exercise as is assumed in the calorie calculations.

Healthy Approaches to Weight Management

The most successful fat losers are the ones who shed body fat and keep it off over the long haul. Many people have experienced remarkable short-term weight loss only to see it all (or more) return in a few short months. For this reason, weight reduction programs need to be sustained efforts rather than all-at-once approaches. You don't have to get back to your goal weight as fast as you can. Attempting to attain your goal weight as fast as possible will most likely jeopardize your long-term prospects.

■ Q&A ■

What is a safe rate of weight loss?

The effects of rapid weight loss can include a starvation response in which your metabolic rate is lowered more than with normal weight loss. This makes it even harder to maintain that weight loss. The National Institutes of Health recommends weight loss of 0.5 to 1 pound (0.2 to 0.45 kg) per week for those with a BMI 27 to 35, 1 to 2 pounds (0.45 to 0.9 kg) per week for those with a BMI greater than 35.

Losing as little as 10 percent of your current body weight can be beneficial to health. Once you have met this initial goal, you should try to maintain that weight loss for three to six months before deciding whether an additional 5 to 10 percent weight loss is warranted. Weight maintenance between cycles of weight loss is believed to allow the body to adjust to its new weight and gives you time to master the behaviors it took to achieve it. Of course 10 percent is not a magic number, but the general idea is that once you've maintained a modest weight loss for a lengthy period of time, you have likely made permanent lifestyle changes that will support your new lower weight and allow you to attempt further weight loss without overwhelming your resolve. A recommended amount of weight loss is 0.5 to 1 pound (0.23 to 0.45 kg) per week if your BMI is between 27 and 35 kg/m^2 and 1 to 2 pounds (0.45 to 0.9 kg) per week if your BMI is greater than 35 kg/m^2. It is desirable to achieve a moderate weight loss of 5 to 10 percent over approximately six months. This slow and steady approach may be the best way to sustain weight loss and prevent regain (9).

Nutrition and physical activity together are important in weight management. The upcoming sections highlight how you can manage your body weight through dietary choices as well as exercise.

Focusing on Nutrition

Nutrition is an important part of the equation when one is managing weight. The foods and beverages you consume determine the calories you add to your body each day.

Managing Your Weight After Weight Loss

Even after successful weight loss, the challenge remains to avoid regaining the weight. To more fully understand the difficulties associated with weight maintenance, researchers have taken a positive approach by looking at the characteristics of individuals who have lost weight and then successfully maintained the weight loss. The most comprehensive research data on weight management comes from the National Weight Control Registry. This is an ongoing research study that has monitored over 5,000 people who have lost an average of more than 60 pounds (27 kg) and have kept it off for an average of five years. Successful fat losers in this registry tend to do the following (8):

- Consume a low-calorie, low- to moderate-fat diet
- Limit consumption of fast food
- Eat breakfast every morning
- Have consistent food intake from day to day
- Eat smaller meals four or five times per day
- Weigh themselves regularly and take corrective action as needed
- Watch TV less than 10 hours per week
- Participate in moderate-intensity exercise for 60 to 90 minutes per day

Two key points to take away from these findings are the importance of regular physical activity and portion control. Portion control helps ensure that you do not consume excessive calories; this is actually more important than the relative distribution of carbohydrates, proteins, and fats in the diet.

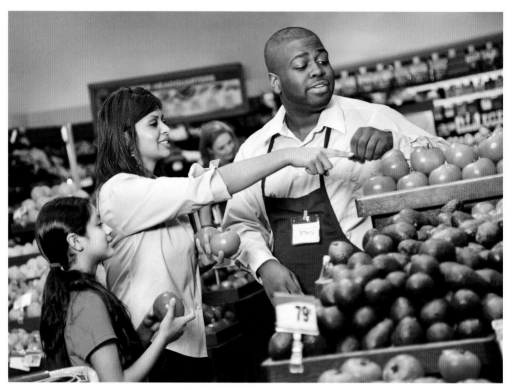

Fruits and vegetables are part of a healthy nutrition plan.

Keeping the calories you consume in balance with the calories you expend helps you maintain your body weight.

Macronutrient Intake

As you learned in chapter 3, the macronutrients (carbohydrates, proteins, and fats) are required in the diet in relatively large amounts. On average, carbohydrates and proteins contain 4 calories per gram, whereas fats contain 9 calories per gram and thus are more energy dense. Keep in mind that all three macronutrients are required for optimal health. No single distribution of calories from carbohydrate, fat, and protein is widely accepted as the most effective for weight management (9). This is reflected in the percentage ranges for each of the macronutrients that are presented in the upcoming sections.

Carbohydrate's Effect on Weight   The primary function of dietary carbohydrate is to fuel body activities. The simplest form of carbohydrate found in the human body is glucose (a sugar). Glucose is the sole fuel source for your brain and central nervous system, so it is absolutely critical in your diet. Glucose also powers skeletal muscle contractions, particularly during intense physical activity. Glucose essentially has three fates in the body: (a) It powers cellular activity; (b) it is stored in the muscles and liver in a different form of carbohydrate called glycogen; and (c) it is converted to fat and stored in adipose tissue throughout the body. Although all three fates occur simultaneously, the third tends to predominate only when carbohydrate ingestion exceeds the body's energy needs. Thus, it is possible to gain fat tissue by overconsuming carbohydrates.

Insulin also has a role in promoting fat storage in the body. Insulin is a hormone released by the pancreas (a small organ located in your abdomen) that helps to store carbohydrate in body cells in response to eating carbohydrates. The higher the concentration of carbohydrate consumed, the greater the amount of insulin secreted into the blood. If you consume a diet high in carbohydrate but not in excess of your energy needs, you will not gain weight. However, a diet high in carbohydrate that exceeds your energy needs creates an environment in which insulin-facilitated fat storage is prominent. You should consume enough carbohydrates to allow your body to perform appropriate levels of physical activity, but not so much that it puts you into positive EB and results in fat storage (10).

The current adult recommendation for carbohydrate is 45 to 65 percent of total energy intake (7). Relatively sedentary people do well at the low end of the range, and very active people require higher amounts of carbohydrate to support elevated energy demands. Many diet books promote a low-carbohydrate diet for weight loss, but current scientific evidence does not support this approach. Most research using low-carbohydrate diets shows significant short-term weight loss, but the long-term success rate is not well established (9). The failure to exhibit sustained success probably is the result of a very restrictive diet coupled with insufficient lifestyle changes.

Protein's Effect on Weight   Normally, dietary carbohydrate and fat supply the body with virtually all the fuel it needs, thereby sparing protein for its other important functions. Protein contributes significantly as a fuel source only when blood glucose drops to very low levels, such as during the late stages of very long-duration exercises. Adults should consume protein equal to 10 to 35 percent of their total energy intake (7). Because dietary protein tends to keep you feeling fuller longer, you should consume protein with each meal and snack in order to curb overeating (10).

Fat's Effect on Weight   Similar to carbohydrates, dietary fat provides the body with fuel. The current recommendation for adults is to consume 20 to 35 percent of total energy intake in the form of dietary fat (1). Also like carbohydrate, fat consumed in the diet has three metabolic roles: (a) It is used to power the body's activities, (b) it is stored in adipose tissue as body fat, and (c) it is converted to an entirely different form called ketones, which some cells can use in place of glucose. The first two roles are the most common; the third tends to occur only when dietary carbohydrate intake is too low and blood glucose levels fall below normal levels.

Obesity and Inflammation

Nutrition affects many aspects of health, including body weight and chronic diseases. Consider the choices you make and how they can promote better health.

- New scientific evidence suggests that there may be a relationship between obesity and inflammation.
- Anti-inflammatory eating is probably a good idea for the prevention and management of many chronic diseases.
- Anti-inflammatory eating includes choosing healthy fats like olive oil, canola oil, nuts, seeds, fatty fish, and omega-3–enhanced products and consuming whole grains, legumes, fruits, and vegetables.

Because dietary fat is the most energy-dense macronutrient and is easily converted to body fat, consuming a low-fat diet seems to be an obvious approach to take to modify your body weight. Furthermore, reduced-fat diets may have beneficial effects on other health conditions such as high blood lipids (9). A low-fat diet can be a useful strategy as long as you are not overconsuming other macronutrients. For example, it is easy to find fat-free foods at the grocery store, but many of these foods contain an abundance of carbohydrates and calories. A word of caution about low-fat diets: Low fat does not mean no fat! Some dietary fats are absolutely essential to human life; without them, body cells would literally break apart. This is why current recommendations set a floor at 20 percent of total energy intake.

Other Nutritional Strategies for Successful Weight Management

Successful weight management can be a challenge. In addition to the balanced approach to nutrition already discussed, additional considerations are to avoid fad diets, to set goals, and to pay attention to portion size.

Avoid Fad Diets   New diet books appear on the market regularly. If the diets were as easy as promised and resulted in weight loss and long-term maintenance, obesity would not be such a problem. Many of these efforts are just marketing gimmicks without any credible scientific research to support the claims. If the diet seems too good to be true, it probably is.

No single macronutrient distribution works best for everybody. If you find a plan that eliminates or severely limits one of the macronutrients, it is probably a fad diet that will likely fail in the long term. For example, some popular diets on the market advocate eating only foods that have a low glycemic index, which is basically a measure of the extent to which a food causes blood glucose levels to rise. As the body senses increases in blood glucose, insulin is released. The diet is based on the idea that insulin promotes fat storage, so eating only low glycemic index foods will minimize insulin's effect. This sounds reasonable except that it doesn't work (9). This oversimplified explanation of insulin's action ignores many aspects of the process, including whether the person is in positive or negative EB and the effect that consuming various combinations of foods has on the glycemic index. See How to Identify a Fad Diet for information on recognizing a fad diet.

Focus on developing positive dietary habits that are sustainable for a lifetime, as quick fixes do not work. The following are components of sound weight management plans (10):

- They promote a reasonable rate of weight loss.
- They recognize a reduced or controlled energy intake as part of your regular mindset.
- They promote regular physical activity.
- They incorporate behavior management.
- They acknowledge the need for lifelong changes to maintain healthy weight.
- They provide flexibility for eating out or in social settings.
- They promote all aspects of health, not just weight loss.
- They include advice from qualified nutrition professionals such as Registered Dietitians.

How to Identify a Fad Diet

In general, fad diet plans have the following characteristics (10):

- They tend to advertise quick and easy weight loss.
- They have limited food selections or eliminate entire food groups altogether.
- They use testimonials instead of discussing and referencing sound scientific studies.
- They are promoted as a cure for many ailments.
- They may recommend expensive supplements.
- They are hard to plan for and follow since they require change in habits overnight.
- They ignore the need to make permanent lifestyle changes.
- They criticize credentialed health professionals or the scientific community.

Set Realistic Goals   Both weight loss and weight maintenance take work and planning, so be sure to set and regularly reevaluate your goals in order to succeed. When establishing your goals, refer to the discussion in chapter 4 of SMARTS goals, which reflect the characteristics of effective goals in that they are specific, measurable, action-oriented, realistic, timely, and self-determined (1). Instead of "I will try and make better food choices," consider the specific goal "This week I will bring lunch from home three times." To keep goals measurable, replace the general goal "I will drink less soda" with "I will replace my afternoon soda with plain iced tea." An action-oriented and realistic goal might be "I will preplan three breakfasts, lunches, and dinners this week" rather than "I will eat perfectly for the next seven days without a mistake." Maintaining a time line is also valuable. For example, instead of "I will search the Internet for recipes when I get a chance," consider "I will find five healthy recipes that I will try over the next two weeks." Determining the right goals for yourself will help you achieve success. Once you have met your SMARTS goals, you can establish new ones for future use, and eventually you will develop some positive habits.

Pay Attention to Portions   There is much evidence that portion control is an effective method for weight loss and maintenance (9). At first it may seem burdensome to weigh or measure items, but eventually it becomes a habit. A great place to start learning about portions is the Choose MyPlate website (www.choosemyplate.gov), which provides information about appropriate portion sizes for each food group. You should also pay attention to the portions (serving sizes) on food labels. A food item that looks like a single serving may actually comprise several portions. At home, weigh and measure for a while and use the same dishes consistently. With practice, you will be able to easily estimate the portions without the use of a scale or measuring device. Check your portion sizes over time because they tend to creep up.

Focusing on Physical Activity

Physical activity is important for overall health as well as for long-term weight management. This section highlights some differences from the general recommendations previously outlined in this book and points out specifically how much exercise is recommended as part of a weight management plan.

Portion Control Made Practical

To gain a better understanding of portion control, try to master the skill of reading food labels and apply that knowledge to the amount of food you normally eat. Learn how many calories there are in a typical serving of the foods that you eat most often. Actually visualize what a standard serving of your favorite food looks like on the plates you have at home. You may be surprised at how small a single serving appears on your plate or in your bowl and realize that you are likely eating two or three servings instead of only one.

A couple of simple tips to help with portion control are to put food on your plate in the preparation area and bring only that serving to the table (box up the leftovers immediately for another day) and to serve meals using smaller plates or bowls. Both of these techniques will help you more accurately visualize the amount of food you consume.

Precautions for Exercise

Before starting an exercise program, refer to the preparticipation screening process in chapter 2 and consult with your physician or health care provider as needed based on this screening (1).

Physical Activity Recommendations

For many years now, it has been widely accepted that physical activity is an important part of any weight management program; however, recent research suggests that more physical activity than previously thought may be required to modify body weight. In 2001 and again in 2009, the ACSM published landmark position stands that summarize scientifically supported strategies for weight loss, prevention of weight gain, and weight maintenance (6). Both publications stress the benefits of physical activity; the only question is precisely how much physical activity is needed.

Aerobic Exercise   People desiring simply to prevent weight gain over the long term should engage in moderate-intensity physical activity roughly 150 to 250 minutes per week. This is equal to about 1,200 to 2,000 calories per week. From a practical standpoint, this means exercising at a moderate intensity for 30 to 50 minutes five days per week, burning 240 to 400 calories in each session. Note that this level of physical activity prevents weight gain only if you are consuming the same amount of energy you are expending.

With respect to the goal of losing weight, a dose-response relationship exists between the quantity of exercise and the amount of weight loss exhibited. This means that the more exercise you do and the higher the intensity, the greater the weight loss. Physical activity of 150 minutes per week provides some benefit, but additional benefits can be realized with physical activity levels of 225 to 420 minutes per week. This is equal to about 1,800 to 3,360 calories per week. From a practical standpoint, this means exercising at a moderate intensity for 45 to 90 minutes five days per week, burning 360 to 720 calories in each session. If you tolerate higher-intensity exercise well, then you can burn the same number of calories by working harder for a shorter period of time; but there are risks associated with very strenuous efforts and you may want to consult with a certified fitness professional before engaging in more vigorous activity. Also, because weight loss requires that you be in a state of negative EB, your diet must provide fewer calories than you are expending. You can further enhance the rate of weight loss by combining physical activity with food restriction, but be careful not to consume too few calories, which makes it difficult to take in sufficient vitamins and minerals, does not give you the energy you need to fuel exercise, and may lower your metabolic rate. As a general rule, you should never consumer fewer calories than required to fuel your resting metabolism.

Finally, if your goal is to maintain your body weight after weight loss, approximately 200 to 300 minutes per week of physical activity is probably sufficient. This can usually be accomplished by walking about 60 minutes per day at a brisk pace. Remember, you must maintain neutral EB by eating only as many calories as you expend (6).

Resistance Training The physical activity guidelines discussed in this section pertain to aerobic activities, such as walking or cycling, but resistance training activities are a very important component of physical fitness that should not be ignored. Although a session of resistance training burns far fewer calories than a session of aerobic exercise does, resistance training has the

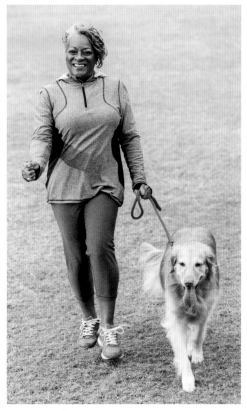

Physical activity is an important part of any weight management program.

potential to promote skeletal muscle growth, which contributes to resting metabolism. Although the addition of resistance training to dietary restrictions may not have a major impact, resistance training may improve your muscular strength and physical function, as well as conferring other health benefits as discussed in detail in chapter 6 (1, 6). The recommended amount of resistance training is not particular to weight management, so you should follow the guidance presented in chapter 6, performing resistance training two to three days per week.

Flexibility and Neuromotor Training Flexibility training and neuromotor exercises have more to do with daily functioning than with weight management. Thus, following the general guidelines in chapter 7 and 8 will help you maintain or improve these fitness components.

Influence of Supplements and Medications

When you want to lose weight, it is easy to fall prey to quick-fix promises. Evaluate any weight loss plan or supplement and use your common sense before implementing a program. If a diet seems too good to be true, it will likely not result in long-term success. Successful weight management includes not only weight loss but also weight maintenance. A program that loudly proclaims rapid weight loss but mentions nothing about sustainability is probably one that you should avoid.

As with some diet plans, many promoters of dietary supplements promise easy weight loss. A dietary supplement is defined by the Food and Drug Administration (FDA) as "a product (other than tobacco) added to the total diet that contains at least one of the following: a vitamin, mineral, amino acid, herb, botanical, or concentrate, metabolite, constituent, or extract of such ingredients or combination of any ingredient described above" (11). Dietary supplements are regulated by the FDA and are considered foods, not food additives or drugs. This means that the tests for efficacy and public safety are not as extensive as they are for food additives or drugs. Food additives and drugs must be tested for years to prove that they work and are safe before they are approved by the FDA. In contrast, supplements are not approved before they are placed on the market for sale.

Whereas nutrient content and health claims must be approved by the FDA, structure–function claims do not. But how do you tell the difference between these claims? The only way to tell for sure is to read the label and package carefully. If the package bears the warning "This statement has not been evaluated by the Food and Drug Administration. This product is not intended to diagnose, treat, cure, or prevent any disease," the claim has not been investigated and approved by the FDA. Be wary in this case because there may not be an extensive amount of research data to support the claims or promises made by the manufacturer (11, 12).

It would be amazing if you could lose body fat simply by swallowing a pill. If this were possible, the obesity epidemic would suddenly be history, the pill would be acclaimed worldwide, and the manufacturer would likely win a Nobel Prize. Because none of this has happened to date, you should be skeptical when evaluating the merits of any weight loss supplement. Even without an exhaustive review of every supplement on the market, it is pretty clear that no currently existing supplement definitively produces significant weight loss and long-term safe weight maintenance. Until sound scientific evidence supports the use of a particular weight loss supplement, you would do better investing in healthy foods and pursuing a physically active lifestyle.

Overweight and obesity is a growing problem. Both genetic and environmental factors contribute to body weight and body fat patterns. A key concept in weight management is energy balance—you must tailor your food intake to your energy expenditure to achieve your goals. No single macronutrient distribution is best for everyone trying to maintain or lose body weight. Carbohydrates, fats, and proteins are all important nutrients that play a role in health and wellness. Based on the current scientific data, the best strategy for successful long-term weight management is food portion control and regular physical activity. It is easy to say that you are going to eat less and exercise more, but it takes quite a bit of effort to make this part of a long-term lifestyle. Behavior modification involves restructuring your environment to reduce actions and habits that contribute to weight gain. Registered Dietitians with expertise and training in weight management, certified exercise professionals, and cognitive behavioral therapists are great resources to help you learn and use these strategies.

NINETEEN

Pregnancy and Postpartum

Historically, pregnancy was often thought of as a time requiring rest and limited physical activity, but today the majority of pregnant women in the United States choose to engage in at least some exercise (13). If you are currently pregnant or thinking about becoming pregnant soon, the good news is that exercise can improve your health outcomes during pregnancy and postpartum (i.e., the first year after birth) (22). Even better, research also indicates that exercising during pregnancy may improve child health outcomes too.

This chapter touches on some nutritional areas to consider as well as highlighting the benefits of different types of exercise during pregnancy, goes over common concerns about exercise during pregnancy and some precautions, and gives tips about how to incorporate exercise and healthy nutrition into your life during pregnancy and the postpartum period.

Maintaining Health During Pregnancy

What makes a healthy pregnancy? Certainly most pregnant women are primarily concerned with the appropriate growth and development of their baby. To ensure appropriate fetal development, it's important to optimize mom's health during pregnancy. Important factors during pregnancy include the mom's weight, fasting glucose levels, and blood pressure.

Starting pregnancy with a healthy weight (i.e., body mass index [BMI] between 18.5 and 25 kg/m²) and gaining an appropriate amount of weight helps to ensure a pregnancy with fewer complications (31). Even if you start pregnancy underweight or overweight or obese, gaining an amount that is within the recommended weight ranges will improve your chances of experiencing a normal pregnancy with a healthy baby (see table 19.1 for recommended weight gain during pregnancy) (31).

The two most common pregnancy complications are gestational diabetes and hypertension (i.e., gestational hypertension or preeclampsia). Gestational diabetes affects 5 to 9 percent of U.S. pregnancies and is diagnosed as abnormally high blood glucose (sugar) occurring for the first time during pregnancy (17). Women who have a family history of diabetes, who are overweight or obese, or who previously delivered a large infant (i.e., greater than 4.5 kilograms [10 lb]) are at higher risk for developing gestational diabetes. Gestational diabetes increases the risk of delivering a large infant, who then has a higher risk of being obese during childhood (36). Women diagnosed with gestational diabetes should work closely with a Registered Dietician or other health care provider to control their blood glucose level while ensuring that optimal nutrients are available for the developing baby.

Gestational hypertension or preeclampsia affects 2 to 7 percent of U.S. pregnancies. Gestational hypertension is diagnosed as high blood pressure occurring for the first time during pregnancy, while preeclampsia is a more severe condition characterized by hypertension combined with excess protein in the urine (3). Both conditions increase the risk of delivering an infant who is small or premature. Women with a family history of hypertension who are African American, are overweight or obese, have gestational diabetes, or are carrying multiples (e.g., twins, triplets) are at higher risk for gestational hypertension or preeclampsia.

Healthy Approaches to Pregnancy

Physical activity and eating a healthy diet are two important lifestyle behaviors for pregnant women that can help them avoid or treat the pregnancy complications highlighted next.

Focusing on Nutrition

Nutrition during pregnancy takes on special importance since it affects both maternal and fetal health. The Academy of Nutrition and Dietetics (AND) states that the key components of a healthy pregnancy include appropriate weight gain, healthy nutrition, and safe food handling (30).

Appropriate Weight Gain

Recommended amounts of weight gain during pregnancy are based on prepregnancy weight status to optimize infant birth weight, avoid excessive postpartum weight retention for mom, and reduce the risk of later chronic disease development for mom and baby. Gaining either not enough or too much is associated with poorer birth outcomes. To find out how much weight you should gain during a singleton pregnancy (i.e., resulting in the birth of one infant), first calculate your BMI from your weight and height before pregnancy (see chapter 18 for details on determining your BMI) and then check table 19.1 (31). For multiple births (e.g., twins, triplets), higher weight gains are needed to improve infant birth weight and length of pregnancy: Weight gain should be 40 to 54 pounds (18 to 25 kg) for women who are normal weight, more for those who are underweight (50 to 62 pounds or 23 to 28 kg), and less for those who are overweight or obese (as little as 29 to 38 pounds or 13 to 17 kg) (31).

Consumption of a Variety of Foods

The Dietary Guidelines, as discussed in chapter 3, are appropriate during pregnancy. The daily energy needs of pregnant women increase in the second and third trimester

TABLE 19.1   **Recommended Ranges for Total Weight Gain During Singleton Pregnancy by Prepregnancy Weight Status**

Prepregnancy BMI (kg/m²)	Recommended weight gain
Underweight (<18.5)	28 to 40 lb (13 to 18 kg)
Normal weight (18.5 to 24.9)	25 to 35 lb (11 to 16 kg)
Overweight (25.0 to 29.9)	15 to 25 lb (7 to 11 kg)
Obese (>30.0)	11 to 20 lb (5 to 9 kg)

Adapted by permission from Institute of Medicine and National Research Council of the National Academies, 2009, p. 2.

by about 340 calories and 450 calories, respectively, but calories add up quickly so it's important to eat nutrient-packed foods like fruits, vegetables, and whole grains. Multiple births require additional calorie intake, but researchers have not precisely determined these energy requirements (30).

Appropriate Vitamin and Mineral Supplementation

Many women of childbearing age do not maintain healthy enough eating habits to meet their nutrient needs, and this continues to be a concern during pregnancy. For this reason, and because of the role folic acid plays in preventing specific birth defects when taken very early in pregnancy, all women who are capable of becoming pregnant (including adolescents) should supplement with folic acid. This includes consuming 400 micrograms of synthetic folic acid from dietary supplements or fortified foods (e.g., bread, pasta, and some breakfast cereals) in addition to eating foods like green leafy vegetables that are a good source of natural folate; pregnant women are encouraged to consume a total of 600 micrograms from all sources (35). Iron requirements are also higher during pregnancy. Iron supplementation is recommended to meet the increased demands during pregnancy and is particularly important for anemic women (18). Pregnant and breastfeeding women should ask their health care provider about taking these and other prenatal supplements, including omega-3 fatty acids, vitamins B_{12} and D, choline, calcium, iodine, and zinc, which may be warranted for women with poor diets or those who exclude entire food groups like meat or dairy from their usual diets (30).

Avoidance of Alcohol, Tobacco, and Other Harmful Substances

Pregnant women should not consume alcohol; drinking during pregnancy is associated with developmental and neurological birth defects (30). Smoking should also be avoided because it limits the oxygen available for the baby and increases the risk of spontaneous abortion, preterm birth, and sudden infant death syndrome, among other concerns (30).

Safe Food Handling

Pregnant women and their babies have a higher risk of developing food-borne illnesses. Therefore, it is recommended that pregnant women avoid soft cheeses not made with pasteurized milk, cold smoked fish, and cold deli salads. For any deli meats, luncheon meats, bologna, or frankfurters, the items should be reheated to steaming hot. Pregnant women should avoid any unpasteurized products or raw or undercooked eggs or meat.

■Q&A

Where can I get healthy meal plans for pregnancy and postpartum?

You can use www.choosemyplate.gov/moms-pregnancy-breastfeeding to help you devise a healthy meal plan during your pregnancy and postpartum. All women of childbearing age should be sure to eat foods high in folic acid (green leafy vegetables and fortified grains). During pregnancy and postpartum, talk to your health care provider about other dietary supplements.

Due to mercury levels in fish, do not eat shark, swordfish, king mackerel, or tilefish if you're pregnant. Lower mercury content seafood (e.g., shrimp, canned light tuna, salmon, pollock, catfish) is considered safe and encouraged because of its beneficial fatty acid content at 8 to 12 ounces (225-340 g; about three servings) per week.

Thus, although good nutrition is always important for your health, dietary choices are especially important during pregnancy when your body needs extra energy and nutrients to ensure that both you and your baby stay healthy. In addition to the recommendations regarding iron and folate supplements to ensure healthy birth outcomes, you should consume at least 8 to 10 cups (64-80 fl oz) of fluid per day to stay hydrated (30). You can use the Daily Food Plan for Moms (see www.choosemyplate.gov/moms-pregnancy-breastfeeding) to create food plans that meet energy needs (i.e., ~2200 to 2900 calories per day for most pregnant women) while ensuring that all food groups are covered.

Women who exercise during pregnancy should take additional care to make sure to balance energy expenditure with energy intake. In other words, make sure to eat extra calories to make up for the ones you burn while exercising—pregnancy is not the time to lose weight! More details on calculating calories burned for an activity based on your body weight are found in chapter 5. Recall that once you know the MET value (metabolic equivalent; a unit of measure reflecting the amount of oxygen used) you can also determine the calories burned per minute during the activity using the equations on page 93. Your total number of calories burned depends on how long you exercise at a given intensity. If you choose to exercise vigorously during pregnancy or pursue athletic training for competition, you may wish to meet with a Registered Dietitian to make sure you and your developing baby's energy and nutrient needs are being met. For more information on general nutrition recommendations see chapter 3, which includes details on the Dietary Guidelines recommendations.

Focusing on Physical Activity

The original 1985 guidelines for physical activity during pregnancy published by the American College of Obstetricians and Gynecologists (ACOG) were cautious, advising pregnant women that heart rate "should not exceed 140 bpm" (1); however, there was actually no scientific basis for that recommendation. Heart rate limitations have never been mentioned in pregnancy exercise guidelines since that time, and a broad range of health benefits associated with exercise during pregnancy have been documented (22). The ACOG guidelines now state that "women with uncomplicated pregnancies should be encouraged to engage in aerobic and strength-conditioning exercises

■ **Q&A**

What are examples of "moderate" and "vigorous" activities?

It is recommended that pregnant and postpartum women engage in 150 minutes per week (30 minutes, five days per week) of moderate aerobic physical activity. Moderate activities you might like include walking, swimming, bicycling (10 to 13 miles per hour [16 to 21 km]), dancing, and aerobics. Women who are already vigorously active can most often maintain those activities. Vigorous activities include jogging, fast bicycling (14 miles per hour [22.5 km] or faster), hiking, and singles tennis. You can use the talk test to help determine your intensity: During moderate activities, you are able to talk in complete sentences, while during vigorous activities you may be able to say only a few words at a time (2). Talk to your health care provider and listen to your body to adjust the intensity of your physical activity.

before, during, and after pregnancy" (2). The *Physical Activity Guidelines for Americans* recommends the following (34):

- Healthy women who are not already highly active or doing vigorous-intensity activity should get at least 150 minutes (2 hours and 30 minutes) of moderate-intensity aerobic activity per week during pregnancy and the postpartum period. Preferably, this activity should be spread throughout the week.

- Pregnant women who habitually engage in vigorous-intensity aerobic activity or are highly active can continue physical activity during pregnancy and the postpartum period, provided that they remain healthy and discuss with their health care provider how and when activity should be adjusted over time.

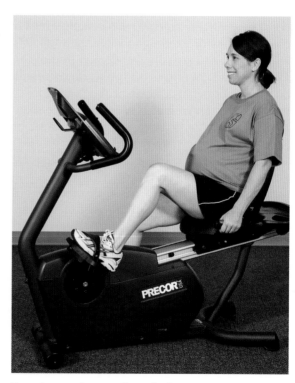

Exercise, such as cycling, during pregnancy provides many benefits.

Benefits of Exercise

Exercise before as well as during pregnancy is associated with lower risk for excessive gestational weight gain, gestational diabetes, preeclampsia, and preterm delivery (22). Exercise during pregnancy also appears to be a safe and effective way to maintain blood glucose within normal limits among women who are already diabetic or who become so during pregnancy (32). Importantly, women reporting the recommended amount of physical activity during pregnancy (i.e., at least 150 minutes per week) also seem to deliver babies with healthier birth weights (23). Exercising women have a lower risk of delivering a large infant (i.e., over 4.5 kilograms [10 lb]) without changing their risk of delivering a small infant (i.e., less than 2.5 kilograms [5.5 lb]). This is important since both low and high birth weight have been linked to increased risk of heart disease and obesity later in life. A few small studies have shown that children of women who exercised during pregnancy had less body fat or reduced risk of obesity compared to children of women who did not exercise (9, 19, 24). Thus, participation in aerobic exercise during pregnancy not only improves maternal health; it may also contribute to better child health outcomes.

These results were based on self-reported physical activity and likely largely reflect values for women who were active before pregnancy and continued their routines, since most women do not choose to start exercise when they become pregnant. Unfortunately, research studies that have previously inactive women either start exercising (most often walking) or participate in a control group (like a health education class) have largely failed to show significant effects of exercise on risk of pregnancy complications or excessive weight gain (20, 25, 27). Importantly, most of these studies also failed to actually get women in the exercise groups to exercise regularly (20). Thus, the lack of effects on health outcomes most likely reflects the difficulty of getting people to change their health behaviors. More studies are needed to determine whether women who start exercising once they become pregnant will enjoy the same health benefits as women who were active beforehand and continue their activity levels during their pregnancy.

The benefits of exercise continue during the postpartum period. The 2015 ACOG guidelines recommend that women resume prepregnancy exercise routines gradually after birth as soon as it is physically and medically safe (2). The exact amount of time needed to recover after birth varies from woman to woman depending on the difficulty of labor, type of delivery (cesarean versus vaginal), preexisting fitness level, and other medical complications. Typically women can resume exercise within days of delivery if no complications are present, although women who experience cesarean deliveries should not start exercising before four to six weeks postpartum. Consulting with your health care provider will allow you to determine what is best for you and your situation.

Exercising during the postpartum period helps with weight loss and appears to have psychological benefits. Women reporting greater amounts of exercise have less weight

■ Q&A

How to stay active after baby's birth?

Home-based activities might include walking around the neighborhood or on a treadmill to promote aerobic fitness or using resistance bands for muscular fitness. In addition, community-based activity programs can provide social aspects in addition to opportunities to be active. For example, some communities have exercise programs specifically for mothers and their babies at shopping malls. With babies happily riding in their strollers, the moms power walk, resistance train with tubing or bands, and stretch. Not only are these exercise sessions invigorating, they also provide a chance to chat with other new mothers.

retention at six weeks and one year postpartum compared to less active women (26, 34). While being active during pregnancy or the postpartum period (or both) does not seem to reduce the occurrence of postpartum depression, exercise prescriptions have been effective at alleviating depressive symptoms among women with postpartum depression (33, 34).

Therefore, current recommendations endorse regular exercise as part of a healthy pregnancy and postpartum period. Research shows that exercise is both safe and beneficial during pregnancy. While it is recommended that women get at least 150 minutes per week of moderate activity during pregnancy, more specific recommendations for aerobic fitness, muscular fitness, and flexibility training are not available (34). Some women choose to continue running 50+ miles (80+ km) per week during pregnancy with no ill effect, while others choose to start walking or swimming during pregnancy. Women who already have an exercise program before pregnancy are advised to continue the same program until they feel the need to modify it by decreasing intensity, frequency, or duration of exercise. Women who are not already active are advised to begin moderate exercise during pregnancy to improve their own health as well as their child's health. As outlined throughout this book, a balanced exercise program includes aerobic and muscular fitness, along with flexibility. This section outlines some special considerations for pregnant women regarding exercise.

Precautions for Pregnancy Conditions Before Exercise

During pregnancy, women are encouraged to discuss physical activity with their health care provider since some women may have contraindications to exercise. Table 19.2 includes a list of relative and absolute contraindications to exercise during pregnancy (2). Women with absolute contraindications should not exercise until those health conditions are resolved. A woman with relative contraindications may participate

TABLE 19.2   Absolute and Relative Contraindications to Aerobic Exercise During Pregnancy

Absolute contraindications	Relative contraindications
• Hemodynamically significant heart disease	• Anemia
• Restrictive lung disease	• Unelevated maternal cardiac arrhythmia
• Incompetent cervix or cerclage	• Chronic bronchitis
• Multiple gestation at risk for premature labor	• Poorly controlled type 1 diabetes
• Persistent bleeding in second or third trimester	• Extreme morbid obesity
• Placenta previa after 26 weeks gestation	• Extreme underweight
• Premature labor in current pregnancy	• History of extremely sedentary lifestyle
• Ruptured membranes	• Intrauterine growth restriction in current pregnancy
• Preeclampsia or pregnancy-induced hypertension	• Poorly controlled hypertension
• Severe anemia	• Orthopedic limitations
	• Poorly controlled seizure disorder
	• Poorly controlled hyperthyroidism
	• Heavy smoker

Reprinted with permission from Physical activity and exercise during pregnancy and the postpartum period. Committee Opinion No. 650. American College of Obstetricians and Gynecologists. *Obstet Gynecol* 2015; 126: e135–e142.

in physical activities as long as she checks with her health care provider first. More intensive monitoring of maternal and fetal health may be warranted for women with relative contraindications.

Pregnant women face unique barriers to exercise, including fatigue, lack of time, morning sickness, increasing physical and joint discomfort, and lack of child care for other children (12, 22). In order to overcome these barriers, you should seek to incorporate exercise into your daily life. Exercise sessions can be broken up into smaller bouts to ease fatigue and time constraints. If you experience low back or joint pain, you may wish to pursue non–weight-bearing activities like swimming, cycling, or water aerobics. An abdominal support band can also help to support the pregnant belly during weight-bearing exercise and ease discomfort. In the postpartum, you may choose to include your baby in your workout by using a jogging stroller. It is also a good idea to try exercising with a friend or a group, especially during postpartum when many women encounter feelings of depression or feel shut off from the outside world.

Exercise prescription during pregnancy and postpartum does not differ from exercise prescription at any other time, except for the need to avoid or modify certain activities and monitor the baby's well-being (see table 19.3). You should maintain open communication about your exercise program with your health care provider. Additionally, you can check on your baby's health by monitoring weight gain during pregnancy to ensure that you are gaining recommended amounts and by recording your baby's activity patterns, such as kicking or rolling, during the day. Knowing normal activity patterns can help you determine whether a change occurs with exercise. In general, the baby should move several times within the first half hour after exercise in the second and third trimesters (10). If the baby stops moving or decreases the amount of usual activity throughout the day, you should contact your health care provider.

If you were already doing vigorous activities before becoming pregnant, you can feel good about continuing those activities throughout pregnancy, although you may choose to make some practical changes to your exercise routine later in pregnancy. If you are not already an exerciser when you become pregnant, research supports that starting a moderate aerobic exercise program like walking or swimming is both safe and beneficial.

Women often ask "How much do I need to exercise?" or "How much is too much?" during pregnancy. While the guidelines provide direction for a minimum amount of exercise (i.e., 150 minutes per week of at least moderate activity), they do not address an upper limit for exercise during pregnancy (34). Instead, women who were already active before pregnancy are advised to continue normal exercise routines until symptoms tell them to stop. Basically, if it feels good, it's probably OK to keep doing it during pregnancy. The ACOG also gives a list of warning signs that call for terminating exercise during pregnancy (2):

- Vaginal bleeding
- Regular painful contractions
- Amniotic fluid leakage
- Dizziness or headache
- Chest pain
- Muscle weakness affecting balance
- Calf pain or swelling
- Shortness of breath (before exercise)

Symptoms don't always need to be dramatic. Warning signs are relative to each woman and should be interpreted in light of your exercise and medical history. Many women simply report the need to decrease exercise intensity, duration, or frequency later in pregnancy. Now, more than ever, it is important to listen to your body!

Some women fear that exercise might hurt their baby and perceive vigorous or high-impact activities as unsafe (21). While such fears are unwarranted based on current research results, precautions should still be followed. Specifically, you should not engage in contact sports (e.g., ice hockey, boxing, soccer, basketball), activities with a high risk of falling (e.g., downhill skiing, waterskiing, surfing, off-road cycling, gymnastics, horseback riding), scuba diving, or sky diving (2). You should also be cautious about trying new activities that require balance and coordination, like lifting free weights, since the risk of falling increases due to a changing center of gravity and increases in joint laxity. Maintaining a normal body temperature during activity can also be harder during pregnancy, so avoid exercising in hot and humid conditions (including "Hot yoga" or "Hot Pilates"), and use a fan when exercising indoors on a treadmill or other exercise machine. Table 19.3 summarizes common exercise concerns during pregnancy and suggests modifications to lessen any risk (28).

In the postpartum period, many women are concerned about how exercise might affect breastfeeding. From a comfort perspective, enlarged breasts from lactation pose a problem for exercise; thus it takes some effort and planning to coordinate breast-feeding and exercise. Breastfeeding also requires a lot of water, so drinking plenty of water before, during, and after exercise is important. Feeding or pumping immediately before working out can ease discomfort associated with enlarged breasts. Also, many women choose to wear two sport bras or use an elastic bandage wrap to give more support while exercising. Importantly, research shows that milk volume and nutrient content are not negatively affected by exercise (4). So you can choose to be active during the postpartum period and reap the many benefits associated with exercise while knowing you are not depriving your infant in any way.

TABLE 19.3   **Exercise Risks and Suggested Modifications During Pregnancy**

Exercise risk	Suggested modifications
Fetal harm because of blunt trauma	Avoid activities like waterskiing and downhill skiing and contact sports.
Falling because of changing center of gravity	Switch to weight machines rather than free weights; use a treadmill or track with even footing rather than a sidewalk.
Overheating during intense exercise	Do not exercise in hot and humid conditions; use a fan when exercising indoors; wear clothes that allow heat to dissipate, and drink plenty of water.
Reduced blood return to the heart during supine exercise	Avoid prolonged exercises lying on the back; use an incline bench to do crunches with the head higher than the feet.
Feeling excessively tired or fatigued during or after exercise	Do not exercise to exhaustion; be sure to consume extra calories (pregnancy requires ~300 extra calories a day); have a snack right before exercising to avoid hypoglycemia.

Adapted by permission from J.M. Pivarnik and L. Mudd, 2009, p. 11.

Physical Activity Recommendations

Physical activity can provide benefits for you and your baby, with consideration given to the previously described precautions. This section highlights recommendations for aerobic exercise, resistance training, and flexibility.

Aerobic Exercise   Most of the research on physical activity during pregnancy has focused on aerobic exercise. Among active women, the most commonly reported activity during pregnancy is walking for exercise (~50 percent), followed by swimming (~12 percent) and aerobics (~12 percent). Fewer women choose to participate in more vigorous activities like running (~6 percent) or team sports (~1 percent), and participation in vigorous exercise tends to decrease from the first to the third trimester (13).

Although most women do not choose to do vigorous activity, those who do so experience healthy pregnancies (14). Some active females may worry that their aerobic fitness levels will decrease during pregnancy. Actually, research shows that aerobic fitness declines very little during pregnancy when women continue to exercise, and their fitness rebounds quickly in the postpartum to prepregnancy levels or better (29).

Aerobic exercise is discussed in detail in chapter 5. During pregnancy you can follow general adult population guidelines for exercise, with the caveat that you should monitor your symptoms, discomforts, and abilities and make any necessary adjustments. Regular aerobic activity is the target so shoot for at least three days per week rather than sporadic exercise. For women just starting to exercise, work up gradually to 30 minutes per day of accumulated activity with a weekly goal of 150 minutes. Examples of these activities are found in chapter 5. If you are already doing more, that's great. Just continue to monitor your body's individual response to exercise and be willing to fine-tune the workout.

A moderate level of intensity is appropriate for most women. It is important to realize that resting heart rate tends to increase during pregnancy, so heart rate is not a good measure of exercise intensity at this time. Rather, you should monitor intensity using your perception of effort (5). During exercise, an intensity corresponding to a level 5 or 6 on a 10-point scale is recommended for moderate-intensity activity (see chapter 5 for details on exercise intensity). The talk test also helps to ensure that you are staying at appropriate exercise intensities, as long as you can continue talking while exercising.

Walking is a popular form of exercise during pregnancy because it is low stress (physiologically), and easy to do at home or with friends. You may want to wear a pedometer or activity tracker to track the distance you walk each day and set goals

---

■ Q&A

What is a good way to encourage physical activity?

Realizing the benefits of physical activity for mom and baby provides a strong incentive to make exercise a priority. One simple way to help track activity is to purchase a simple pedometer or activity tracker to count daily steps. Wear the pedometer for several typical days to determine your baseline level of activity and then develop a plan to increase activity toward 10,000 steps per day. Many smartphones now have step counting capabilities and mobile apps that can track your activity too. It can be fun to use these to see your activity level over time, work toward goals, and even compete against friends and family members.

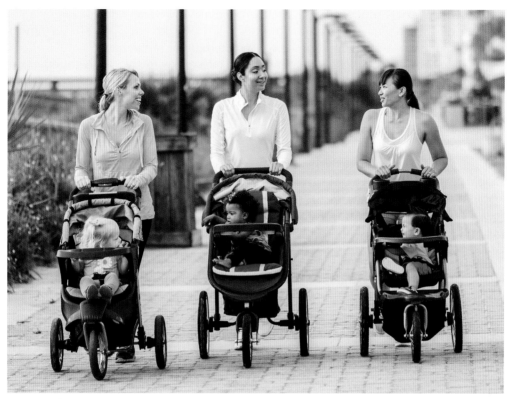

Exercise during the postpartum period is highly encouraged.

for yourself. Pedometer-based programs (like walking 10,000 steps/day) have been effective at helping overweight women stay within recommended weight gain ranges during pregnancy (32).

Resistance Training   Very little research has considered resistance training and muscular fitness during pregnancy, which is reflected by the lack of recommendations for resistance training. In theory, heavy lifting could reduce blood flow to the developing baby and result in poorer growth; however, this has not been documented. Rather, the few research studies examining resistance training compared to no exercise during pregnancy found no differences in length of gestation or birth weight (6, 7). One small study found that pregnant women with gestational diabetes assigned to resistance exercise training with elastic bands had better glucose control than women assigned to the control group, but these findings need to be replicated in a larger study (11). Thus, although it likely isn't harmful, the possible benefits of resistance training during pregnancy have yet to be determined.

Past studies on resistance training during pregnancy involved light to moderate weightlifting programs that used machines, resistance bands, or body weight activities rather than free weights. For details on the various methods of resistance training, see chapter 6. Typically, lifting free weights during pregnancy is not advised due to increasing instability associated with changes in the center of gravity and increased joint laxity as pregnancy progresses. To avoid balance issues, you may want to modify programs to use weight machines or resistance bands in place of free weights. Given the lack of research studies about possible benefits or adverse effects of resistance training during pregnancy, you should work with a health care provider or fitness professional to develop an appropriate resistance training program.

In general, resistance training programs should include low-resistance, high-repetition exercises for the major muscle groups rather than powerlifting activities, which are contraindicated during pregnancy. As outlined in chapter 6, resistance training on two to three days per week is recommended, including exercises for the major muscle groups and completing 12 to 15 repetitions to the point of moderate fatigue (5). Extra care should be taken to avoid breath holding (called the Valsalva maneuver) while lifting. Instead, exhale during the exertion or muscle-shortening phase of each exercise. You should also modify exercises to avoid lying on your back (supine position), especially late in pregnancy when the weight and location of the baby may decrease the normal return of blood to the heart (2). This can ultimately cause an unwanted drop in blood pressure. Although not traditionally thought of as strength training, Kegel exercises (voluntarily squeezing muscles of the pelvic floor) are recommended during pregnancy and postpartum to reduce pregnancy-related urinary incontinence (4).

Recently, prenatal yoga and Pilates classes have grown in popularity. While systematic research on the efficacy of yoga or Pilates to improve pregnancy outcomes is still scarce, no adverse effects have been reported. Yoga and Pilates may improve pregnancy outcomes by helping to strengthen core muscles that help with labor and delivery and by improving maternal stress and mood. There is growing evidence that participation in yoga during pregnancy is associated with decreased symptoms of maternal stress, anxiety, and depression (15). A smaller body of literature supports decreases in low back and pelvic pain associated with yoga during pregnancy; however, effects on birth weight and preterm delivery have been mixed (16). More research is needed to determine what types of yoga have the best effects and whether effects are driven by mindfulness or breathing techniques, physical stances, or a combination of factors. It should be noted that Bikram yoga (aka "Hot yoga") and "Hot Pilates" are not recommended during pregnancy due to concerns about increased maternal core temperature possibly leading to neural tube defects in the fetus and increased risk of muscle damage, dizziness, and fainting in the mother (2, 8). In addition, some yoga positions, such as those lying on the floor, may need to be modified in order to avoid loss of blood flow return to the heart (2).

Flexibility

Joint laxity (i.e., the feeling of joint "looseness" and flexibility) increases throughout pregnancy in preparation for labor and delivery. As a result, the risk for injury to joints and surrounding tissues (ligaments) is higher in pregnancy, and you should be cautious about rapidly changing direction during exercise to avoid ankle or knee sprains and other injuries. As with any exercise program, it is important to include proper warm-up and cool-down periods when exercising during pregnancy. All major muscle groups should be stretched during the cool-down when the muscles are warm.

As with any healthy adult, pregnant women should target at least 10 minutes of stretching including four or more repetitions of individual stretches on at least two to three days per week. Chapter 7 provides information on stretching programs.

Although these general recommendations on stretching are appropriate, some special considerations should be noted. Due to greater joint laxity, pregnant women should be especially careful not to "overstretch" past the point of discomfort. Some stretching exercises, especially those for the lower body, might also need to be modified later in pregnancy to account for the "baby bump" and to avoid lying on the back for too long (see "Lower Body Stretches for Pregnancy" for several suggested stretches). In addition to being an important part of an exercise routine, regular stretching may also help lessen low back pain during pregnancy.

———————————

Pregnancy is an exciting time of life for a woman, and it's the perfect time to make changes to nutrition and activity patterns not only to improve your own health, but also to ensure a healthy start for your infant. For women who already exercise, there is no reason to make drastic changes to your routine as long as you talk with your health care provider. Common sense should be used, however, and you should listen to your body and modify activities as needed. Women who don't already exercise can begin at any time, but it's important to start slow and progress as appropriate. Just as at any other time in life, consultation with your personal health care provider before starting an exercise program can help ensure that you are proceeding in the best manner possible.

LOWER BODY STRETCHES FOR PREGNANCY

Lower Back Stretch 1

Begin on your hands and knees, with hands directly below shoulders and knees directly below hips (a). Your back should be flat. Inhale, drawing your chin into your chest, pulling your stomach into your spine, and rounding your back to make a hump (b). Exhale and return your back to a flat line. Slowly repeat several times.

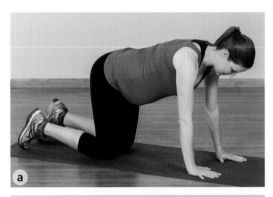

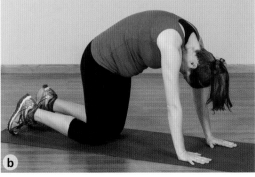

Lower Back Stretch 2

Stand up tall with your back against a wall. Exhale while pushing the small of your back against the wall. Inhale and relax. Repeat several times.

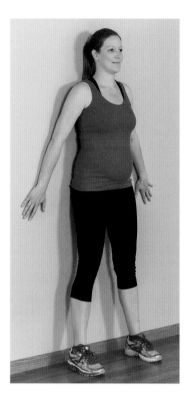

Lower Back Stretch 3

Sit up with your legs folded underneath you or cross-legged with your right side next to a wall (a). Maintaining good posture, slowly twist your upper body to face the wall (b). Press your palms or upper arms into the wall to support your body twist while keeping your legs on the floor. You should feel a stretch in your lower back. Sit facing the opposite direction and repeat on the left side.

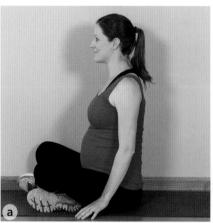
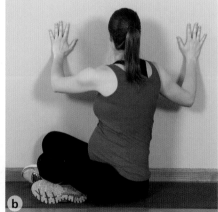

Hamstring and Buttock Stretch

Begin on your hands and knees *(a)*. Slide your right knee up so that it is on the floor under your right shoulder and twist your lower leg so that your right foot is on the floor under your left hip. Exhale while slowly lowering your hips toward the floor and sliding your left knee back so that your left leg is extended and lying on the floor *(b)*. Feel the stretch in the back of your right leg and buttock. For a deeper stretch once your back leg is extended, slowly lower your upper body to lie on top of your bent leg and place your arms on the floor. Repeat with your left leg bent under.

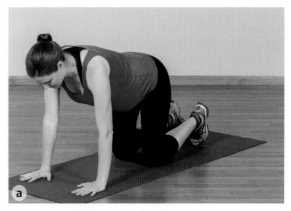

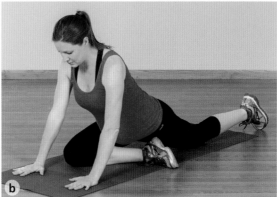

Inner Thigh Stretch

Sit on the floor with your back straight against a wall and your legs out in front. Slowly bend knees out to the side while sliding feet in toward your body until the soles of your feet touch. Keep sitting up tall and exhale while gently pushing down on knees until you feel the stretch in your inner thighs.

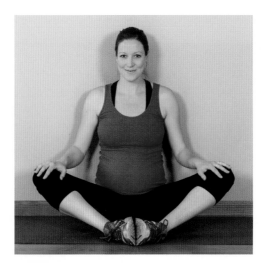

Calf Stretch

Stand an arm's length away from a wall and extend arms until the palms are flat on the wall, slightly above shoulder height *(a)*. Step back with the right foot, straighten the right leg, and bend the left leg toward the wall *(b)*. Both feet should be flat and pointed toward the wall. Weight should be balanced between feet and hands. You should feel the stretch in your right calf. Switch leg positions and repeat on the left side.

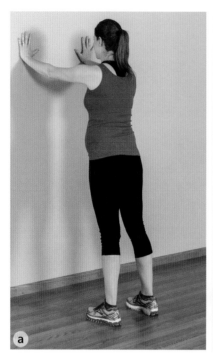
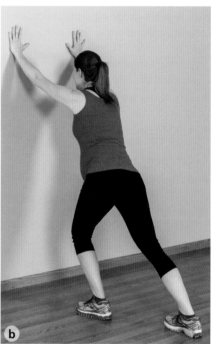

Hip Flexor Stretch

Begin by kneeling on the floor with your body upright. Place your left foot in front of you, flat on the floor with the knee bent directly over the ankle *(a)*. Place hands on top of the left knee and slowly shift forward, keeping your back straight, so that your left knee moves over your left toe, and lean your hips forward *(b)*. You should feel a stretch on the top of your right thigh (the hip flexor). Switch leg positions and repeat.

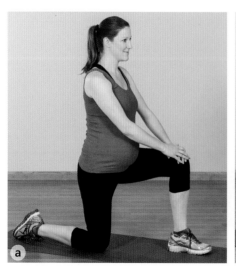
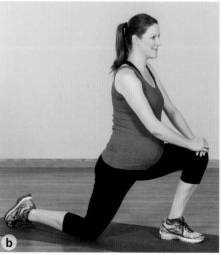

TWENTY

Depression

Feeling down or sad occasionally is a typical response to situations in life; in contrast, in depression, such feelings become persistent and affect routine activities. Depression is a common chronic health condition that negatively affects physical, emotional, and social health and significantly interferes with daily functioning. In addition, the potential economic consequences and public health burden of depression are substantial. As with many other health conditions described in this book, research supports a beneficial role of physical activity in the prevention and treatment of depressive disorders.

Depression is more common than one might expect. Major depressive disorder, also referred to as unipolar depression or clinical depression, is the most common psychiatric disorder. Worldwide, 350 million people suffer from depression (36). Estimates suggest that approximately 7 percent of adults report a major depressive episode in the past year, and one in five U.S. adults has a mood disorder over the course of life, with major depression the most common (29, 30). According to the World Health Organization, depression is the leading cause of disability and global disease burden in industrialized nations (36). In addition to the tremendous impact of depression on individuals and families, the financial drain is immense. The economic costs of depression include medical costs such as increased frequency of medical visits, longer hospital stays, greater risk and severity of chronic health conditions, and premature death due to both suicide and poor medical outcomes (8), as well as workplace costs including absenteeism and reduced productivity while one is at work (also referred to as presenteeism) (53).

What Is Depression?

While everyone feels sad or down on occasion, someone with clinical depression has persistent symptoms that interfere with daily functioning. Symptoms of depression include these:

- Depressed mood or feelings of sadness
- Loss of interest or pleasure in previously enjoyed activities

- Changes in appetite (increase or decrease) or body weight (loss or gain)
- Changes in sleeping habits (sleeping too much or problems falling or staying asleep)
- Fatigue or loss of energy
- Feelings of hopelessness, worthlessness, or guilt
- Difficulty thinking or concentrating or not being able to make decisions
- Agitation, restlessness, or slowed movements
- Thoughts of suicide or death

To receive a diagnosis of depression, an individual must experience either low mood or loss of interest (first two items in the preceding list) and four or more of the remaining symptoms. In addition, these symptoms must be severe enough to affect daily activities, must persist for a period of two weeks or more, and must not be due to a physical illness or a substance (either drug of abuse or medication) (2).

Other mood disorders include persistent depressive disorder (dysthymia), bipolar disorder, and premenstrual dysphoric disorder (see table 20.1 for more information on each of these types) (2). Additionally, the childbearing period is a high-risk time for depression in women, so it is important to watch for signs of peripartum depression (occurring during pregnancy or within four weeks of delivery) and postpartum depression. Depression also frequently co-occurs with many chronic medical illnesses. Because depression may last for a long period of time and symptoms may be mistakenly attributed to stress or illness, it is important to talk to your doctor if you think you could be experiencing symptoms of depression.

TABLE 20.1 Types of Depressive Disorders

Major depressive disorder	Major depressive disorder (MDD) is a condition characterized by depressed mood or loss of interest in activities (or both) as well as changes in appetite-weight, sleep, or motor activity; fatigue; feelings of worthlessness or guilt; difficulty concentrating; and thoughts of death or suicide.
Persistent depressive disorder	Persistent depressive disorder (PDD) encompasses the formerly known dysthymia and chronic major depression diagnoses. This is a more chronic type of depression in which symptoms are persistent, lasting for at least two years.
Premenstrual dysphoric disorder	Premenstrual dysphoric disorder is characterized by the presence of five symptoms, one of which is significant mood alterations, irritability-anger, depressed mood, or anxiety-tension, as well as one or more of the following: decreased interest, difficulty concentrating, reduced energy, sleep and appetite changes, feeling overwhelmed, or physical symptoms such as breast tenderness and swelling. These symptoms are present in the week before onset of menses and begin to resolve shortly thereafter, and this pattern characterizes the majority of menstrual cycles.
Bipolar disorder	Bipolar disorder was previously known as manic depression. People with bipolar disorder experience shifting mood and behavior, with depressive episodes alternating with episodes of mania (elevated mood and energy). The cycles in mood can vary in length from days to months.

Depression and Health

As previously mentioned, chronic health conditions have been associated with a higher likelihood of developing depression. People with chronic medical conditions, such as cardiovascular disease, stroke, diabetes, cancer, and pulmonary disease, commonly experience elevated symptoms of depression (26); and depression is also associated with increased risk for many chronic illnesses (28). Depression can interfere with glycemic control (i.e., maintaining normal glucose levels in the body), reduce immunity, and negatively affect the cardiovascular system (27). Because the symptoms of several chronic diseases may overlap with symptoms of depression, diagnosis can be problematic. However, depression that is not treated can lead to worse medical outcomes due to both psychological and physiological factors. Taking medication properly, seeking medical care, quitting smoking, eating a healthy diet, and getting adequate sleep are all more difficult if you are experiencing symptoms of depression (26). Individuals with a medical illness who may have symptoms of depression should speak with a doctor or a mental health professional to better understand the symptoms and how they might affect illness and treatment.

While anyone can be affected by depression at any time, certain factors are associated with increased risk of developing depression:

- Being female
- Having a family history of depression
- Having experienced a previous bout of depression
- Having low social support or social isolation
- Having a chronic health condition
- Experiencing stressful life events
- Low levels of physical activity

Women are about twice as likely to suffer depression as men. People who have a family history of depression are more likely to suffer depression themselves. In addition, someone who has had a prior episode of depression is significantly more likely than others to experience a subsequent episode. Other risk factors include stressful life events, social isolation, and having a chronic health condition (40). Finally, being physically inactive has been shown to increase risk for depression, providing further support for the important role of physical activity in promoting mental as well as physical health (19). Having these risk factors does not mean that you will become depressed; however, if you are aware of the risk factors, you can be more alert to the signs and symptoms for yourself or loved ones.

Treatment for Depression

There are a variety of treatments for depression, including antidepressant medications and psychotherapy. Antidepressants are not habit-forming drugs but work by correcting chemical imbalances in the brain. However, the exact mechanism of antidepressant medications is not fully known. Common antidepressant medications work to influence the brain in various ways. Some affect chemicals in the brain, including norepinephrine, serotonin, and dopamine. These medications include the older and now less commonly used monoamine oxidase inhibitors and tricyclic antidepressants, as well as the newer, safer selective serotonin reuptake inhibitors (SSRIs) and serotonin and norepinephrine reuptake inhibitors (SNRIs) (49). Newer medications that have unique mechanisms of action (atypical antidepressants) or that combine different mechanisms of action (multimodal antidepressants) are commonly used. More recently, the use of antidepressant medications that target other brain chemicals, such as glutamate, or that target brain communication pathways related to depression has increased, with the hope of improving treatment outcomes (49).

Clinical and research experience has revealed that not every medication is effective for every person. Unfortunately, medication selection is often a "trial and error" approach, with challenges in matching individuals with the antidepressant medication that is most likely to benefit them. If you take an antidepressant medication, you may feel some improvement in the first couple of weeks, but the full benefits are not generally seen for a couple of months. It may take several attempts or even a combination of medications to find a prescription that fully relieves depression, so it is important to talk with your doctor about your medication and symptoms. Even after you get better, your doctor will want you to continue medication for a period of time to maintain improvement and protect against relapse (8).

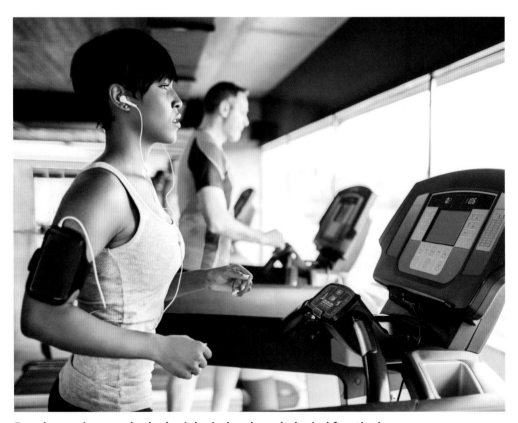

Exercise can improve both physiological and psychological functioning.

In addition to potential difficulties of identifying the appropriate medication and dosage to relieve symptoms, side effects can be a frequent problem of medications, and they are often noticed before people feel relief of depression symptoms. Commonly reported side effects of antidepressant medications include changes in weight or appetite, headache, dizziness, nausea, sexual dysfunction, and sleep disturbances, although the type and severity of these symptoms vary depending upon the type of medication (4). Thus, if you are using a medication, it is important to have ongoing monitoring of the medication, side effects, and symptoms to ensure that successful remission is achieved and maintained (54). Routine and consistent monitoring of symptoms is recognized as very important in the management of other chronic diseases, and depression should be no exception. In what is referred to as "measurement-based care" (38), standardized scales are used to quantify the frequency and severity of symptoms, side effects, and adherence in order to aid in treatment.

Psychotherapy, including cognitive behavioral therapy and interpersonal therapy, can also effectively treat depression. Cognitive behavioral therapy focuses on developing problem-solving skills and changing negative or unhelpful thinking, and has been shown to be particularly effective as a psychological treatment for depression. Interpersonal therapy assists individuals through life transitions, grief, and other difficulties. As with medication, it may take some time to see significant improvement, and ongoing maintenance sessions may be necessary. There are different options for counseling formats, and family or group counseling may be helpful in addition to individual sessions. Finding a well-trained, experienced therapist or counselor is an important factor in the effectiveness of psychotherapy (32).

For more severe depression or when other treatments have not been adequate, electroconvulsive therapy may be indicated. This medical treatment involves stimulating the brain under anesthesia over a series of sessions and can be effective when other treatments have not been successful. Additional medical treatments involving specific stimulation of certain brain areas include vagus nerve stimulation, transcranial magnetic stimulation, and deep brain stimulation (8, 40). It is important for individuals to partner with their mental health professional to select a treatment that is appropriate for them and their individual situation.

Although more attention has been given to depression in recent years, adequate treatment remains problematic (36). Barriers include difficulty in finding an effective treatment and full relief of symptoms (8), as well as the cost of health care visits, medication, or psychotherapy. Thus, many avoid seeking treatment or discontinue treatment before full remission. Despite a greater understanding of depression, social stigma and accessibility to treatment are other commonly reported barriers to seeking treatment (8). Even among those who seek and receive treatment, many do not achieve full relief of symptoms. Without full relief of symptoms (remission), the risk of future episodes is increased (22). Therefore, the role of exercise in the prevention and treatment of depression is an important health issue.

Healthy Approaches to Managing Depression

Lifestyle factors can have a potential role in the prevention and treatment of depression. The value of a healthy diet and regular physical activity are discussed in the upcoming sections.

Mental Health Resources

Help is available from many community resources, including these:

- Mental health professionals: psychiatrists (MD, DO), psychologists (PhD, PsyD), social workers (LSW, LCSW), and mental health counselors (LPC, MFT, LMHC)
- Physicians including family medicine, internal medicine, and obstetrics and gynecology
- Community mental health centers and clinics
- Social service agencies
- Religious organizations and clergy

Focusing on Nutrition

Balanced nutrition is an important consideration in the treatment and prevention of depression. However, because changes in appetite and weight are a symptom of depression, nutrition can be particularly problematic. In addition, people with depression often have low motivation and difficulty planning and problem solving, which makes maintaining a healthy diet even more difficult. People who are feeling down, anxious, or stressed may make poor food choices for comfort, while other people may skip meals altogether. Some antidepressant medications are associated with weight gain, which is another reason physical activity is important.

For purposes of mental health, people should generally follow the recommended guidelines for nutrition according to their age and calorie needs (56) (see chapter 3 for dietary guidance). In addition, some evidence indicates that people with depression may have lower levels of omega-3 fatty acids, B vitamins (B_{12}, folate), and other minerals and amino acids that affect brain function (48). A health professional or dietitian may recommend a vitamin supplement if your diet is not providing adequate nutrients.

Focusing on Physical Activity

Exercise is valuable for the prevention and treatment of a variety of medical conditions. Exercise can improve both physiological and psychological functioning. Exercise has also been shown to improve depressive symptoms in individuals with other chronic diseases including cancer (11), neurologic diseases such as Alzheimer's disease and multiple sclerosis (1), and heart disease (42).

Several benefits of physical activity play a role in the interrelationship between mental and physical health. For example, feeling troubled or distressed is related to increased risk for mental illness as well as physical illnesses such as heart disease, and such feelings have a negative impact on one's quality of life. Physical activity and exercise training are generally associated with less distress and enhanced feelings of well-being (43). The benefits include these:

- Reduced depressive symptoms
- Reduced likelihood of future episodes of depression
- Improved sleep quality and reduced fatigue
- Improved cognitive function

- Decreased pain and somatic complaints
- Improved self-esteem and self-efficacy
- Improved quality of life and daily functioning

Exercise as a Treatment for Depression

Although the role of exercise in alleviating symptoms of depression has been proposed for centuries, researchers have accumulated evidence within the past several decades supporting the health benefits of exercise. Even for individuals who do not have clinical levels of depressive symptoms, consistent evidence shows a positive effect on mood with both acute bouts of exercise and longer-term exercise training. Exercisers often report feeling more energy, greater self-esteem, and less stress (43). However, people with depression tend to be less active and to have high amounts of sedentary time, and few achieve adequate levels of physical activity (23).

Physical activity such as walking has been found to be associated with a lower risk of developing depression (35). People who are more active report fewer depressive symptoms and reduced incidence of physician-diagnosed depression (15, 19). However, this type of research examines relationships, showing that higher levels of activity are associated with lower risk of depression. The direction of the relationship—does physical activity reduce depression or does depression result in less activity?—cannot be determined by associations alone. To answer this question, clinical research studies in which exercise is prescribed and risk of depression is then determined provide better insights on how physical activity can be used as an antidepressant therapy.

Overall, clinical research studies that use exercise as a treatment for depression show a clinically meaningful positive effect of exercise as an antidepressant therapy (31, 33, 37). Most of the research has used aerobic-type activities such as walking, jogging, or cycling, but there is evidence that resistance training and even yoga might be helpful. Several studies have reported that exercise alone can reduce depression symptoms comparably to traditional pharmacotherapy or psychotherapy in individuals with mild to moderate major depressive disorder (6, 18, 44, 51). However, only a few studies have examined the appropriate "dose" of exercise to achieve a reduction in symptoms. Available evidence suggests that the dose of exercise recommended for general health benefits, as described throughout this book, may also be effective to reduce depression symptoms (18, 43).

Achieving full relief of symptoms can be a challenge in the treatment of depression, and adding exercise to other treatments may be effective (55). Given the difficulty in obtaining full remission of depressive symptoms and the likelihood of future episodes, the use of exercise in combination with traditional therapies is promising but requires further study.

Supporting the inclusion of exercise, evidence suggests that exercise may directly improve particular symptoms of depression, specifically sleep, fatigue, and cognitive function. Sleep disturbances are a key feature of depression and can negatively affect health and daily functioning. Some evidence indicates that exercise may increase sleep time and sleep quality (41), and single bouts of exercise have been shown to enhance feelings of energy and reduce fatigue (16). Exercise training may be helpful in reducing symptoms of fatigue for both healthy adults and those with health conditions (45). Recent evidence also suggests that, when added to an antidepressant, various levels of exercise improve sleep quality and reduce awakening in the middle of the night and early morning (46). These benefits are in addition to the effects of exercise on the overall symptoms of depression. The following are other benefits:

- Low cost
- Convenience
- Accessibility
- Fitness and health benefits
- Few negative side effects
- Alterability of the routine to meet needs and goals
- Greater individual control

Cognitive function, such as learning, remembering, and using information, is frequently disrupted in depression and can create significant and persistent difficulties in daily functioning. Similar to the observations of exercise effects on sleep, various levels of exercise have been shown to directly improve cognitive functions, independent of changes in overall depressive symptoms. Higher levels of exercise have been associated with additional benefits, particularly with respect to spatial working memory, or tasks that measure how one works with visual and spatial information (21). However, there are few studies in this area, so more research is needed.

How Exercise May Affect Mental Health

The exact mechanisms by which physical activity improves mental health are largely unknown. But this is also the case for psychotherapy and medications. It is likely that antidepressant therapies work due to a combination of effects, including changes in thoughts, feelings, and brain pathways. There may also be a type of placebo or expectancy effect, with treatments working, in part, because patients believe that they will help. For example, if you are confident that exercise will lower depression, you may be more likely to see that outcome when engaging in exercise. Physical activity may also provide a distraction from worries or symptoms and reduce stress by offering a "time-out" from daily concerns, which can be very important in the management of depression and anxiety. Individuals who are successful in becoming more physically active commonly report improved self-confidence and enhanced self-esteem, and this can also enhance feelings of control. In a study of older adults, increases in self-esteem predicted decreases in depression symptoms after treatment with physical activity (39). Exercise may also provide additional opportunities for social support and interaction, which can be helpful for those suffering from depression (7).

In addition, biological adaptations in brain systems may contribute to the antidepressant effect of physical activity. Exercise appears to enhance the way the brain functions. Positive effects on mood and depression may be due to the impact of exercise on the brain chemicals norepinephrine and serotonin (10, 13, 14, 17, 20). Other studies have focused on proteins in the brain, called nerve growth factors, which promote growth and connectivity of nerve cells in the brain. Whether with reference to a single exercise session or to an established exercise routine, benefits have been identified related to various proteins in the brain that enhance mental health and function (e.g., brain-derived neurotrophic factor [BDNF] and VGF nerve growth factor) (24, 47). In addition, researchers continue to examine other substances (e.g., brain opioids) that may play a role in regulating mood and affecting mental disorders (7).

Physical Activity Recommendations

Although more research is needed to help guide exercise recommendations specific to the management of depression, there is good evidence that physical activity of different types and doses can be beneficial for mental health. Aerobic exercise, resistance training, and yoga have all been shown to help manage depressive symptoms.

Aerobic Exercise   The current evidence suggests that an exercise program that meets the recommendations in chapter 5 is also beneficial for mental health (5, 18, 43). Most research regarding exercise and depression has focused on aerobic modes of exercise, including walking, jogging, and stationary cycling. A good initial target for aerobic physical activity is 150 minutes a week of moderate-intensity physical activity or 75 minutes a week of vigorous-intensity exercise (43).

A range of exercise intensities have been used in research on depression, with most studies using a moderate or self-selected pace. Moderate-intensity physical activity is comparable to brisk walking, while vigorous-intensity exercise includes jogging or running. For individuals with depression, a more moderate pace may seem less daunting, especially for those not used to exercise. If you are physically active at a moderate pace, the exercise will feel "somewhat hard" and you will notice a slight increase in breathing and heart rate. However, the pace will seem easy enough that you could continue for a while. Research suggests that moderate to high intensities, compared to lower intensities, are more effective at reducing depression (18). Remember, as your fitness increases, physical activity will be easier, and you will be able to work harder with less effort.

Calories burned during exercise, or energy expenditure, is another way to measure exercise dose. This method is most helpful for people who like to use exercise equipment like elliptical trainers, treadmills, or stationary bicycles. Smartphone apps can also

Yoga and Mindful Exercise

Yoga has a long history of improving mood, and most existing research, despite some limitations, supports improved mood with yoga practice. In addition, there is support for improvement in residual symptoms, such as anxiety, with yoga (12). For example, Sudarshan Kriya yoga, which consists of rhythmic breathing, has been assessed in individuals with both depression and dysthymia and compared to drug therapy or electroconvulsive therapy. Remission rates were comparable for individuals engaged in the yoga and those receiving drug therapy, although the remission rate was highest for the electroconvulsive therapy (25). Mindfulness techniques have been used in stress reduction programs for decades (34). Mindful Hatha yoga is a formal meditation technique composed of gentle stretching and strengthening exercises that are completed slowly, with awareness of breathing. Preliminary research supports reduction of depression and anxiety with Hatha yoga and meditation (57). Meditation, which is often incorporated into the practice of yoga but has been studied as a sole practice as well, has also been associated with improvements in mood and reduced anxiety (3). Tai chi is another form of mind–body exercise that incorporates a series of slowly performed martial arts movements with meditation and breathing. Tai chi has been found to reduce stress, anxiety, and depression and enhance well-being and self-efficacy (58). Thus, it may be helpful to include yoga or other mindful exercises in physical activity plans for mental health (12). However, these types of exercises have not been as widely studied and do not offer all of the benefits of traditional fitness-based physical activity.

help you calculate calories you burn during exercise. Expending about 1,000 calories per week has been shown to have beneficial health effects and provide mental and physical health benefits (5, 18).

Other considerations for exercise dose are frequency and duration. Most research on exercise and depression has used a traditional exercise format of three to four times per week for 30 to 45 minutes per session (52). However, benefits have been seen with a variety of exercise programs. Research has shown that exercising for a shorter duration but more frequently (five days per week) and for a longer duration less frequently (three days per week) both result in a reduction of depression symptoms and remission of depression (18). Thus, there are many effective options. Some people prefer doing longer-duration exercise a few days a week while others prefer performing shorter bouts more often. People who have trouble finding time for exercise may prefer to break their sessions into shorter 10- to 15-minute bouts over the course of the day (43). You may find that more frequent bouts are less intimidating while still helping to reduce stress, improve thinking, and energize you.

It is important for people with symptoms of depression who would like to begin exercise to gradually increase their physical activity level over a period of a few weeks until they reach an adequate dose. This helps one develop physical fitness, prevents

Building Behavioral Skills for Physical Activity

Being physically active can be challenging for anyone, but for individuals who struggle with depression, developing an exercise routine can be particularly difficult. Low motivation, lack of enjoyment, difficulty planning, and fatigue are real barriers to physical activity. However, simple behavioral strategies or skills can help you incorporate more physical activity into your daily life (9).

Set Yourself Up for Success

Use positive cues to help you be more active, and remove cues that cause you to be less active. Examples of positive cues are posted notes, athletic shoes placed in a highly visible location, and notes on your calendar. Activity trackers or phone apps can help track movement and provide information such as steps, distance, calories, and sleep in order to prompt and monitor activity levels.

Have a Goal

Although many options for physical activity can help you on your journey to physical and mental health, set goals that meet your needs, preferences, and schedule. Goals provide direction and motivation. Make sure you set small, short-term goals that are realistic. For someone with depression, motivation is likely to be a problem. A realistic goal such as walking for 15 minutes a day can help you get started. Make sure you don't try to set too many goals at once. Focus on one type of physical activity first; then you can try new activities as you reach your goals.

Reward Yourself, and Find Some Fun

Positive reinforcement helps you establish a behavior, especially when you don't feel like doing it. Rewards don't have to be big, but they are important to mark small steps toward

frustration, and assists in planning and problem solving. While you may notice some improvement in mood when you first begin exercising, significant improvements in depression usually take several weeks, similarly to what is seen with pharmacotherapy and psychotherapy. Full relief of symptoms may take several months of consistent exercise.

Resistance Training Although not as widely studied as aerobic exercise, resistance exercise or strength training has been shown to have beneficial effects with regard to reducing depression (50). General recommendations for strength training as outlined in chapter 6 are to do resistance exercises two to three days per week, including the major muscle groups of the chest, back, arms, shoulders, hips, legs, and core, performing two to three sets of each exercise for 8 to 12 repetitions (43). One study using resistance training as a depression intervention reported greater symptom reduction at higher intensity (80 percent one-repetition maximum [1RM]) compared to lower intensity (20 percent 1RM) in an exercise program of three days per week for eight weeks (51). Generally, studies using resistance training have included two to three sessions per week with a duration of approximately 45 to 60 minutes, similar to the time spent in aerobic exercise programs (50).

success. Also, pairing physical activity with something you like such as listening to your favorite music, watching a television show, or spending time with a friend can help you find enjoyment in exercise.

Recruit Social Support

Social support is especially important because a lack of support is a risk factor for depression. Having social support has also been shown to help people adopt healthy habits such as physical activity. Support can come in many forms, including having someone with whom to be active, having someone who encourages you, or having someone who can help you with your physical activity plans. Having several different sources of social support is ideal.

Identify Resources

Creating or making use of an environment that supports your physical activity can help you be more active and reach your goals. Examples include community resources like parks, trails, and fitness centers; mobile apps and technology; and educational information such as DVDs, social media, and magazines. Many businesses and malls have courses mapped out to help promote activity and help you track how far you've walked.

Plan Ahead, and Stay Positive

Everyone experiences barriers to exercise and interruptions to exercise plans. If you prepare for times when physical activity is more difficult (e.g., travel, illness, holidays), you will be more likely to get back on track. Often people drop out when they experience lapses because they tend to think negatively ("I'm a failure" or "I blew it"). This is particularly true for someone who struggles with depression. Changing negative thoughts to positive ones can help prevent a slip from becoming a relapse into old habits of inactivity.

As to types of exercise, you have a variety of options for mental health promotion, including aerobic, resistance, and mindful exercise. Although this topic is not as widely studied in relation to depression, you can also be active by playing sports and enjoying other lifestyle activities such as walking and gardening. Consider doing your physical activity at a moderate pace, and aim for 150 minutes per week. But doing any physical activity is better than none; you can start at a lower level and then work your way toward a healthy dose of exercise that fits with recommendations. It is often useful to have a fitness professional help you plan your exercise routine and provide supervision as you get started. Most of the studies on depression have given participants exercise treatment using supervised exercise programs or a combined program of supervised and home-based exercise. If you are concerned about depression or another health condition, it is important that you consult with your health care provider to ensure that your symptoms do not get worse and to receive advice about the safest, most appropriate type of exercise for you.

Depression is a very common disorder that can occur at any time throughout the lifespan, and it significantly affects daily functioning in many areas. A variety of treatments are available, including medication and psychotherapy, and communication with a health care provider is important to monitor depressive symptoms and other concurrent health conditions. Exercise can also be an effective intervention for depression, both as a stand alone treatment and when added to other therapy. Using behavioral strategies can help promote adherence to exercise and should be incorporated as a part of physical activity adoption and maintenance.

REFERENCES

Chapter 1

1. American College of Sports Medicine. *ACSM's Guidelines for Exercise Testing and Prescription.* 10th ed. Philadelphia (PA): Lippincott Williams & Wilkins; in press.
2. American Diabetes Association. Standards of medical care in diabetes–2014. *Diabetes Care.* 2014;37:S14-S80.
3. American Psychological Association Web site [Internet]. Stress effects on the body. American Psychological Association; Washington, DC [cited 2015 August 26]. Available at www.apa.org/helpcenter/stress-body.aspx.
4. American Psychological Association Web site [Internet]. Stress in America: Paying with our health. American Psychological Association; Washington, DC [released February 4, 2015; cited 2015 August 26]. Available at www.apa.org/news/press/releases/stress/index.aspx.
5. American Psychological Association Web site [Internet]. Types of stress. American Psychological Association; Washington, DC [cited 2015 August 26]. Available at www.apa.org/helpcenter/stress-kinds.aspx.
6. American Psychological Association Web site [Internet]. Understanding chronic stress. American Psychological Association; Washington, DC [cited 2015 August 26]. Available at www.apa.org/helpcenter/understanding-chronic-stress.aspx.
7. Arthritis Foundation Web site [Internet]. Arthritis Facts. Arthritis Foundation; Atlanta (GA) [cited 2015 August 18]. Available at www.arthritis.org/about-arthritis/understanding-arthritis/arthritis-statistics-facts.php.
8. Becker C, McPeck W. Web site [Internet]. Creating positive health: it's more than risk reduction. National Wellness Institute White Paper. National Wellness Institute; Stevens Point (WI); 2013 [cited 2015 August 26]. Available at www.nationalwellness.org/?page=WhitePapers.
9. Chodzko-Zajko W, Proctor D, Fiatarone Singh M, Minson C, Nigg C, Salem G, Skinner J. American College of Sports Medicine position stand. Exercise and physical activity for older adults. *Med Sci Sports Exerc.* 2009;41:1510-1530.
10. Garber CE, Blissmer B, Deschenes MR, et al. American College of Sports Medicine position stand. Quantity and quality of exercise for developing and maintaining cardiorespiratory, musculoskeletal, and neuromotor fitness in apparently healthy adults: guidance for prescribing exercise. *Med Sci Sports Exerc.* 2011;43(7):1334-1359.
11. Hettler B. Web site [Internet]. Six dimensions of wellness. National Wellness Institute; Stevens Point, (WI); 1976 [cited 2015 August 26]. Available at www.nationalwellness.org/?page=Six_Dimensions.
12. Kottler JA, Chen DD. *Stress Management and Prevention: Application to Everyday Life.* 2nd ed. New York (NY): Routledge Taylor & Francis; 2011. 407 p.
13. Long BC, Van Stavel R. Effects of exercise training on anxiety: a meta-analysis. *J Appl Sport Psychol.* 1995;7:167-189.
14. Mosca L, Manson JE, Sutherland SE, Langer RD, Manolio T, Barrett-Conner E. Cardiovascular disease in women: a statement for healthcare professionals from the American Heart Association. *Circulation.* 1997;96:2468-2482.
15. National Heart, Lung, and Blood Institute. U.S. Department of Health and Human Services; National Institutes of Health Web site [Internet]. Your Guide to Healthy Sleep. NIH publication no. 11-5271. National Heart Lung and Blood Institute; Bethesda (MD); 2011 [cited 2015 August 18]. Available at www.nhlbi.nih.gov/health/public/sleep/healthy_sleep.htm.
16. National Institute of Mental Health Web site [Internet]. Q&A on stress for adults: how it affects your health and what you can do about it. National Institute of Mental Health; Bethesda (MD) [cited 2015 August 26]. Available at www.nimh.nih.gov/health/publications/stress/index.shtml.

17. National Sleep Foundation Web site [Internet]. 2013 Sleep in America poll: exercise and sleep. National Sleep Foundation; Arlington (VA); 2013 [cited 2015 August 18]. Available at http://sleep-foundation.org/sleep-polls-data/sleep-in-america-poll/2013-exercise-and-sleep.

18. National Sleep Foundation Web site [Internet]. How much sleep do we really need? National Sleep Foundation; Arlington (VA); 2013 [cited 2015 August 18]. Available at http://sleepfounda-tion.org/how-sleep-works/how-much-sleep-do-we-really-need.

19. Owen N. Sedentary behavior: understanding and influencing adults' prolonged sitting time. *Prev Med.* 2012;55(6):535-539.

20. Patel AV, Bernstein L, Deka A, Feigelson HS, Campbell PT, Gapstur SM, Colditz GA, Thun MJ. Leisure time spent sitting in relation to total mortality in a prospective cohort of U.S. adults. *Am J Epidemiol.* 2010;172(4):419-429.

21. Penedo FJ, Dahn JR. Exercise and well-being: a review of mental and physical health benefits associated with physical activity. *Curr Opin Psychiatr.* 2005;18(2):189-193.

22. President's Council on Fitness, Sports & Nutrition Web site [Internet]. Presidential Youth Fitness Program. President's Council on Fitness, Sports & Nutrition; Rockville (MD) [cited 2015 August 18]. Available at www.pyfp.org/.

23. Staiano AE, Harrington DM, Barreira TV, Katzmarzyk PT. Sitting time and cardiometabolic risk in U.S. adults: associations by sex, race, socioeconomic status and activity level. *Br J Sports Med.* 2014;48(3):213-219.

24. Stults-Kolehmainen MA, Sinha R. The effects of stress on physical activity and exercise. *Sports Med.* 2014;44:81-121.

25. U.S. Department of Health and Human Services Web site [Internet]. 2008 Physical Activity Guidelines for Americans. USDHHS; Atlanta (GA) [cited 2015 August 18]. Available at http://health.gov/paguidelines/.

26. U.S. Department of Health and Human Services Web site [Internet]. Healthy People 2020. USDHHS; Washington, DC; 2014 [cited 2015 September 2]. Available at www.healthypeople.gov/2020/How-to-Use-DATA2020.

27. U.S. Department of Health and Human Services Web site [Internet]. Physical Activity and Health: A Report of the Surgeon General. USDHHS; Washington, DC; 1999 [cited 2015 September 2]. Available at www.cdc.gov/nccdphp/sgr/index.htm.

28. U.S. Department of Health and Human Services and U.S. Department of Agriculture Web site [Internet]. Dietary Guidelines for Americans 2015. USDHHS; Atlanta (GA) [cited 2016 January 13]. Available at http://health.gov/dietaryguidelines/2015/guidelines/.

29. U.S. Department of Health and Human Services and U.S. Department of Agriculture Web site [Internet]. Scientific Report of the 2015 Dietary Guidelines Advisory Committee. USDHHS; Atlanta (GA) [cited 2015 August 19]. Available at http://health.gov/dietaryguidelines/2015-scientific-report/.

Chapter 2

1. American College of Sports Medicine. *ACSM's Guidelines for Exercise Testing and Prescription.* 10th ed. Philadelphia (PA): Lippincott Williams & Wilkins; in press.

2. Canadian Society for Exercise Physiology Web site [Internet]. The Physical Activity Readiness Questionnaire for Everyone. CSEP; Ottawa, ON, Canada; [cited 12 October 2015]. Available at: http://www.csep.ca/en/publications.

3. Garber CE, Blissmer B, Deschenes MR, et al. American College of Sports Medicine Position Stand. Quantity and quality of exercise for developing and maintaining cardiorespiratory, musculo-skeletal, and neuromotor fitness in apparently healthy adults: guidance for prescribing exercise. *Med Sci Sports Exerc.* 2011;43(7):1334-1359.

4. U.S. Department of Health and Human Services, Office of Disease Prevention and Health Promotion Web site [Internet]. 2008 Physical Activity Guidelines for Americans. USDHHS; Atlanta (GA); [cited 2015 August 18]. Available at: http://health.gov/paguidelines/

Chapter 3

1. American College of Sports Medicine. *ACSM's Guidelines for Exercise Testing and Prescription.* 10th ed. Philadelphia (PA): Lippincott Williams & Wilkins; in press.

2. American College of Sports Medicine. *ACSM's Resource Manual for Guidelines for Exercise Testing and Prescription.* 6th ed. Philadelphia (PA): Lippincott Williams & Wilkins; 2010. 868 p.

3. American College of Sports Medicine, American Dietetic Association, and Dietitians of Canada. Position stand: nutrition and athletic performance. *Med Sci Sports Exerc.* 2009;41:709-731.

4. American Heart Association Web site [Internet]. Heart Disease and Stroke Statistics – 2007 Update At-a-Glance [cited 2010 May 26]. Available from: www.americanheart.org/downloadable/heart/1166712318459HS_StatsInsideText.pdf.

5. Casa DJ, Armstrong LE, Hillman SK, et al. National Athletic Trainers' Association position statement: fluid replacement for athletes. *J Athl Train.* 2000;35(2):212-224.

6. Curhan GC, Willett WC, Speizer FE, Spiegelman D, Stampfer MJ. Comparison of dietary calcium with supplemental calcium and other nutrients as factors affecting the risk for kidney stones in women. *Ann Int Med.* 1997;126:497-504.

7. Curhan GC, Willett WC, Speizer FE, Stampfer MJ. Beverage use and risk for kidney stones in women. *Ann Int Med.* 1999;128:534-540.

8. Flegal KM, Carroll MD, Ogden CL, Curtin LR. Prevalence and trends in obesity among US adults, 1999-2008. *JAMA.* 2010;303(3):235-241.

9. Food and Nutrition Board of the Institute of Medicine. *Dietary Reference Intakes for Water, Potassium, Sodium, Chloride, and Sulfate.* Washington, DC: National Academy Press; 2005.

10. Food and Nutrition Board of the Institute of Medicine. *Dietary Reference Intakes for Energy, Carbohydrate, Fiber, Fat, Fatty acids, Cholesterol, Protein, and Amino Acids.* Washington, DC: National Academy Press; 2005.

11. Food and Nutrition Board, Institute of Medicine Web site [Internet]. Dietary Reference Intakes. IOM; Washington, DC [accessed 2015 October 28]. Available from: http://fnic.nal.usda.gov/dietary-guidance/dietary-reference-intakes.

12. Hamada K, Doi T, Sakura M, et al. Effects of hydration on fluid balance and lower-extremity blood viscosity during long airplane flights. *JAMA.* 2002;287:844-845.

13. Harris J, Benedict F. *A Biometric Study of Basal Metabolism in Man.* Washington, DC: Carnegie Institute of Washington; 1919. Publication no. 279.

14. Hulston CJ, Jeukendrup AE. No placebo effect from carbohydrate intake during prolonged exercise. *Int J Sport Nutr Exerc Metab.* 2009;19(3):275-284.

15. Jones JM, Anderson JW. Grain foods and health: a primer for clinicians. *Phys Sportsmed.* 2008;36(1):18-33.

16. Math MV, Rampal PM, Faure XR, Delmont JP. Gallbladder emptying after drinking water and its possible role in prevention of gallstone formation. *Singapore Med J.* 1986;27:531-532.

17. Maughan RJ, Dargavel LA, Hares R, Shirreffs SM. Water and salt balance of well-trained swimmers in training. *Int J Sport Nutr Exerc Metab.* 2009;19(6):598-606.

18. McGinnis JM, Foege WH. Actual causes of death in the United States. *JAMA.* 1993;270(18):2207-2212.

19. Mifflin MD, St Jeor ST, Hill LA, Scott BJ, Daughterty SA, Koh YO. A new predictive equation for resting energy expenditure in healthy individuals. Am J Clin Nutr. 1990;51:241-247.

20. Minino A, Smith L. Deaths: preliminary data for 2000. *Natl Vital Stat Rep.* 2001;49(12):1-40.

21. Mokdad AH, Marks JS, Stroup DF, Gerberding JL. Actual causes of death in the United States, 2000. *JAMA.* 2004;291:1238-1245.

22. Centers for Disease Control and Prevention. *National Diabetes Statistics Report: Estimates of Diabetes and Its Burden in the United States.* Atlanta (GA): CDC; 2014.

23. National Osteoporosis Foundation Web site [Internet]. What Is Osteoporosis? Washington, DC; National Osteoporosis Foundation [cited 2010 May 26]. Available from; www.nof.org/.

24. Ogden CL, Carroll MD, Curtin LR, Lamb MM, Flegal KM. Prevalence of high body mass index in US children and adolescents, 2007-2008. *JAMA.* 2010;303(3):242-249.

25. Pereira MA, Kottke TE, Jordan C, O'Connor PJ, Pronk NP, Carreón R. Preventing and managing cardiometabolic risk: the logic for intervention. *Int J Environ Res Public Health.* 2009;6(10):2568-2584.

26. Sawka MN, Burke LM, Eichner ER, Maughan RJ, Montain SJ, Stachenfield NS. American College of Sports Medicine position stand: exercise and fluid replacement. *Med Sci Sports Exerc.* 2007;39(2):377-390.

27. Slattery ML, Caan BJ, Anderson KE, Potter JD. Intake of fluids and methylxantine-containing beverages: association with colon cancer. *Int J Cancer*. 1999;81:199-204.

28. U.S. Department of Agriculture Web site [Internet]. ChooseMyPlate. USDA; Alexandria (VA) [accessed 4 November 2015]. Available from; www.choosemyplate.gov/.

29. U.S. Department of Agriculture, Agricultural Research Services Web site [Internet]. Nutrient Data Laboratory. USDA-ARS; Beltsville (MD) [accessed 5 October 2015]. Available from: http://ndb.nal.usda.gov/.

30. U.S. Department of Health and Human Services Web site [Internet]. Dietary Guidelines for Americans 2015-2020. 8th ed. Atlanta (GA): USDHHS [cited 2016 January15]. Available from; http://health.gov/dietaryguidelines/2015/guidelines/.

31. U.S. Department of Health and Human Services Web site [Internet]. How to Understand and Use the Nutrition Facts Label. Atlanta (GA): USDHHS [cited 2015 October 15]. Available from: www.fda.gov/food/ingredientspackaginglabeling/labelingnutrition/ucm274593.htm.

32. U.S. Department of Health and Human Services and U.S. Department of Agriculture Web site [Internet]. Scientific Report of the 2015 Dietary Guidelines Advisory Committee [cited 2016 January 15]. Available from: http://health.gov/dietaryguidelines/2015-scientific-report/.

33. U.S. Food and Drug Administration Web site [Internet]. Changes to the Nutrition Facts Label. Silver Spring (MD): USFDA [cited 2016 May 21]. Available from: www.fda.gov/Food/GuidanceRegulation/GuidanceDocumentsRegulatoryInformation/LabelingNutrition/ucm385663.htm.

34. U.S. National Library of Medicine, U.S. Department of Health and Human Services, and National Institutes of Health Web site [Internet]. National Library of Medicine; Bethesda (MD) [cited 2015 October 5]. Available from: www.nlm.nih.gov/medlineplus/.

Chapter 4

1. American College of Sports Medicine. Nigg CR, ed. *ACSM's Behavioral Aspects of Physical Activity and Exercise*. Philadelphia (PA): Lippincott Williams & Wilkins; 2014. 284 p.

2. American College of Sports Medicine. *ACSM's Guidelines for Exercise Testing and Prescription*. 10th ed. Philadelphia (PA): Lippincott Williams & Wilkins; in press.

3. Buckworth J. Behavior change. In: Howley ET, Thompson DL, *Fitness Professional's Handbook*, 6th ed. Champaign (IL): Human Kinetics; 2012. 596 p.

4. Health Canada Web site [Internet]. Overcoming barriers: Canada's Food Guide. Ottawa, ON; Health Canada [cited 2015 November 14]. Available from: www.hc-sc.gc.ca/fn-an/food-guide-aliment/maintain-adopt/obstacles-eng.php.

5. Norcross JC, Mrykalo MS, Blagys MD. Auld Lang Syne: success predictors, change processes, and self-reported outcomes of New Year's resolvers and nonresolvers. *J Clin Psychol*. 2002;54(4):397-405.

6. Norcross JC, Vangarelli DJ. The resolution solution: longitudinal examination of New Year's change attempts. *J Subst Abuse*. 1989;1:127-134.

7. U.S. Department of Agriculture Web site [Internet]. ChooseMyPlate. USDA; Alexandria (VA) [accessed 4 November 2015]. Available from: www.choosemyplate.gov/.

8. U.S. Department of Health and Human Services, Centers for Disease Control and Prevention, Division of Nutrition, Physical Activity, and Obesity Web site [Internet]. Adding Physical Activity to Your Life. USDHHS, CDC; Atlanta (GA)[accessed 16 November 2015]. Available from; www.cdc.gov/physicalactivity/basics/adding-pa/barriers.html.

9. U.S. Department of Health and Human Services, Office of Disease Prevention and Health Promotion Web site [Internet]. 2008 Physical Activity Guidelines for Americans. Atlanta (GA): USDHHS [cited 2015 August 18]. Available from: http://health.gov/paguidelines/.

10. U.S. Department of Health and Human Services and U.S. Department of Agriculture Web site [Internet]. Scientific Report of the 2015 Dietary Guidelines Advisory Committee [cited 2015 August 19]. Available from: http://health.gov/dietaryguidelines/2015-scientific-report/.

11. Zimmerman GL, Olsen CG, Bosworth MF. A "stages of change" approach to helping patients change behavior. *Am Fam Physician*. 2000;61(5):1409-1416.

Chapter 5

1. Ainsworth BE, Haskell WL, Herrmann SD, Meckes N, Bassett Jr DR, Tudor-Locke C, Greer JL, Vezina J, Whitt-Glover MC, Leon AS. The Compendium of Physical Activities Tracking Guide Web site [Internet]. Healthy Lifestyles Research Center, College of Nursing & Health Innovation, Arizona State University [cited 2015 September 21]. Available from: https://sites.google.com/site/compendiumofphysicalactivities/.
2. American College of Sports Medicine. *ACSM's Guidelines for Exercise Testing and Prescription.* 10th ed. Philadelphia (PA): Lippincott Williams & Wilkins; in press.
3. Cooper Institute. Meredith MD, Welk GJ, eds. *FitnessGram/Activitygram Test Administration Manual,* updated 4th ed. Champaign (IL): Human Kinetics; 2013. 142 p.
4. Cooper Institute Web site [Internet]. Health Fitness Zone Standards v10. The Cooper Institute; Dallas (TX) [cited 2015 September 16]. Available from: www.cooperinstitute.org/healthyfitnesszone.
5. Cureton KJ, Sloniger MA, O'Bannon JP, Black DM, McCormack WP. A generalized equation for prediction of VO2peak from 1-mile run/walk performance. *Med Sci Sports Exerc.* 1995;27:445-451.
6. Garber CE, Blissmer B, Deschenes MR, et al. American College of Sports Medicine position stand. Quantity and quality of exercise for developing and maintaining cardiorespiratory, musculoskeletal, and neuromotor fitness in apparently healthy adults: guidance for prescribing exercise. *Med Sci Sports Exerc.* 2011;43(7):1334-1359.
7. Rikli RE, Jones CJ. *Senior Fitness Test Manual.* 2nd ed. Champaign (IL): Human Kinetics; 2013. 186 p.
8. U.S. Department of Health and Human Services, Office of Disease Prevention and Health Promotion Web site [Internet]. 2008 Physical Activity Guidelines for Americans. USDHHS; Atlanta (GA) [cited 2015 August 18]. Available from: http://health.gov/paguidelines/.

Chapter 6

1. American College of Sports Medicine. *ACSM's Guidelines for Exercise Testing and Prescription.* Baltimore (MD): Lippincott Williams & Wilkins; in press.
2. Artero E, Lee D, Lavie C, España-Romero V, Sui X, Church T, Blair S. Effects of muscular strength on cardiovascular risk factors and prognosis. *J Cardiopulm Rehabil Prev.* 2012;32:351-358.
3. Chodzko-Zajko W, Proctor D, Fiatarone Singh M, Minson C, Nigg C, Salem G, Skinner J. American College of Sports Medicine position stand. Exercise and physical activity for older adults. *Med Sci Sports Exerc.* 2009;41:1510-1530.
4. Cooper Institute Web site [Internet]. Health Fitness Zone Standards v10. The Cooper Institute; Dallas (TX); [cited 2015 September 16].Available from: http://www.cooperinstitute.org/healthyfitnesszone
5. Cooper Institute, ed. *FitnessGram/ActivityGram Test Adminstration Manual.* Champaign (IL): Human Kinetics; 2013. 141 p.
6. Faigenbaum A, Westcott W. *Youth Strength Training.* Champaign (IL): Human Kinetics; 2009. 235 p.
7. Fleck S, Kraemer W. *Designing Resistance Training Programs.* Champaign (IL): Human Kinetics; 2014. 520 p.
8. Giangregorio L, Papaioannou A, Macintyre N, Ashe M, Heinonen A, Shipp K, Wark J, McGill S, Keller H, Jain R, Laprade J, Cheung A. Too Fit to Fracture: exercise recommendations for individuals with osteoporosis or osteoporotic vertebral fracture. *Osteoporos Int.* 2014;25:821-835.
9. Gómez-Cabello A, Ara I, González-Agüero A, Casajús J, Vicente-Rodríguez G. Effects of training on bone mass in older adults: a systematic review. *Sports Med.* 2012;42:301-325.
10. Granacher U, Gollhofer A, Hortobágyi T, Kressig R, Muehlbauer T. The importance of trunk muscle strength for balance, functional performance, and fall prevention in seniors: a systematic review. *Sports Med.* 2013;43:627-641.
11. Guadalupe-Grau A, Fuentes T, Guerra B, Calbet A. Exercise and bone mass in adults. *Sports Med.* 2009;39:439-468.
12. Hurley B, Hanson E, Sheaff A. Strength training as a countermeasure to aging muscle and chronic disease. *Sports Med.* 2011;41:289-306.

13. Kerr Z, Collins C, Comstock R. Epidemiology of weight training-related injuries presenting to United States emergency departments, 1990 to 2007. *Am J Sports Med.* 2010;38:765-771.

14. Krieger J. Single versus multiple sets of resistance exercise: a meta-regression. *J Strength Cond Res.* 2009;23:1890-1901.

15. Marcell T. Sarcopenia: causes, consequences, and preventions. *J Gerontol A Biol Med Sci.* 2003;58:M911-M916.

16. Mazzetti SA, Kraemer WJ, Volek JS, Duncan ND, Ratamess NA, Gomez AL, Newton RU, Hakkinen K, Fleck SJ. The influence of direct supervision of resistance training on strength performance. *Med Sci Sports Exerc.* 2000;32:1175-1184.

17. Myer G, Quatman C, Khoury J, Wall E, Hewett T. Youth vs. adult "weightlifting" injuries presented to United States emergency rooms: accidental vs. non-accidental injury mechanisms. *J Strength Cond Res.* 2009;23:2054-2060.

18. Peterson M, Rhea M, Sen A, Gordon P. Resistance exercise for muscular strength in older adults: a meta-analysis. *Ageing Res Rev.* 2010;9:226-237.

19. Radaelli R, Fleck S, Leite T, Leite R, Pinto R, Fernandes L, Simão R. Dose-response of 1, 3, and 5 sets of resistance exercise on strength, local muscular endurance, and hypertrophy. *J Strength Cond Res.* 2015;29:1349-1358.

20. Ratamess N. *ACSM's Foundations of Strength Training and Conditioning.* Philadelphia (PA): Lippincott Williams & Wilkins; 2012. 560 p.

21. Ratamess N, Alvar B, Evetoch T, Housh T, Kibler WB, Kraemer WJ, Triplett T. Progression models in resistance training in healthy adults. *Med Sci Sports Exerc.* 2009;41:687-708.

22. Ratamess NA, Faigenbaum AD, Hoffman JR, Kang J. Self-selected resistance training intensity in healthy women: the influence of a personal trainer. *J Strength Cond Res.* 2008;22:103-111.

23. Reid K, Fielding R. Skeletal muscle power: a critical determinant of physical functioning in older adults. *Exerc Sport Sci Rev.* 2012;40:4-12.

24. Rikli R, Jones C. *Senior Fitness Test Manual.* Champaign (IL): Human Kinetics; 2013.

25. Ruiz JR, Sui X, Lobelo F, Morrow JR Jr, Jackson AW, Sjöström M, Blair S. Association between muscular strength and mortality in men: prospective cohort study. *BMJ.* 2008;337:92-95.

26. Strasser B, Schobersberger W. Evidence of resistance training as a treatment therapy in obesity. *J Obesity.* 2011, 2011: 482564.

27. Trombetti A, Reid K, Hars M, Herrmann F, Pasha E, Phillips E, Fielding R. Age-associated declines in muscle mass, strength, power, and physical performance: impact on fear of falling and quality of life. *Osteoporos Int.* 2016;27(2):463-71.

28. U.S. Department of Health and Human Services Web site [Internet]. 2008 Physical Activity Guidelines for Americans. USDHHS; Atlanta (GA) [cited 2015 August 15]. Available at http://health.gov/paguidelines/.

29. Weinsier R, Schutz Y, Bracco D. Reexamination of the relationship of resting metabolic rate to fat-free mass and to the metabolically active components of fat-free mass in humans. *Am J Clin Nutr.* 1992;55:790-794.

30. Westcott W. Resistance training is medicine: effects of strength training on health. *Curr Sports Med Rep.* 2012;11:209-216.

31. Westcott W, Baechle T. *Strength Training Past 50.* Champaign (IL): Human Kinetics; 2015. 264 p.

32. Williams M, Stewart K. Impact of strength and resistance training on cardiovascular disease risk factors and outcomes in older adults. *Clin Geriatr Med.* 2009;25:703-714.

33. World Health Organization. *Global Recommendations on Physical Activity for Health.* Geneva: WHO Press; 2010. 60 p.

Chapter 7

1. Alter MJ. *Science of Flexibility.* Champaign (IL): Human Kinetics; 1996. 373 p.

2. American College of Sports Medicine. American College of Sports Medicine position stand. The recommended quantity and quality of exercise for developing and maintaining cardiorespiratory and muscular fitness, and flexibility in healthy adults. *Med Sci Sports Exerc.* 1998;30(6):975-991.

3. American College of Sports Medicine. *ACSM's Guidelines for Exercise Testing and Prescription.* Philadelphia (PA): Lippincott Williams & Wilkins; in press.

4. American College of Sports Medicine. *ACSM's Resources for the Personal Trainer.* Baltimore (MD): Lippincott Williams & Wilkins; 2014. 627 p.

5. Behm DG, Blazevich AJ, Kay AD, McHugh M. Acute effects of muscle stretching on physical performance, range of motion, and injury incidence in healthy active individuals: a systematic review. *Appl Physiol Nutr Metab.* 2016;41:1-11.

6. Christmas C, Andersen RA. Exercise and older patients: guidelines for the clinician. *J Am Geriatr Soc.* 2000;48(3):318-324.

7. Covert CA, Alexander MP, Petronis JJ, Davis DS. Comparison of ballistic and static stretching on hamstring muscle length using an equal stretching dose. *J Strength Cond Res.* 2010;24(11):3008-3014.

8. Deslandes A, Moraes H, Ferreira C, et al. Exercise and mental health: many reasons to move. *Neuropsychobiology.* 2009;59(4):191-198.

9. Doriot N, Wang X. Effects of age and gender on maximum voluntary range of motion of the upper body joints. *Ergonomics.* 2006;49(3):269-281.

10. Golding LA, Myers CR. *Y's Way to Physical Fitness: The Complete Guide to Fitness Testing and Instruction.* Champaign (IL): Human Kinetics; 1989. 192 p.

11. Herbert RD, Gabriel M. Effects of stretching before and after exercising on muscle soreness and risk of injury: systematic review. *BMJ.* 2002;325(7362):468 p.

12. McMillian DJ, Moore JH, Hatler BS, Taylor DC. Dynamic vs. static-stretching warm up: the effect on power and agility performance. *J Strength Cond Res.* 2006;20(3):492-499.

13. Milani RV, Lavie CJ. Reducing psychosocial stress: a novel mechanism of improving survival from exercise training. *Am J Med.* 2009;122(10):931-938.

14. Mosca L, Manson JE, Sutherland SE, Langer RD, Manolio T, Barrett-Connor E. Cardiovascular disease in women: a statement for healthcare professionals from the American Heart Association. Writing Group. *Circulation.* 1997;96(7):2468-2482.

15. Nieman D. *Exercise Testing & Prescription.* New York (NY): McGraw-Hill Education; 2011. 652 p.

16. Rikli RE, Jones CJ. *Senior Fitness Test Manual.* 2nd ed. Champaign (IL): Human Kinetics; 2013. 186 p.

17. Shin G, Shu Y, Li Z, Jiang Z, Mirka G. Influence of knee angle and individual flexibility on the flexion-relaxation response of the low back musculature. *J Electromyogr Kinesiol.* 2004;14(4):485-494.

18. The Cooper Institute. *FitnessGram/ActivityGram Test Administration Manual.* Updated 4th ed. Champaign (IL): Human Kinetics; 2013. 142 p.

19. van der Heijden MM, van Dooren FE, Pop VJ, Pouwer F. Effects of exercise training on quality of life, symptoms of depression, symptoms of anxiety and emotional well-being in type 2 diabetes mellitus: a systematic review. *Diabetologia.* 2013;56(6):1210-1225.

20. Woolstenhulme MT, Griffiths CM, Woolstenhulme EM, Parcell AC. Ballistic stretching increases flexibility and acute vertical jump height when combined with basketball activity. *J Strength Cond Res.* 2006;20(4):799-803.

Chapter 8

1. Adkins D, Boychuk J, Remple M, Kleim J. Motor training induces experience-specific patterns of plasticity across motor cortex and spinal cord. *J Appl Physiol.* 2006;101:1776-1782.

2. Aman J, Elangovan N, Konczak J. The effectiveness of proprioceptive training for improving motor function: a systematic review. *Front Hum Neurosci.* 2015;8(1075):1-18.

3. American College of Sports Medicine. *ACSM's Guidelines for Exercise Testing and Prescription.* 10th ed. Philadelphia (PA): Lippincott Williams & Wilkins; in press.

4. Brach J, Lowry K, Perera S, Hornyak V, Wert D, Studenski S, VanSwearingen J. Improving motor control in walking: a randomized clinical trial in older adults with subclinical walking difficulty. *Arch Phys Med Rehabil.* 2015;96(3):388-394.

5. Centers for Disease Control and Prevention Web site [Internet]. STEADI (Stopping Elderly Accidents, Deaths & Injuries) materials for health care providers: the 4-stage balance test. April 20, 2015 [cited 2015 June 10]. Available at www.cdc.gov/injury/STEADI.

6. Chin A, van Uffelen J, Riphagen I, van Mechelen W. The functional effects of physical exercise training in frail older people: a systematic review. *Sports Med.* 2008;38(9):781-793.

7. Duncan PW, Weiner DK, Chandler J, Studenski S. Functional reach: a new clinical measure of balance. *J Gerontol.* 1990;45(6):M192-M197.

8. Edgren H. An experiment in the testing of agility and progress in basketball. *Res Q.* 1932;3(1):159-171.

9. Farlie M, Robins L, Keating J, Molloy E, Haines T. Intensity of challenge to the balance system is not reported in the prescription of balance exercises in randomised trials: a systematic review. *J Physiother.* 2013;59:227-235.

10. Forman D, Fleg J. Special populations: aging. In: Ehrman J, et al. *Clinical Exercise Physiology.* Human Kinetics: Champaign (IL); 2013, p. 589-604.

11. Garber C, Blissmer B, Deschenes M, Franklin B, Lamonte M, Lee I, Nieman D, Swain D. Quantity and quality of exercise for developing and maintaining cardiorespiratory, musculoskeletal, and neuromotor fitness in apparently healthy adults: guidance for prescribing exercise. *Med Sci Sports Exerc.* 2011;1334-1359.

12. Gatts A. Neural mechanics underlying balance control in Tai Chi. *Med Sports Sci.* 2008;52:87-103.

13. Gillespie L, Robertson M, Gillespie W. Interventions for preventing falls in older people living in the community. *Cochrane Database Syst Rev.* 2009;2:CD007146.

14. Hewett T, Myer G, Ford K. Reducing knee and anterior cruciate ligament injuries among female athletes: a systematic review of neuromuscular training interventions. *J Knee Surg.* 2005;18(1):82-88.

15. Hubscher M, Refshauge K. Neuromuscular training strategies for preventing lower limb injuries: what's new and what are the practical implications of what we already know? *Br J Sports Med.* 2013;47(15):939-940.

16. Jones C, Rikli R, Beam W. A 30-s chair-stand test as a measure of lower body strength in community-residing older adults. *Res Q Exerc Sport.* 1999;70(2):113-119.

17. Liu H, Frank A. Tai Chi as a balance improvement exercise for older adults: a systematic review. *J Geriatr Phys Ther.* 2010;33(3):103-109.

18. Pauole K, Madole K, Garhammer J, Lacourse M, Rozenek R. Reliability and validity of the T-test as a measure of agility, leg power, and leg speed in college-aged men and women. *J Strength Cond Res.* 2000;14(4):443-450.

19. Rikli R, Jones C. Development and validation of criterion-referenced clinically relevant fitness standards for maintaining physical independence in later years. *Gerontologist.* 2013;53(2):255-267.

20. Rikli R, Jones C. *Senior Fitness Test Manual.* 2nd ed. Champaign (IL): Human Kinetics; 2013. 186 p.

21. Semenick D. The T-test. *Natl Strength Cond Assoc J.* 1990;12(1):36-37.

22. Springer B, Marin R, Cyhan T, Roberts H, Gill N. Normative values for the unipedal stance test with eyes open and closed. *J Geriatr Phys Ther.* 2007;30(1):8-15.

23. Theou O, Stathokostas L, Roland K, Jakobi J, Patterson C, Vandervoort A, Jones G. The effectiveness of exercise interventions for the management of frailty: a systemtaic review. *J Aging Res.* 2011;2011;1-19.

24. Umphred D. *Neurological Rehabilitation.* Burton G, Rolando T, Roller M, eds. 5th ed. St. Louis (MO): Mosby/Elsevier; 2007. 1257 p.

25. Wayne P, Berkowitz D, Litrownik D, Buring J, Yeh G. What do we really know about the safety of Tai Chi?: a systematic review of adverse event reports in randomized trials. *Arch Phys Med Rehabil.* 2015;95(12):2470-2483.

26. Weiner DK, Duncan PW, Chandler J, Studenski SA. Functional reach: a marker of physical frailty. *J Am Geriatr Soc.* 1992;40(3):203-207.

27. Wolpaw J. Spinal cord plasticity in acquisition and maintenance motor skills. *Acta Physiol.* 2007;189:155-169.

Chapter 9

1. Adolph KE, Joh AS. Motor development: how infants get into the act. In: Slater A, Lewis M, eds. *Introduction to Infant Development.* New York (NY): Oxford University Press; 2007, p. 63-80.

2. Adolphus K, Lawton CL, Dye L. The effects of breakfast on behavior and academic performance in children and adolescents. *Front Hum Neurosci.* 2013;7:425.

3. American College of Sports Medicine. *ACSM's Guidelines for Exercise Testing and Prescription*. 10th ed. Philadelphia (PA): Lippincott Williams & Wilkins; in press.

4. American College of Sports Medicine. *ACSM's Resource Manual for Guidelines for Exercise Testing and Prescription*. 6th ed. Philadelphia (PA): Lippincott Williams & Wilkins; 2010. 896 p.

5. Behm DG, Faigenbaum AD, Falk B, Klentrou P. Canadian Society for Exercise Physiology position paper: resistance training in children and adolescents. *Appl Physiol Nutr Metab*. 2008;33:547-561.

6. Belcher BR, Berrigan D, Dodd KW, et al. Physical activity in U.S. youth: effect of race/ethnicity, age, gender, and weight status. *Med Sci Sports Exerc*. 2010;42:2211-2221.

7. Briefel RR., Johnson CL. Secular trends in dietary intake in the United States. *Annu Rev Nutr*. 2004;24:401-431.

8. Centers for Disease Control and Prevention Web site [Internet]. The association between school based physical activity, including physical education, and academic performance. CDC; Atlanta (GA); [accessed 15 November 2015]. Available from:www.cdc.gov/healthyyouth/health_and_academics/pdf/pa-pe_paper.pdf.

9. Centers for Disease Control and Prevention. Youth risk behavior surveillance—United States, 2007. *MMWR*. 2008;57(SS04):1-131.

10. Centers for Disease Control and Prevention Web site [Internet]. About child and teen BMI. CDC; Atlanta (GA); [cited 2015 November 16]. Available from: www.cdc.gov/healthyweight/assessing/bmi/childrens_bmi/about_childrens_bmi.html.

11. Centers for Disease Control and Prevention Web site [Internet]. Childhood overweight and obesity. CDC; Atlanta (GA); [cited 2010 May 15]. Available from: www.cdc.gov/obesity/childhood/index.html.

12. Chung AE, Skinner AC, Steiner MJ, et al. Physical activity and BMI in a national representative sample of children and adolescents. *Clin Pediatr (Phila)*. 2012;51:122-129.

13. Faigenbaum AD, Kraemer WJ, Blimkie CJR, et al. Youth resistance training: updated position statement paper from the National Strength and Conditioning Association. *J Strength Cond Res*. 2009;23(suppl 5):S60-S79.

14. Faigenbaum AD, Micheli LJ. Youth strength training. ACSM current comment [Internet] ACSM; Indianapolis (IN); [cited 3 June 2010]. Available at www.acsm.org/AM/Template.cfm?Section=Current_Comments1.

15. Ferraro KF, Thorpe RJ, Wilkinson JA. The life course of severe obesity: does childhood overweight matter? *J Gerontol*. 2003;58B(2):S110-S119.

16. Forshee RA, Anderson PA, Storey ML. Changes in calcium intake and association with beverage consumption and demographics: comparing data from CSFII 1994–1996, 1998 and NHANES 1999–2002. *J Am Coll Nutr*. 2006;25:108-116.

17. Freedman DS, Khan LK, Dietz WH, Srinivasan SR, Berenson GS. Relationship of childhood obesity to coronary heart disease risk factors in adulthood: the Bogalusa Study. *Pediatrics*. 2001;108(3):712-718.

18. Fulkerson JA, Story M, Mellin A, Leffert N, et al. Family dinner meal frequency and adolescent development: relationships with developmental assets and high-risk behaviors. *J Adolesc Health*.2006;39:337-345.

19. Giddings SS, Dennison BA, Birch LL, et al. Dietary recommendations for children and adolescents: a guide for practitioners. Consensus statement from the American Heart Association. *Circulation*. 2005;112(13):2061-2075.

20. Haskell WL, Lee I-M, Pate RR, et al. Physical activity and public health: updated recommendation for adults from the American College of Sports Medicine and the American Heart Association. *Med Sci Sports Exerc*. 2007;39:1423-1434.

21. Janssen I, LeBlanc AG. Systematic review of the health benefits of physical activity and fitness in school-aged children and youth. *Int J Behav Nutr Phys Act*. 2010;7:40.

22. MacKelvie KJ, Khan KM, McKay HA. Is there a critical period for bone response to weight-bearing exercise in children and adolescents? A systematic review. *Br J Sports Med*. 2002;36:250-257.

23. Morgan DW. Right from the start: promotion of health-related fitness in toddlers and preschoolers. *Kinesiol Rev*. 2013;2:88-92.

24. National Association for Sport and Physical Education. *Active Start: A Statement of Physical Activity Guidelines for Children from Birth to Five Years*. 2nd ed. Reston (VA): NASPE; 2009. 48 p.

25. National Association for Sport and Physical Education. *Physical Activity for Children: A Statement of Guidelines for Children Ages 5-12.* 2nd ed. Reston (VA): NASPE; 2004. 28 p.

26. National Heart, Lung, and Blood Institute Web site [Internet]. NHLBI; Bethesda (MD); [cited 2015 November 16]. Available from: www.nhlbi.nih.gov/health/health-topics/topics/obe/risks.

27. National Physical Activity Plan Alliance Web site [Internet]. 2014 United States Report Card on Physical Activity for Children and Youth. NPAP; Columbia (SC); [cited 2015 November 16] Available from: www.physicalactivityplan.org/reportcard/NationalReportCard_longform_final%20 for%20web.pdf.

28. Ogden CL, Carroll MD, Flegal KM. High body mass index for age among U.S. children and adolescents 2003-2006. *JAMA.* 2008;299(20):2401-2405.

29. Paredes AZ, Persaud E, Shelnutt KP. Raising healthy children: the importance of family meals. University of Florida IFAS Extension Web site [Internet] IFAS-IT; Gainesville (FL); [cited 2015 November 16]. Available from: https://edis.ifas.ufl.edu/fy1195.

30. Pate RR, Baranowski T, Dowda M, et al. Tracking of physical activity in young children. *Med Sci Sports Exerc.* 1996;28:92-96.

31. Reedy J, Krebs-Smith SM. Dietary sources of energy, solid fats, and added sugars among children and adolescents in the United States. *J Am Diet Assoc.* 2010;110:1477-1484.

32. Shay CM, Ning H, Daniels SR, et al. Status of cardiovascular health in U.S. adolescents: prevalence estimates from the National Health and Nutrition Examination Surveys (NHANES) 2005–2010. *Circulation.* 2013;127:1369-1376.

33. Strong WB, Malina RM, Blimke CJR, et al. Evidence based physical activity for school-aged youth. *J Pediatr.* 2005;146:732-737.

34. Telema R. Tracking of physical activity from childhood to adulthood: a review. *Obes Facts.* 2009;3:187-195.

35. Thune I, Furberg A-S. Physical activity and cancer risk: dose-response and cancer, all sites, and site-specific. *Med Sci Sports Exerc.* 2001;33(supp 6):S530-S550.

36. Timmons BW, Naylor, P-J, Pfeiffer KA. Physical activity for preschool children – how much and how? *Appl Physiol Nutr Metab.* 2007;32:S122-S134.

37. Troiano RP, Berrigan D, Dodd KW, et al. Physical activity in the United States measured by accelerometer. *Med Sci Sports Exerc.* 2008;40:181-188.

38. U.S. Department of Agriculture Website [Internet]. Alexandria (VA); USDA [cited 2015 November 16]. Available from: www.ChooseMyPlate.gov/.

39. U.S. Department of Agriculture Web site [Internet]. Agriculture Research Service. 2010. Nutrient intakes from food: mean amounts consumed per individual, by gender and age. What We Eat in America, NHANES 2007-2008. Available from: www.ars.usda.gov/ba/bhnrc/fsrg.

40. U.S. Department of Health and Human Services Web site [Internet]. 2008 Physical Activity Guidelines for Americans. USDHHS; Atlanta (GA);[cited 2010 January 1]. Available from: www. health.gov/paguidelines.

41. U.S. Department of Health and Human Services and U.S. Department of Agriculture Web site [Internet]. Dietary Guidelines for Americans 2010 and Report of the Dietary Guidelines Advisory Committee on the Dietary Guidelines for Americans 2010 Washington DC; USDHHS; [cited 2011 February 1]. Available from: https://health.gov/dietaryguidelines/2010/.

42. U.S. Department of Health and Human Services and U.S. Department of Agriculture website [Internet]. Dietary Guidelines for Americans 2015. USDHHS; Atlanta (GA) [cited 2016 August 11]. Available at http://health.gov/dietaryguidelines/2015/guidelines/.

43. U.S. National Library of Medicine Web site [Internet]. Causes and risks for obesity – children [cited 2015 November 16]. Available from: www.nlm.nih.gov/medlineplus/ency/patientinstruc-tions/000383.htm.

Chapter 10

1. American College of Sports Medicine. *ACSM's Guidelines for Exercise Testing and Prescription.* 10th ed. Philadelphia: Lippincott Williams & Wilkins; in press.

2. American College of Sports Medicine. *ACSM's Resource Manual for Guidelines for Exercise Testing and Prescription.* 6th ed. Philadelphia (PA): Lippincott Williams & Wilkins; 2010. 868 p.

3. Garber CE, Blissmer B, Deschenes MR, et al. American College of Sports Medicine position stand. Quantity and quality of exercise for developing and maintaining cardiorespiratory, musculoskeletal, and neuromotor fitness in apparently healthy adults: guidance for prescribing exercise. *Med Sci Sports Exerc.* 2011;43(7):1334-1359.

4. U.S. Department of Health and Human Services Web site [Internet]. Dietary Guidelines for Americans. Atlanta (GA): USDHHS [cited 2010 January 4]. Available from: www.health.gov/dietaryguidelines/dga2005/default.htm#2.

5. U.S. Department of Health and Human Services Web site [Internet]. Physical Activity Guidelines for Americans. Atlanta (GA): USDHHS [cited 2015 November 4]. Available from: http://health.gov/paguidelines/.

6. U.S. Department of Health and Human Services Web site [Internet]. Healthy People 2020. Washington, DC; USDHHS; 2014 [cited 2015 September 2]. Available at www.healthypeople.gov/2020/How-to-Use-DATA2020.

7. U.S. Department of Health and Human Services, National Institutes of Health, Office of Dietary Supplements Web site [Internet]. Vitamin and mineral supplement fact sheets. Bethesda (MD); NIH, Office of Dietary Supplements [cited 2015 October 29]. Available from: https://ods.od.nih.gov/factsheets/list-VitaminsMinerals/.

8. U.S. Department of Health and Human Services and U.S. Department of Agriculture Web site [Internet]. Dietary Guidelines for Americans 2015. Atlanta (GA): USDHHS [cited 2016 January 13]. Available from: http://health.gov/dietaryguidelines/2015/guidelines/.

9. U.S. Department of Health and Human Services and U.S. Department of Agriculture Web site [Internet]. Scientific Report of the 2015 Dietary Guidelines Advisory Committee. Atlanta (GA): USDHHS [cited 2016 January 20]. Available from: http://health.gov/dietaryguidelines/2015-scientific-report/.

10. U.S. Food and Drug Administration Web site [Internet]. Sodium in Your Diet: Using the Nutrition Facts Label to Reduce Your Intake. Silver Spring (MD); FDA [cited 2015 November 2]. Available from: www.fda.gov/Food/ResourcesForYou/Consumers/ucm315393.htm.

Chapter 11

1. Alzheimer's Association Web site [Internet]. Alzheimer's Disease Facts and Figures. 2013. Alzheimer's Association; Chicago (IL); [cited 2015 August 15]. Available from www.alz.org/downloads/facts_figures_2013.pdf.

2. Arem H, Moore SC, Patel A, et al. Leisure time physical activity and mortality: a detailed pooled analysis of the dose-response relationship. *JAMA Intern Med.* 2015;175(6):959-967.

3. Barnes JN. Exercise, cognitive function, and aging. *Adv Physiol Educ.* 2015;39:55-62.

4. Bay SL, Baxter AS, Leite GF. Prevalence of self-reported sleep disorders among older adults and the association of disturbed sleep with service demand and medical conditions. *Int Psychogeriatr.* 2008;20(3):582-595.

5. Bell AJ, Talbot-Stern JK, Hennessy A. Characteristics and outcomes of older patients presenting to the emergency department after a fall: a retrospective analysis. *Med J Aust.* 2000;173(4):176-177.

6. Booth FW, Roberts CK, Laye MJ. Lack of exercise is a major cause of chronic diseases. *Compr Physiol.* 2012;2(2):1143-1211.

7. Brown AD, McMorris CA, Longman RS, et al. Effects of cardiorespiratory fitness and cerebral blood flow on cognitive outcomes in older women. *Neurobiol Aging.* 2010;31:2047-2057.

8. Centers for Disease Control and Prevention, National Center for Injury Prevention and Control Web site [Internet] Web-based Injury Statistics Query and Reporting System (WISQARS). CDC; Atlanta (GA); [cited 2015 August 15]. Available from: http://www.cdc.gov/injury/wisqars/index.html.

9. Chen KM, Chen MH, Chao HC, et al. Sleep quality, depression state, and health status of older adults after silver yoga exercises: cluster randomized trial. *Int J Nurs Stud.* 2009;46(2):154-163.

10. Cho J, Shin MK, Kim D, et al. Treadmill running reverses cognitive declines due to Alzheimer's disease. *Med Sci Sports Exerc.* 2015;47(9):1814-1824.

11. Chodzko-Zajko WJ, Proctor DN, Fiatarone MA, et al. American College of Sports Medicine position stand. Exercise and physical activity for older adults. *Med Sci Sports Exerc.* 2009;41:1510-1530.

12. Cricco M, Simonsick EM, Foley DJ. The impact of insomnia on cognitive functioning in older adults. *J Am Geriatr Soc.* 2001;49(9):1185-1189.

13. Garber CE, Blissmer B, Deschenes MR, et al. American College of Sports Medicine position stand. Quantity and quality of exercise for developing and maintain cardiorespiratory, musculoskeletal, and neuromotor fitness in apparently healthy adults: guidance for prescribing exercise. *Med Sci Sports Exerc.* 2011;43(7):1334-1359.

14. Gebel K, Ding D, Chey T, et al. Effects of moderate to vigorous physical activity on all-cause mortality in middle-aged and older Australians. *JAMA Intern Med.* 2015;175(6):970-977.

15. King AC, Pruitt LA, Woo S, et al. Effects of moderate-intensity exercise on polysomnographic and subjective sleep quality in older adults with mild to moderate sleep complaints. *J Gerontol A Biol Sci Med Sci.* 2008;63(9):997-1004.

16. Magaziner J, Hawkes W, Hebel JR, Zimerman SI, Fox KM, Dolan M, et al. Recovery from hip fracture in eight areas of function. *J Gerontol Med Sci.* 2000;55A(9):M498-M507.

17. Marks R, Allegrante JP, MacKenzie CR, Lane JM. Hip fractures among the elderly: causes, consequences and control. *Aging Res Rev.* 2003;2:57-93.

18. National Institute on Aging Web site [Internet]. Exercise & Physical Activity: Your Everyday Guide. 2011. NIA; Bethesda (MD); [cited 2015 August 15]. Available from www.nia.nih.gov/health/publication/exercise-physical-activity/introduction.pdf.

19. Reid KJ, Baron KG, Lu B, et al. Aerobic exercise improves self-reported sleep and quality of life in older adults with insomnia. *Sleep Med.* 2010;11:934-940.

20. Rikli RE, Jones CJ. *Senior Fitness Test Manual.* 2nd ed. Champaign (IL): Human Kinetics; 2013. 186 p.

21. Stewart R, Besset A, Bebbington P, et al. Insomnia comorbidity and impact and hypnotic use by age group in a national survey population aged 16 to 74 years. *Sleep.* 2006;29(11):1391-1397.

22. Suzuki T, Shimada H, Makizako H, et al. A randomized controlled trial of multicomponent exercise in older adults with mild cognitive impairment. *PLoS One.* 2013;8:e61483.

23. Thompson PD, Buchner D, Pina IL, et al. Exercise and physical activity in the prevention and treatment of atherosclerotic cardiovascular disease. *Circulation.* 2003;107:3109-3116.

24. Trappe S, Hayes E, Galpin A, et al. New records in aerobic power among octogenarian lifelong endurance athletes. *J Appl Physiol.* 2013;114(1):3-10.

25. Tromp AM, Pluijm SMF, Smit JH, et al. Fall-risk screening test: a prospective study on predictors for falls in community-dwelling elderly. *J Clin Epidemiol.* 2001;54(8):837-844.

26. U.S. Department of Health and Human Services and U.S. Department of Agriculture Web site [Internet]. Dietary Guidelines for Americans 2015. USDHHS; Atlanta (GA) [cited 20 January 2016]. Available from: http://health.gov/dietaryguidelines/2015.asp.

27. van der Ploeg HP, Chey T, Korda RJ, Banks E, Bauman A. Sitting time and all-cause mortality risk in 222 497 Australian adults. *Arch Intern Med.* 2012;172(6):494-500.

28. Wright KP, Frey DJ. Age related changes in sleep and circadian physiology: from brain mechanisms to sleep behavior. In: Avidan AY, Alessi C, *Geriatric Sleep Medicine.* New York (NY): CRC Press; 2009, p. 1-18.

Chapter 12

1. Aburto NJ, Hanson S, Gutierrez H, Hooper L, Elliott P, Cappuccio FP. Effect of increased potassium intake on cardiovascular risk factors and disease: systematic review and meta-analyses. *BMJ.* 2013;346:f1378.

2. American College of Sports Medicine. *ACSM's Guidelines for Exercise Testing and Prescription.* 10th ed. Baltimore (MD): Lippincott Williams & Wilkins; in press.

3. American Heart Association Web site [Internet]. Alcohol and Heart Health [updated January 12, 2015] Dallas (TX); AHA; [cited September 2, 2015]. Available from: www.heart.org/HEARTORG/GettingHealthy/NutritionCenter/HealthyEating/Alcohol-and-Heart-Health_UCM_305173_Article.jsp.

4. American Heart Association Web site [Internet]. Fish and Omega-3 Fatty Acids [updated June 15, 2015] Dallas (TX); AHA; [cited September 2, 2015]. Available from: www.heart.org/HEARTORG/GettingHealthy/NutritionCenter/HealthyEating/Fish-and-Omega-3-Fatty-Acids_UCM_303248_Article.jsp.

5. American Heart Association Web site [Internet]. Saturated fats [updated January 12, 2015] Dallas (TX): AHA; [cited September 2, 2015]. Available from: www.heart.org/HEARTORG/Getting-Healthy/NutritionCenter/HealthyEating/Saturated-Fats_UCM_301110_Article.jsp.

6. American Heart Association Web site [Internet]. Trans fat [updated August 5, 2015] Dallas (TX): AHA; [cited September 2, 2015]. Available from: www.heart.org/HEARTORG/GettingHealthy/NutritionCenter/HealthyEating/Trans-Fats_UCM_301120_Article.jsp.

7. American Heart Association Web site [Internet]. Understand Your Risk of Heart Attack. Dallas (TX); AHA;[cited November 21, 2015]. Available from: www.heart.org/HEARTORG/Conditions/HeartAttack/UnderstandYourRiskofHeartAttack/Understand-Your-Risk-of-Heart-Attack_UCM_002040_Article.jsp - .VlEMPq6rT-Y.

8. Appel LJ, Brands MW, Daniels SR, et al. Dietary approaches to prevent and treat hypertension: a scientific statement from the American Heart Association. *Hypertension*. 2006;47(2):296-308.

9. Appel LJ, Moore TJ, Obarzanek E, et al. A clinical trial of the effects of dietary patterns on blood pressure. DASH Collaborative Research Group. *N Engl J Med*. 1997;336(16):1117-1124.

10. Chobanian AV, Bakris GL, Black HR, et al. The Seventh Report of the Joint National Committee on Prevention, Detection, Evaluation, and Treatment of High Blood Pressure: the JNC 7 report. *JAMA*. 2003;289(19):2560-2572.

11. Eckel RH, Jakicic JM, Ard JD, et al. 2013 AHA/ACC guideline on lifestyle management to reduce cardiovascular risk: a report of the American College of Cardiology/American Heart Association Task Force on Practice Guidelines. *Circulation*. 2014;129(25 suppl 2):S76-S99.

12. Expert Panel on Detection, Evaluation, and Treatment of High Blood Cholesterol in Adults. Executive Summary of the Third Report of the National Cholesterol Education Program (NCEP) Expert Panel on Detection, Evaluation, and Treatment of High Blood Cholesterol in Adults (Adult Treatment Panel III). *JAMA*. 2001;285(19):2486-2497.

13. Hansson GK. Inflammation, atherosclerosis, and coronary artery disease. *N Engl J Med*. 2005;352(16):1685-1695.

14. Libby P, Theroux P. Pathophysiology of coronary artery disease. *Circulation*. 2005;111(25):3481-3488.

15. Mozaffarian D, Benjamin EJ, Go AS, et al. Heart disease and stroke statistics—2015 update: a report from the American Heart Association. *Circulation*. 2015;131(4):e29-e322.

16. National Heart, Lung, and Blood Institute. *Your Guide to Lowering Your Cholesterol With TLC*. Bethesda (MD): U.S. Department of Health and Human Services; 2005.

17. National Heart, Lung, and Blood Institute Web site [Internet]. What Is the DASH eating plan? Bethesda (MD); NHLBI; [cited September 2, 2015]. Available from: www.nhlbi.nih.gov/health/health-topics/topics/dash.

18. Pescatello LS, MacDonald HV, Ash GI, et al. Assessing the existing professional exercise recommendations for hypertension: a review and recommendations for future research priorities. *Mayo Clin Proc*. 2015;90(6):801-812.

19. Rosendorff C, Lackland DT, Allison M, et al. Treatment of hypertension in patients with coronary artery disease: a scientific statement from the American Heart Association, American College of Cardiology, and American Society of Hypertension. *Circulation*. 2015;131(19):e435-e470.

20. Sacks FM, Svetkey LP, Vollmer WM, et al. Effects on blood pressure of reduced dietary sodium and the Dietary Approaches to Stop Hypertension (DASH) diet. DASH-Sodium Collaborative Research Group. *N Engl J Med*. 2001;344(1):3-10.

21. Stone NJ, Robinson JG, Lichtenstein AH, et al. 2013 ACC/AHA guideline on the treatment of blood cholesterol to reduce atherosclerotic cardiovascular risk in adults: a report of the American College of Cardiology/American Heart Association Task Force on Practice Guidelines. *Circulation*. 2014;129(25 suppl 2):S1-S45.

22. U.S. Department of Agriculture and U.S. Department of Health and Human Services. Scientific Report of the 2015 Dietary Guidelines Advisory Committee Part A. Executive Summary. Cross-Cutting Topics of Public Health. USDA and USDHHS; 2015.

23. U.S. Department of Health and Human Services Web site [Internet]. Physical Activity Guidelines for Americans 2008. Atlanta (GA): USDHHS [cited September 11, 2015]. Available at http://health.gov/paguidelines/guidelines/.

24. U.S. Department of Agriculture, Agricultural Research Service. *Nutrient Intakes from Food and Beverages: Mean Amounts Consumed per Individual, by Gender and Age.* USDA, ARS; 2014.

25. U.S. Food and Drug Administration Web site [Internet]. Sodium in Your Diet: Using the Nutrition Facts Label to Reduce Your Intake [updated September 3, 2015]. Silver Spring (MD); USFDA; [cited September 11, 2015]. Available from: www.fda.gov/Food/ResourcesForYou/Consumers/ucm315393.htm.

26. U.S. Department of Health and Human Services, National Institutes of Health, National Heart, Lung, and Blood Institute. *Your Guide to Lowering Cholesterol with Therapeutic Lifestyle Changes.* NIH publication no. 06-5235, December 2005.

Chapter 13

1. American College of Sports Medicine. *ACSM's Guidelines for Exercise Testing and Prescription.* Philadelphia (PA): Lippincott Williams & Wilkins; in print.

2. American Diabetes Association. Classification and diagnosis of diabetes. *Diabetes Care.* 2016;39 suppl:S13-S22.

3. American Diabetes Association. Foundations of care: education, nutrition, physical activity, smoking cessation, psychosocial care, and immunization. *Diabetes Care.* 2016;39 suppl:S23-S35.

4. American Diabetes Association. Glycemic targets. *Diabetes Care.* 2016;398 suppl:S39-S46.

5. American Diabetes Association. Microvascular complications and foot care. *Diabetes Care.* 2016. 39 suppl:S72-S80.

6. American Diabetes Association. Children and adolescents. *Diabetes Care.* 2016;39 suppl:S86-S93.

7. Balducci S, Iacobellis G, Parisi L, Di Biase N, Calandriello E, Leonetti F, Fallucca F. Exercise training can modify the natural history of diabetic peripheral neuropathy. *J Diabetes Complications.* 2006;20:216-223.

8. Brand-Miller J, McMillan-Price J, Steinbeck K, Caterson I. Dietary glycemic index: health implications. *J Am Coll Nutr.* 2009;28 suppl:446s-449s.

9. Brazeau AS, Leroux C, Mircescu H, Rabasa-Lhoret R. Physical activity level and body composition among adults with type 1 diabetes. *Diabetes Med.* 2012;29:e402-e408. doi: 410.1111/j.1464-5491.2012.03757.x.

10. Burge MR, Garcia N, Qualls CR, Schade DS. Differential effects of fasting and dehydration in the pathogenesis of diabetic ketoacidosis. *Metabolism.* 2001;50:171-177.

11. Chiang JL, Kirkman MS, Laffel LM, Peters AL. Type 1 diabetes through the lifespan: a position statement of the American Diabetes Association. *Diabetes Care.* 2014;37:2034-2054.

12. Chimen M, Kennedy A, Nirantharakumar K, Pang TT, Andrews R, Narendran P. What are the health benefits of physical activity in type 1 diabetes mellitus? A literature review. *Diabetologia.* 2012;55:542-551.

13. Chu L, Hamilton J, Riddell MC. Clinical management of the physically active patient with type 1 diabetes. *Phys Sportsmed.* 2011;39:64-77.

14. Colberg SR, ed. *Diabetic Athlete's Handbook.* Champaign (IL): Human Kinetics; 2009. 284 p.

15. Colberg SR, Albright AL, Blissmer BJ, Braun B, Chasan-Taber L, Fernhall B, Regensteiner JG, Rubin RR, Sigal RJ; American College of Sports Medicine; American Diabetes Association. Exercise and type 2 diabetes: American College of Sports Medicine and the American Diabetes Association: joint position statement. *Med Sci Sports Exerc.* 2010;42:2282-2303.

16. Colberg SR, Sigal RJ. Prescribing exercise for individuals with type 2 diabetes: recommendations and precautions. *Phys Sportsmed.* 2011;39:13-26.

17. Colberg SR, Vinik AI. Exercising with peripheral or autonomic neuropathy: what health care providers and diabetic patients need to know. *Phys Sportsmed.* 2014;42:15-23.

18. Colberg SR, Zarrabi L, Bennington L, Nakave A, Thomas Somma C, Swain DP, Sechrist SR. Postprandial walking is better for lowering the glycemic effect of dinner than pre-dinner exercise in type 2 diabetic individuals. *J Am Med Dir Assoc.* 2009;10:394-397.

19. Cooper AR, Sebire S, Montgomery AA, Peters TJ, Sharp DJ, Jackson N, Fitzsimons K, Dayan CM, Andrews RC. Sedentary time, breaks in sedentary time and metabolic variables in people with newly diagnosed type 2 diabetes. *Diabetologia.* 2012;55:589-599.

20. Delvecchio M, Zecchino C, Salzano G, Faienza MF, Cavallo L, De Luca F, Lombardo F. Effects of moderate-severe exercise on blood glucose in Type 1 diabetic adolescents treated with insulin pump or glargine insulin. *J Endocrinol Invest.* 2009;32:519-524.

21. D'Hooge R, Hellinckx T, Van Laethem C, Stegen S, De Schepper J, Van Aken S, Dewolf D, Calders P. Influence of combined aerobic and resistance training on metabolic control, cardiovascular fitness and quality of life in adolescents with type 1 diabetes: a randomized controlled trial. *Clin Rehabil.* 2011;25:349-359.

22. Farmer A, Balman E, Gadsby R, Moffatt J, Cradock S, McEwen L, Jameson K. Frequency of self-monitoring of blood glucose in patients with type 2 diabetes: association with hypoglycemic events. *Curr Med Res Opin.* 2008;24:3097-3104.

23. Garber CE, Blissmer B, Deschenes MR, Franklin BA, Lamonte MJ, Lee IM, Nieman DC, Swain DP, American College of Sports Medicine. American College of Sports Medicine position stand. Quantity and quality of exercise for developing and maintaining cardiorespiratory, musculoskeletal, and neuromotor fitness in apparently healthy adults: guidance for prescribing exercise. *Med Sci Sports Exerc.* 2011;43:1334-1359.

24. Grossman E, Messerli FH. Management of blood pressure in patients with diabetes. *Am J Hypertens.* 2011;24:863-875.

25. Hawley JA, Lessard SJ. Exercise training-induced improvements in insulin action. *Acta Physiol (Oxf).* 2008;192:127-135.

26. Herriott MT, Colberg SR, Parson HK, Nunnold T, Vinik AI. Effects of 8 weeks of flexibility and resistance training in older adults with type 2 diabetes. *Diabetes Care.* 2004;27:2988-2989.

27. Houmard JA, Tanner CJ, Slentz CA, Duscha BD, McCartney JS, Kraus WE. Effect of the volume and intensity of exercise training on insulin sensitivity. *J Appl Physiol.* 2004;96:101-106.

28. Jimenez C, Santiago M, Sitler M, Boden G, Homko C. Insulin-sensitivity response to a single bout of resistive exercise in type 1 diabetes mellitus. *J Sport Rehabil.* 2009;18:564-571.

29. Johansen KL. Exercise and chronic kidney disease: current recommendations. *Sports Med.* 2005;35:485-499.

30. Kalergis M, Schiffrin A, Gougeon R, Jones PJ, Yale JF. Impact of bedtime snack composition on prevention of nocturnal hypoglycemia in adults with type 1 diabetes undergoing intensive insulin management using lispro insulin before meals: a randomized, placebo-controlled, crossover trial. *Diabetes Care.* 2003;26:9-15.

31. Kilbride L, Charlton J, Aitken G, Hill GW, Davison RC, McKnight JA. Managing blood glucose during and after exercise in Type 1 diabetes: reproducibility of glucose response and a trial of a structured algorithm adjusting insulin and carbohydrate intake. *J Clin Nurs.* 2011;20:3423-3429.

32. Knowler WC, Barrett-Connor E, Fowler SE, Hamman RF, Lachin JM, Walker EA, Nathan DM. Reduction in the incidence of type 2 diabetes with lifestyle intervention or metformin. *N Engl J Med.* 2002;346:393-403.

33. Kones R. Primary prevention of coronary heart disease: integration of new data, evolving views, revised goals, role of rosuvastatin in management. A comprehensive survey. *Drug Des Devel Ther.* 2011;5:325-380.

34. Kuritzky L, Samraj GP. Enhanced glycemic control with combination therapy for type 2 diabetes in primary care. *Diabetes Ther.* 2011;2:162-177.

35. McBride PE, Einerson JA, Grant H, Sargent C, Underbakke G, Vitcenda M, Zeller L, Stein JH. Putting the Diabetes Prevention Program into practice: a program for weight loss and cardiovascular risk reduction for patients with metabolic syndrome or type 2 diabetes nellitus. *J Nutr Health Aging.* 2008;12:745s-749s.

36. McMahon SK, Ferreira LD, Ratnam N, Davey RJ, Youngs LM, Davis EA, Fournier PA, Jones TW. Glucose requirements to maintain euglycemia after moderate-intensity afternoon exercise in adolescents with type 1 diabetes are increased in a biphasic manner. *J Clin Endocrinol Metab.* 2007;92:963-968.

37. Mitri J, Hamdy O. Diabetes medications and body weight. *Expert Opin Drug Saf.* 2009;8:573-584.

38. Morrison S, Colberg SR, Parson HK, Vinik AI. Exercise improves gait, reaction time and postural stability in older adults with type 2 diabetes and neuropathy. *J Diabetes Complications.* 2014;28:715-722.

39. Otles S, Ozgoz S. Health effects of dietary fiber. *Acta Sci Pol Technol Aliment.* 2014;13:191-202.

40. Rognmo O, Moholdt T, Bakken H, Hole T, Molstad P, Myhr NE, Grimsmo J, Wisloff U. Cardiovascular risk of high- versus moderate-intensity aerobic exercise in coronary heart disease patients. *Circulation.* 2012;126:1436-1440.

41. Shahar J, Hamdy O. Medication and exercise interactions: considering and managing hypoglycemia risk. *Diabetes Spectr.* 2015;28:64-67.

42. Sharma MD. Potential for combination of dipeptidyl peptidase-4 inhibitors and sodium-glucose co-transporter-2 inhibitors for the treatment of type 2 diabetes. *Diabetes Obes Metab.* 2015;17(7):616-621.

43. Stephenson EJ, Smiles W, Hawley JA. The relationship between exercise, nutrition and type 2 diabetes. *Med Sport Sci.* 2014;60:1-10.

44. U.S. Department of Health and Human Services, Centers for Disease Control and Prevention. *National Diabetes Statistics Report.* Atlanta (GA): U.S. Department of Health and Human Services; 2014.

45. Williamson DA, Rejeski J, Lang W, Van Dorsten B, Fabricatore AN, Toledo K, Look ARG. Impact of a weight management program on health-related quality of life in overweight adults with type 2 diabetes. *Arch Intern Med.* 2009;169:163-171.

46. Yardley JE, Hay J, Abou-Setta AM, Marks SD, McGavock J. A systematic review and meta-analysis of exercise interventions in adults with type 1 diabetes. *Diabetes Res Clin Pract.* 2014;106:393-400.

47. Yardley JE, Sigal RJ. Exercise strategies for hypoglycemia prevention in individuals with type 1 diabetes. *Diabetes Spectr.* 2015;28:32-38.

Chapter 14

1. American Cancer Society Web site [Internet]. ACS; Atlanta (GA); cited [2016 September 28]. Available from: www.cancer.org.

2. American Cancer Society Web site [Internet]. Cancer facts and figures 2016. In: American Cancer Society, ed. ACS; Atlanta (GA); [2016 September 28]. Available at: www.cancer.org/research/cancerfactsstatistics/cancerfactsfigures2016/index

3. American College of Sports Medicine. *Guidelines for Exercise Testing and Prescription.* 10th ed. Philadelphia (PA): Lippincott Williams & Wilkins; in press.

4. Brown JC, Huedo-Medina TB, Pescatello LS, Pescatello SM, Ferrer RA, Johnson BT. Efficacy of exercise interventions in modulating cancer-related fatigue among adult cancer survivors: a meta-analysis. *Cancer Epidemiol Biomarkers Prev.* 2011;20(1):123-133.

5. Brown JC, Huedo-Medina TB, Pescatello LS, et al. The efficacy of exercise in reducing depressive symptoms among cancer survivors: a meta-analysis. *PLoS One.* 2012;7(1):e30955.

6. Demark-Wahnefried W, Platz EA, Ligibel JA, et al. The role of obesity in cancer survival and recurrence. *Cancer Epidemiol Biomarkers Prev.* 2012;21(8):1244-1259.

7. DeSantis CE, Lin CC, Mariotto AB, et al. Cancer treatment and survivorship statistics, 2014. *CA Cancer J Clin.* 2014;64(4):252-271.

8. Hewitt M, Greenfield, S., Stovall, E. *From Cancer Patient to Cancer Survivor: Lost in Transition.* Washington, DC: National Academies Press; 2006.

9. Kushi LH, Doyle C, McCullough M, et al. American Cancer Society Guidelines on nutrition and physical activity for cancer prevention: reducing the risk of cancer with healthy food choices and physical activity. *CA Cancer J Clin.* 2012;62(1):30-67.

10. Ligibel JA, Denlinger CS. New NCCN guidelines for survivorship care. *J Natl Compr Canc Netwk.* 2013;11(5 suppl):640-644.

11. Mustian KM, Sprod LK, Janelsins M, et al. Multicenter, randomized controlled trial of yoga for sleep quality among cancer survivors. *J Clin Oncol.* 2013;31(26):3233-3241.

12. Rock CL, Doyle C, Demark-Wahnefried W, et al. Nutrition and physical activity guidelines for cancer survivors. *CA Cancer J Clin.* 2012;62(4):242-274.

13. Schmitz K, Ahmed RL, Troxel A, Cheville A, Smith R, Grant LL, Bryan CJ, Williams-Smith CT, Greene QP. Weight lifting in women with breast cancer-related lymphedema. *N Engl J Med.* 2009;361:664-673.

14. Schmitz KH, Ahmed RL, Troxel A, et al. Weight lifting in women with breast-cancer-related lymphedema. *N Engl J Med.* 2009;361(7):664-673.

15. Schmitz KH, Ahmed RL, Troxel AB, et al. Weight lifting for women at risk for breast cancer-related lymphedema: a randomized trial. *JAMA.* 2010;304(24):2699-2705.

16. Schmitz KH, Courneya KS, Matthews C, et al. American College of Sports Medicine roundtable on exercise guidelines for cancer survivors. *Med Sci Sports Exerc.* 2010;42(7):1409-1426.

17. Speck RM, Courneya KS, Masse LC, Duval S, Schmitz KH. An update of controlled physical activity trials in cancer survivors: a systematic review and meta-analysis. *J Cancer Surviv.* 2010;4(2):87-100.

18. Winters-Stone KM, Laudermilk M, Woo K, Brown JC, Schmitz KH. Influence of weight training on skeletal health of breast cancer survivors with or at risk for breast cancer-related lymphedema. *J Cancer Surviv.* 2014;8(2):260-268.

19. Winters-Stone KM, Neil SE, Campbell KL. Attention to principles of exercise training: a review of exercise studies for survivors of cancers other than breast. *Br J Sports Med.* 2014;48(12):987-995.

Chapter 15

1. Academy of Nutrition and Dietetics Web site [Internet]. Choose Healthy Fats. AND; Chicago (IL); [released January 28, 2014; cited 2015 August 28]. Available from: www.eatright.org/resource/food/nutrition/dietary-guidelines-and-myplate/choose-healthy-fats.

2. Afzal S, Bojesen SE, Nordestgaard BG. Reduced 25-hydroxyvitamin D and risk of Alzheimer's disease and vascular dementia. *Alzheimers Dement.* 2014;10:296-302.

3. Ahlskog JE, Geda YE, Graff-Radfrod NR, et al. Physical exercise as a preventive or disease-modifying treatment of dementia and brain aging. *Mayo Clin Proc.* 2011;86:879-884.

4. Akter K, Lanza EA, Martin SA, Myronyuk N, Rua M, Raffa RB. Diabetes mellitus and Alzheimer's disease: shared pathology and treatment?. *Br J Clin Pharmacol.* 2011;71(3):365-376.

5. Alzheimer's Association Web site [Internet]. Alternative Treatments. Alzheimer's Association; Chicago (IL); [cited 2015 August 27]. Available from: www.alz.org/alzheimers_disease_alternative_treatments.asp.

6. Alzheimer's Drug Discovery Foundation Web site [Internet]. Fish and long-chain omega-3 fatty acids, DHA & EPA. Alzheimer's Drug Discovery Foundation; New York (NY) [released September 3, 2014; cited 2015 August 28]. Available from:www.alzdiscovery.org/cognitive-vitality/report/fish-and-long-chain-omega-3-fatty-acids.

7. Alzheimer's Research Center. *Alzheimer's Prevention.* Alzheimer's Research Center; St. Paul, (MN) [cited 2015 August 19].

8. Barnes, JN. Exercise, cognitive function, and aging. *Adv Physiol Educ.* 2015;39:55-62.

9. Bos D, Vernooij MW, Elias-Smale SE, et al. Atherosclerotic calcification relates to cognitive function and to brain changes on magnetic resonance imaging. *Alzheimers Dement.* 2012;(8):S104-S111.

10. Buchman AS, Boyle PA, Yu L, et al. Total daily physical activity and the risk of AD and cognitive decline in older adults. *Neurology.* 2012;78:1323-1329.

11. Carvalho A, Rae IM, Parimon T, Cusack BJ. Physical activity and cognitive function in individuals over 60 years of age: a systematic review. *Clin Interv Aging.* 2014;9:661-662.

12. Chew EY, Clemons TE, Agron E, et al. Effect of omega-3 fatty acids, lutein/zeaxanthin, or other nutrient supplementation on cognitive function: the AREDS2 Randomized Clinic Trial. *JAMA.* 2015;314(8):791-801.

13. Clarke R, Bennet D, Parish S. Effects of homocysteine lowering with B vitamins on cognitive aging: meta-analysis of 11 trials with cognitive data on 22,000 individuals. *Am J Clin Nutr.* 2014;100:657-666.

14. Colby SL, Ortman JM. Projections of the size and composition of the U.S. population: 2014 to 2060. Current Population Reports. U.S. Census Bureau, Washington, DC; 2014:25-1143. Available at www.census.gov.

15. Covell GE, Hoffman-Snyder CR, Wellik KE, Woodruff BK, et al. Physical activity level and future risk of mild cognitive impairment or dementia: a critically appraised topic. *Neurologist.* 2015;19(3):89-91.

16. Crane PK, Walker R, Hubbard RA, et al. Glucose levels and risk of dementia. *N Engl J Med.* 2013;369(6):540-548.

17. Dacks PA, Shineman DW, Fillit HM. Current evidence for the clinical use of long-chain polyunsaturated n-3 fatty acids to prevent age-related cognitive decline and Alzheimer's disease. *J Nutr Health Aging.* 2013;17(3):240-251.

18. Dysken MW, Sano M, Asthana S, et al. Effect of vitamin E and memantine on functional decline in Alzheimer disease: the TEAM-AD VA cooperative randomized trial. *JAMA.* 2014;311(1):33-44.

19. Erten-Lyons D, Woltjer RI, Dodge H, Nixon R, Vorobik R, Calvert JF, Leahy M, Montine T, Kaye J. Factors associated with resistance to dementia despite high Alzheimer disease pathology. *Neurology.* 2009;72:354-360.

20. Farina N, Kareem M, Issac N, Clark AR, Rustad J, Tabet N, et al. Vitamin E for Alzheimer's dementia and mild cognitive impairment. *Cochrane Database Syst Rev.* 2012;11:CD002854.

21. Fleischman DA, Yang J, Arfanakis K, Arvanitakis Z, Leurgans SE, Turner AD, Barnes LL, Bennett DA, Bachman AS. Physical activity, motor function, and white matter hyperintensity burden in healthy older adults. *Neurology.* 2015;84:1294-1300.

22. Hamer M, Chida Y. Physical activity and risk of neurodegenerative disease: a systematic review of prospective evidence. *Psychol Med.* 2009;39(1):3-11.

23. Hu N, Yu J, Tan L, Wang Y, Sun L. Nutrition and the risk of Alzheimer's disease. *BioMed Res Int.* 2013;2013:524820.

24. Kirk-Sanchez NJ, McGough EL. Physical exercise and cognitive performance in the elderly: current perspectives. *Clin Interv Aging.* 2014;9:51-62.

25. Kramer AF, Erickson KI. Capitalizing on cortical plasticity: influence of physical activity on cognition and brain function. *Trends Cogn Sci.* 2007;11(8);342-348.

26. Mazereeuw G, Lanctot KL, Chau SA, Swardfager W, Hermann N. Effects of omega-3 fatty acids on cognitive performance: a meta-analysis. *Neurobiol Aging.* 2012;33(7):1482.e17-e29.

27. MedlinePlus Web site [Internet]. Mediterranean diet. U.S. National Library of Medicine; Bethesda (MD); [released August 12, 2014; cited 2015 June 5]. Available from:www.nlm.nih.gov/medlineplus/ency/patientinstructions/000110.htm.

28. Middleton LE, Manini TM, Simonsick EM, et al. Activity energy expenditure and incident cognitive impairment in older adults. *Arch Intern Med.* 2011;171(14):1251-1257.

29. Morris MC. The role of nutrition in Alzheimer's disease: epidemiological evidence. *Eur J Neurol.* 2009;16(suppl 1):1-7.

30. Morris MC, Tangney CC, Wang Y, Sacks FM, Bennett DA, Aggarwal NT. MIND diet associated with reduced incidence of Alzheimer's disease. *Alzheimers Dement.* 2015;11(9):1007-1014.

31. National Center for Complementary and Integrative Health Web site [Internet]. 5 Things To Know About Complementary Health Practices for Cognitive Function, Dementia and Alzheimer's Disease. National Center for Complementary and Integrative Health; Bethesda (MD); [released 2015 January 30; cited 2015 August 29]. Available from: https://nccih.nih.gov/health/tips/alzheimers.

32. National Center for Complementary and Integrative Health Web site [Internet]. 7 Things To Know About Omega-3 Fatty Acids. National Center for Complementary and Integrative Health; Bethesda (MD); [released 2015 January 30; cited 2015 August 29]. Available from: https://nccih.nih.gov/health/tips/omega.

33. National Center for Complementary and Integrative Health Web site [Internet]. Alzheimer's Disease at a Glance. National Center for Complementary and Integrative Health; Bethesda (MD): [released 2014 November; cited 2015 August 20]. Available from: https://nccih.hih.gov/health/alzheimer/ataglance.

34. National Center for Complementary and Integrative Health Web site [Internet]. Dietary Supplements and Cognitive Function, Dementia, Alzheimer's Disease: What the Science Says. National Center for Complementary and Integrative Health; Bethesda (MD); [released 2013 December; cited 2015 August 19]. Available from: https://nccih.nih.gov/health/providers/digest/alzheimers-science.

35. National Institutes of Health Office of Dietary Supplements Web site [Internet]. Vitamin E Fact Sheet for Health Professionals. National Institutes of Health Office of Dietary Supplements; Bethesda (MD); [released 2013 June 5; cited 2015 August 19]. Available from: https://ods.od.nih.gov/factsheets/VitaminE-HealthProfessional/.

36. National Institute on Aging Web site [Internet]. Alzheimer's Caregiving Tips Healthy Eating. NIA; Bethesda (MD); [cited 2015 August 28]. Available from: www.nia.nih.gov/alzheimers/publication/healthy-eating.

37. National Institute on Aging Web site [Internet]. DASH Eating Plan NIA; Bethesda (MD); [cited 2015 July 27]. Available from: www.nia.nih.gov/health/publication/whats-your-plate/dash-eating-plan.

38. National Institute on Aging Web site [Internet]. Alzheimer's Disease: Unraveling the Mystery [cited 2015 June 5]. Available at www.nia.nih.gov/alzheimers.

39. Paillard T, Rolland Y, de Souto Barreto P. Protective effects of physical exercise in Alzheimer's disease and Parkinson's disease: a narrative review. *J Clin Neurol.* 2015;11(3):212-219.

40. Quinn JF, Raman R, Thomas RG, et al. Docosahexaenoic acid supplementation and cognitive decline in Alzheimer disease: a randomized trial. *JAMA.* 2010;304(17):1903-1911.

41. Shea TB, Remington R. Nutritional supplementation for Alzheimer's disease? *Curr Opin Psychiatr.* 2015;28(2):141-147.

42. Smyth A, Dehghan M, O'Donnell M, et al. Healthy eating and reduced risk of cognitive decline. *Neurology.* 2015;84(22):2258-2265.

43. Stern Y. Cognitive reserve in ageing and Alzheimer's disease. *Lancet Neurol.* 2012;11:1006-1012.

44. Swaminathan A, Jicha GA. Nutrition and prevention of Alzheimer's dementia. *Front Aging Neurosci.* 2014;6:282.

45. Tangney CC, Li H, Wang Y, Barnes L, Schneider JA, Bennett DA, Morris MC. Relation of DASH- and Mediterranean-like dietary patterns to cognitive decline in older persons. *Neurology.* 2014;83(16):1410-1416.

46. U.S. Department of Health and Human Services and U.S. Department of Agriculture website. Dietary Guidelines for Americans 2015. USDHHS; Atlanta (GA); [cited 2016 August 13]. Available at http://health.gov/dietaryguidelines/2015.asp.

47. WebMD Web site [Internet]. Resveratrol Supplements: Side Effects and Benefits. WebMD; Atlanta (GA);[released 2014 July 14; cited 2015 August 30]. Available from: http://webmd.com/heart-disease/resveratrol-supplements.

48. WebMD Web site [Internet]. Understanding Alzheimer's Disease—Prevention WebMD; Atlanta (GA); [released 2015 April 25; cited 2015 August 27]. Available from:www.webmd.com/alzheimers/guide/understanding-alzheimers-disease-prevention.

49. Willette AA, Johnson SC, Birdsill AC, et al. Insulin resistance predicts brain amyloid deposition in late middle-aged adults. *Alzheimers Dement.* 2015;11:504-510.

50. Witte V, Kerti L, Floel A. Effects of omega-3 supplementation on brain structure and function in healthy elderly subjects. *J Alzheimers Assoc.* 2012;8(4):69.

51. Xu W, Ten L, Wang H, Teng J, et al. Meta-analysis of modifiable risk factors for Alzheimer's disease. *Neuro Neurosurg Psychiatr.* 2015;86(12):1299-1306.

52. Yaffe K, Fiocco AJ, Lindquist K, et al. Predictors of maintaining cognitive function in older adults: the Health ABC study. *Neurology.* 2009;72(23):2029-2035.

53. Yurko-Mauro K, McCarthy D, Rom D, et al. Beneficial effects of docosahexaenoic acid on cognition in age-related cognitive decline. *Alzheimers Dement.*2010;6(6):456-464.

Chapter 16

1. Bischoff-Ferrari HA. Optimal serum 25-hydroxyvitamin D levels for multiple health outcomes. *Adv Exp Med Biol.* 2014;810:500-525.

2. Cummings SR, Karpf DB, Harris F, et al. Improvement in spine bone density and reduction in risk of vertebral fractures during treatment with antiresorptive drugs. *Am J Med.* 2002;112(4):281-289.

3. Cummings SR, Nevitt MC, Browner WS, et al. Risk factors for hip fracture in white women. Study of Osteoporotic Fractures Research Group. *N Engl J Med.* 1995;332(12):767-773.

4. Diab DL, Watts NB. Bisphosphonate drug holiday: Who, when and how long. *Ther Adv Musculoskel Dis.* 2013;5(3):107-111.

5. Eastell R. Treatment of postmenopausal osteoporosis. *N Engl J Med.* 1998;338:736-746.

6. Grodstein F, Manson JE, Colditz GA, Willett WC, Speizer FE, Stampfer MJ. A prospective, observational study of postmenopausal hormone therapy and primary prevention of cardiovascular disease. *Ann Intern Med.* 2000;133(12):933-941.

7. Guyatt GH, Cranney A, Griffith L, et al. Summary of meta-analyses of therapies for postmenopausal osteoporosis and the relationship between bone density and fractures. *Endocrinol Metab Clin North Am.* 2002;31(3):659-679, xii.

8. Hauer K, Specht N, Schuler M, Bartsch P, Oster P. Intensive physical training in geriatric patients after severe falls and hip surgery. *Age Ageing.* 2002;31(1):49-57.

9. Heaney RP, Layman DK. Amount and type of protein influences bone health. *Am J Clin Nutr.* 2008;87(suppl):1567S-1570S.

10. Institute of Medicine. *Dietary Reference Intakes for Calcium and Vitamin D.* Washington, DC: National Academies Press; 2011. 1116 p.

11. Institute of Medicine. *Dietary Reference Intakes for Energy, Carbohydrate, Fiber, Fat, Fatty Acids, Cholesterol, Protein, and Amino Acids.* Washington, DC: National Academies Press; 2005. 1332 p.

12. Kannus P, Parkkari J, Sievanen H, Heinonen A, Vuori I, Jarvinen M. Epidemiology of hip fractures. *Bone.* 1996;18(1 suppl):57S-63S.

13. Kohrt WM, Bloomfield SA, Little KD, Nelson ME, Yingling VR. American College of Sports Medicine position stand: physical activity and bone health. *Med Sci Sports Exerc.* 2004;36(11):1985-1996.

14. Martyn-St James M, Carroll S. A meta-analysis of impact exercise on postmenopausal bone loss: the case for mixed loading exercise programmes. *Br J Sports Med.* 2009;43(12):898-908.

15. Martyn-St James M, Carroll S. High-intensity resistance training and postmenopausal bone loss: a meta-analysis. *Osteoporos Int.* 2006;17(8):1225-1240.

16. Martyn-St James M, Carroll S. Progressive high-intensity resistance training and bone mineral density changes among premenopausal women: evidence of discordant site-specific skeletal effects. *Sports Med.* 2006;36(8):683-704.

17. National Osteoporosis Foundation Web site [Internet]. NOF; Arlington (VA); [cited October 2015]. Available from: www.nof.org.

18. Reginster JY, Seeman E, De Vernejoul MC, et al. Strontium ranelate reduces the risk of nonvertebral fractures in postmenopausal women with osteoporosis: Treatment of Peripheral Osteoporosis (TROPOS) study. *J Clin Endocrinol Metab.* 2005;90(5):2816-2822.

19. Sambrook P, Cooper C. Osteoporosis. *Lancet.* 2006;367(9527):2010-2018.

20. Snow CM, Shaw JM, Winters KM, Witzke KA. Long-term exercise using weighted vests prevents hip bone loss in postmenopausal women. *J Gerontol A Biol Sci Med Sci.* 2000;55(9):M489-M491.

21. Stevens JA, Rudd RA. The impact of decreasing U.S. hip fracture rates on future hip fracture estimates. *Osteoporosis Int.* 2013;24:2725-2728.

22. U.S. Department of Health and Human Services. *Bone Health and Osteoporosis: A Report of the Surgeon General.* USDHHS, Office of the Surgeon General; Rockville (MD): 2004.

23. Weatherall M. A meta-analysis of 25 hydroxyvitamin D in older people with fracture of the proximal femur. *N Z Med J.* 2000;113(1108):137-140.

24. Winters KM, Snow CM. Detraining reverses positive effects of exercise on the musculoskeletal system in premenopausal women. *J Bone Miner Res.* 2000;15:2495-2503.

Chapter 17

1. Altman R, Asch E, Bloch D, et al. The American College of Rheumatology criteria for the classification and reporting of osteoarthritis of the knee. *Arthritis Rheum.* 1986;29:1039-1049.

2. American College of Rheumatology Web site [Internet]. Biologic Treatments for Rheumatoid Arthritis. American College of Rheumatology; Atlanta (GA): [cited 2010 January 24]. Available from: www.rheumatology.org/public/factsheets.

3. American College of Sports Medicine. *ACSM's Guidelines for Exercise Testing and Prescription.* 10th ed. Philadelphia (PA): Lippincott Williams & Wilkins; in press.

4. Arnett FC, Edworthy SM, Bloch DA, et al. The American Rheumatism Association 1987 revised criteria for the classification of rheumatoid arthritis. *Arthritis Rheum.* 1988;31:315-324.

5. Baker KR, Nelson ME, Felson DT, Layne JE, Sarno R, Roubenoff R. The efficacy of home based progressive strength training in older adults with knee osteoarthritis: a randomized controlled trial. *J Rheumatol.* 2001;28:1655-1665.

6. Barbour KE, Helmick CG, Theis KA, Murphy LB, Hootman JM, Brady TJ, Cheng YJ. Prevalence of doctor-diagnosed arthritis and arthritis-attributable activity limitation—United States, 2010-2012. *MMWR.* 2013;62(44):869-873.

7. Barker K, Lamb SE, Toye F, Jackson S, Barrington S. Association between radiographic joint space narrowing, function, pain and muscle power in severe osteoarthritis of the knee. *Clin Rehabil.* 2004;18:793-800.

8. Bosch PR, Traustadottir T, Howard P, Matt KS. Functional and physiological effects of yoga in women with rheumatoid arthritis: a pilot study. *Alt Ther Health Med.* 2009;15:24-31.

9. Brandt KD. *Osteoarthritis.* Rheumatic Disease Clinics of North America. 2003;29(4):ix-xiii.

10. Brousseau L, Pelland L, Wells G, et al. Efficacy of aerobic exercises for osteoarthritis (part II): a meta-analysis. *Phys Ther Rev.* 2004;9:125-145.

11. Cochrane T, Davey RC, Matthes Edwards SM. Randomised controlled trial of the cost-effectiveness of water-based therapy for lower limb osteoarthritis. *Health Technol Assess.* 2005;9:iii-76.

12. Darlington LG, Stone TW. Antioxidants and fatty acids in the amelioration of rheumatoid arthritis and related disorders. *Br J Nutr.* 2001;85:251-269.

13. Ettinger WH Jr, Burns R, Messier SP, et al. A randomized trial comparing aerobic exercise and resistance exercise with a health education program in older adults with knee osteoarthritis. The Fitness Arthritis and Seniors Trial (FAST). *JAMA.* 1997;277:25-31.

14. Fitzgerald GK, Childs JD, Ridge TM, Irrgang JJ. Agility and perturbation training for a physically active individual with knee osteoarthritis. *Phys Ther.* 2002;82:372-382.

15. Fitzgerald GK, Piva SR, Gill AB, Wisniewski SR, Oddis CV, Irrgang JJ. Agility and perturbation training techniques in exercise therapy for reducing pain and improving function in people with knee osteoarthritis: a randomized clinical trial. *Phys Ther.* 2011;91:452-469.

16. Häkkinen A, Sokka T, Kotaniemi A, Hannonen P. A randomized two-year study of the effects of dynamic strength training on muscle strength, disease activity, functional capacity, and bone mineral density in early rheumatoid arthritis. *Arthritis Rheum.* 2001;44:515-522.

17. Häkkinen A, Sokka T, Hannonen P. A home-based two-year strength training period in early rheumatoid arthritis led to good long-term compliance: a five-year follow-up. *Arthritis Rheum.* 2004;51:56-62.

18. Hall A, Maher C, Latimer J, Ferreira M. The effectiveness of tai chi for chronic musculoskeletal pain conditions: a systematic review and meta-analysis. *Arthritis Rheum.* 2009;61:717-724.

19. Hauselmann HJ. Nutripharmaceuticals for osteoarthritis. *Best Pract Res Clin Rheumatol.* 2001;15:595-607.

20. Hochberg MC, Dougados M. Pharmacological therapy of osteoarthritis. *Best Pract Res Clin Rheumatol.* 2001;15:583-593.

21. Hurkmans E, van der Giesen FJ, Vliet Vlieland TP, et al. Dynamic exercise programs (aerobic capacity and/or muscle strength training) in patients with rheumatoid arthritis. *Cochrane Database Syst Rev.* 2009;(4):CD006853.

22. Jan M-H, Lin J-J, Liau J-J, Lin Y-F, Lin D-H. Investigation of clinical effects of high- and low-resistance training for patients with knee osteoarthritis: a randomized controlled trial. *Phys Ther.* 2008;88:427-436.

23. Kelley DS, Rasool R, Jacob RA, Kader AA, Mackey BE. Consumption of bing sweet cherries lowers circulating concentrations of inflammation markers in healthy men and women. *J Nutr.* 2006;136:981-986.

24. Mangione KK, McCully K, Gloviak A, Lefebvre I, Hofmann M, Craik R. The effects of high-intensity and low-intensity cycle ergometry in older adults with knee osteoarthritis. *J Gerontol.* 1999;54(A):M184-M190.

25. McAlindon TE, LaValley MP, Gulin JP, Felson DT. Glucosamine and chondroitin for treatment of osteoarthritis: a systematic quality assessment and meta-analysis. *JAMA.* 2000;283:1469-1475.

26. Messier SP, Loeser RF, Miller GD, et al. Exercise and dietary weight loss in overweight and obese older adults with knee osteoarthritis: the Arthritis, Diet, and Activity Promotion Trial. *Arthritis Rheum.* 2004; 50:1501-1510.

27. Millar AL. *Action Plan for Arthritis.* Champaign, IL: Human Kinetics; 2003. 201 p.

28. Minor MA, Hewett JE, Webel RR, et al. Efficacy of physical conditioning exercise in patients with rheumatoid arthritis and osteoarthritis. *Arthritis Rheum.* 1989; 32:1396-1405.

29. Munneke M, deJong Z, Zwinderman AH, et al. Effect of a high-intensity weight-bearing exercise program on radiologic damage progression of the large joints in subgroups of patients with rheumatoid arthritis. *Arthritis Rheum.* 2005;53:410-417.

30. Proudman SM, Cleland LG, James JM. Dietary omega-3 fats for treatment of inflammatory joint disease: efficacy and utility. *Rheum Dis Clin North Am.* 2008;34:469-479.

31. Rosenbaum CC, O'Mathúna DP, Chavez M, Shields K. Antioxidants and anti-inflammatory dietary supplements for osteoarthritis and rheumatoid arthritis. *Alt Ther Health Med.* 2010;16:32-40.

32. Schmitt LC, Fitzgerald GK, Reisman AS, Rudolph KS. Instability, laxity, and physical function in patients with medial knee osteoarthritis. *Phys Ther.* 2008;88:1506-1516.

33. Sharma L, Song J, Felson DT, Cahue S, Samieyeh E, Dunlop DD. The role of knee alignment in disease progression and functional decline in knee osteoarthritis. *JAMA.* 2001;286:188-195.

34. Symmons DP. Epidemiology of rheumatoid arthritis: determinants of onset, persistence and outcome. *Best Pract Res Clin Rheumatol.* 2002;16:707-722.

35. Van den Ende CHM, Vliet Vlieland TPM, Munneke M, Hazes JMW. Dynamic exercise therapy for rheumatoid arthritis. Cochrane Database Syst Rev. 2000;(2):CD000322.

Chapter 18

1. American College of Sports Medicine. *ACSM's Guidelines for Exercise Testing and Prescription.* 10th ed. Philadelphia: Lippincott Williams & Wilkins; in press.

2. Bryant CX, Green DJ, eds. *ACE Lifestyle & Weight Management Consultant Manual.* 2nd ed. San Diego: American Council on Exercise; 2008. 526 p.

3. Centers for Disease Control and Prevention, Division of Nutrition, Physical Activity, and Obesity Web site [Internet]. About Adult BMI. Atlanta (GA): CDC. Available from: www.cdc.gov/healthy-weight/assessing/bmi/adult_bmi/index.html.

4. Centers for Disease Control and Prevention, Division of Nutrition, Physical Activity, and Obesity Web site [Internet]. Adult Obesity Causes & Consequences. Atlanta (GA): CDC [cited July 13, 2015]. Available at www.cdc.gov/obesity/adult/causes.html.

5. Centers for Disease Control and Prevention, Division of Nutrition, Physical Activity, and Obesity Web site [Internet]. Assessing Your Weight. Atlanta (GA): CDC [cited July 13, 2015]. Available at www.cdc.gov/healthyweight/assessing/index.html.

6. Donnelly JE, Blair SN, Jakicic JM, Manore MM, Rankin JW, Smith BK. Appropriate physical activity intervention strategies for weight loss and prevention of weight regain for adults. *Med Sci Sports Exerc.* 2009;41(2):459-471.

7. National Academy of Sciences. Institute of Medicine. Food and Nutrition Board. *Dietary Reference Intakes for Energy, Carbohydrate, Fiber, Fat, Fatty Acids, Cholesterol, Protein, and Amino Acids (Macronutrients).* Washington, DC: National Academies Press; 2005. Available at www.nap.edu. 1332 p.

8. National Weight Control Registry Web site [Internet]. Providence, (RI) [cited September 10, 2015]. Available at www.nwcr.ws/.

9. Seagle HM, Strain GW, Makris A, Reeves RS. Position of the American Dietetic Association: weight management. *J Am Diet Assoc.* 2009 Feb;109(2):330-346.

10. Thompson, JL, Manore, MM, Vaughan, LA. *The Science of Nutrition.* 4th ed. Upper Saddle River, NJ: Pearson; 2017. 773 p.

11. U.S. Food and Drug Administration. Dietary Supplements Web site [Internet]. Silver Spring, (MD): USFDA [cited July 17, 2015]. Available at www.fda.gov/Food/DietarySupplements/default.htm.

12. U.S. Food and Drug Administration. Food Labeling Guide Web site [Internet]. Silver Spring, (MD): USFDA [cited July 17, 2015]. Available at www.fda.gov/food/guidanceregulation/guidancedocumentsregulatoryinformation/labelingnutrition/ucm2006828.htm.

13. U.S. Department of Health and Human Services and U.S. Department of Agriculture website. Dietary Guidelines for Americans 2015. USDHHS; Atlanta (GA) [cited 2016 January 27]. Available at http://health.gov/dietaryguidelines/2015/guidelines/.

Chapter 19

1. American College of Obstetricians and Gynecologists. *Technical Bulletin: Exercise During Pregnancy and the Postnatal Period.* Washington, DC: ACOG; 1985.

2. American College of Obstetricians and Gynecologists. ACOG Committee Opinion No. 650: physical activity and exercise during pregnancy and the postpartum period. *Obstet Gynecol.* 2015;e135-e142.

3. American College of Obstetricians and Gynecologists. Hypertension in pregnancy. Report of the American College of Obstetricians and Gynecologists' task force on hypertension in pregnancy. *Obstet Gynecol.* 2013;122(5):1122-1131.

4. American College of Sports Medicine. Impact of physical activity during pregnancy and postpartum on chronic disease risk. *Med Sci Sports Exerc.* 2006;38(5):989-1006.

5. American College of Sports Medicine. *ACSM's Guidelines for Exercise Testing and Prescription.* 10th ed. Philadelphia (PA): Lippincott Williams & Wilkins; in press.

6. Barakat R, Ruiz JR, Stirling JR, Zakynthinaki M, Lucia A. Type of delivery is not affected by light resistance and toning exercise training during pregnancy: a randomized controlled trial. *Am J Obstet Gynecol.* 2009;201(6):590.e1-e6.

7. Barakat R, Stirling JR, Lucia A. Does exercise training during pregnancy affect gestational age? A randomised controlled trial. *Br J Sports Med.* 2008;42(8):674-678.

8. Chan J, Natekar A, Koren G. Hot yoga and pregnancy: fitness and hyperthermia. *Can Fam Phys.* 2014;60(1):41-42.

9. Clapp JF. The morphometric and neurodevelopmental outcome at five years of the offspring of women who continued exercise throughout pregnancy. *J Pediatr.* 1996;129:856-863.

10. Clapp JF. *Exercising Through Your Pregnancy.* Omaha: Addicus Books; 2002. 256 p.

11. de Barros MC, Lopes MA, Francisco RP, Sapienza AD, Zugaib M. Resistance exercise and glycemic control in women with gestational diabetes mellitus. *Am J Obstet Gynecol.* 2010;203(6):556.e1-e6.

12. Evenson KR, Moos MK, Carrier K, Siega-Riz AM. Perceived barriers to physical activity among pregnant women. *Matern Child Health J.* 2009;13(3):364-375.

13. Evenson KR, Savitz DA, Huston SL. Leisure-time physical activity among pregnant women in the US. *Paediatr Perinat Epidemiol.* 2004;18(6):400-407.

14. Evenson KR, Siega-Riz AM, Savitz DA, Leiferman JA, Thorp JM Jr. Vigorous leisure activity and pregnancy outcome. *Epidemiology.* 2002;13(6):653-659.

15. Gong H, Ni C, Shen X, Wu T, Jiang C. Yoga for prenatal depression: a systematic review and meta-analysis. *BMC Psychiatry.* 2015;15:14.

16. Jiang Q, Wu Z, Zhou L, Dunlop J, Chen P. Effects of yoga intervention during pregnancy: a review for current status. *Am J Perinatol.* 2015;32(6):503-514.

17. Jiwani A, Marseille E, Lohse N, Damm P, Hod M, Kahn JG. Gestational diabetes mellitus: results from a survey of country prevalence and practices. *J Matern Fetal Neonatal Med.* 2012;25(6):600-610.

18. Kaiser LL, Campbell CG. Practice Paper of the Academy of Nutrition and Dietetics: nutrition and lifestyle for a healthy pregnancy outcome. *J Acad Nutr Diet.* 2014;114(7):1099-1112.

19. Mattran K, Mudd LM, Rudey RA, Kelly JS. Leisure-time physical activity during pregnancy and offspring size at 18 to 24 months. *J Phys Act Health.* 2011;8(5):655-662.

20. McDonald SM, Liu J, Wilcox S, Lau EY, Archer E. Does dose matter in reducing gestational weight gain in exercise interventions? A systematic review of literature. *J Sci Med Sport.* 2016;19(4):323-335.

21. Mudd LM, Nechuta S, Pivarnik JM, Paneth N. Factors associated with women's perceptions of physical activity safety during pregnancy. *Prev Med.* 2009;49(2-3):194-199.

22. Mudd LM, Owe KM, Mottola MF, Pivarnik JM. Health benefits of physical activity during pregnancy: an international perspective. *Med Sci Sports Exerc.* 2013;45(2):268-277.

23. Mudd LM, Pivarnik J, Holzman CB, Paneth N, Pfeiffer K, Chung H. Leisure-time physical activity in pregnancy and the birth weight distribution: where is the effect? *J Phys Act Health.* 2012;9(8):1168-1177.

24. Mudd LM, Pivarnik JM, Pfeiffer KA, Paneth N, Chung H, Holzman C. Maternal physical activity during pregnancy, child leisure-time activity, and child weight status at 3 to 9 years. *J Phys Act Health.* 2015;12(4):506-514.

25. Nobles C, Marcus BH, Stanek EJ III, et al. Effect of an exercise intervention on gestational diabetes mellitus: a randomized controlled trial. *Obstet Gynecol.* 2015;125(5):1195-1204.

26. Olson CM, Strawderman MS, Hinton PS, Pearson TA. Gestational weight gain and postpartum behaviors associated with weight change from early pregnancy to 1 y postpartum. *Int J Obes Relat Metab Disord.* 2003;27(1):117-127.

27. Oostdam N, van Poppel MN, Wouters MG, et al. No effect of the FitFor2 exercise programme on blood glucose, insulin sensitivity, and birthweight in pregnant women who were overweight and at risk for gestational diabetes: results of a randomised controlled trial. *BJOG.* 2012;119(9):1098-1107.

28. Pivarnik JM, Mudd LM. Oh Baby! Exercise during pregnancy and the postpartum period. *ACSM Health Fit J.* 2009;13(3):8-13.

29. Pivarnik JM, Perkins CD, Moyerbrailean T. Athletes and pregnancy. *Clin Obstet Gynecol.* 2003;46(2):403-414.

30. Procter SB, Campbell CG. Position of the Academy of Nutrition and Dietetics: nutrition and lifestyle for a healthy pregnancy outcome. *J Acad Nutr Diet.* 2014;114(7):1099-1103.

31. Rasmussen KM, Catalano PM, Yaktine AL. New guidelines for weight gain during pregnancy: what obstetrician/gynecologists should know. *Curr Opin Obstet Gynecol.* 2009;21(6):521-526.

32. Ruchat SM, Mottola MF. The important role of physical activity in the prevention and management of gestational diabetes mellitus. *Diabetes Metab Res Rev.* 2013;29(5):334-346.

33. Teychenne M, York R. Physical activity, sedentary behavior, and postnatal depressive symptoms: a review. *Am J Prev Med.* 2013;45(2):217-227.

34. U.S. Department of Health and Human Services Web site [Internet]. Physical Activity Guidelines for Americans. USDHHS; Atlanta (GA); [cited 2016 August 16]Available from: www.health.gov/paguidelines.

35. U.S. Department of Health and Human Services and U.S. Department of Agriculture Web site [Internet]. Dietary Guidelines for Americans 2015. USDHHS; Atlanta (GA) [cited 2016 January 13]. Available from: http://health.gov/dietaryguidelines/2015/guidelines.

36. Wendland EM, Torloni MR, Falavigna M, et al. Gestational diabetes and pregnancy outcomes—a systematic review of the World Health Organization (WHO) and the International Association of Diabetes in Pregnancy Study Groups (IADPSG) diagnostic criteria. *BMC Pregnancy Childbirth.* 2012;12:23.

Chapter 20

1. Adamson BC, Ensari I, Motl RW. Effect of exercise on depressive symptoms in adults with neurologic disorders: a systematic review and meta-analysis. *Arch Phys Med Rehabil.* 2015 Jul;96(7):1329-1338.

2. American Psychiatric Association. *Diagnostic and Statistical Manual of Mental Disorders.* 5th ed. Arlington (VA): APA; 2013. 991 p.

3. Barrows KA, Jacobs BP. Mind-body medicine. An introduction and review of the literature. *Med Clin North Am.* 2002 Jan;86(1):11-31.

4. Bet PM, Hugtenburg JG, Penninx BW, Hoogendijk WJ. Side effects of antidepressants during long-term use in a naturalistic setting. *Eur Neuropsychopharmacol.* 2013 Nov;23(11):1443-1451.

5. Blair SN, LaMonte MJ, Nichaman MZ. The evolution of physical activity recommendations: how much is enough? *Am J Clin Nutr.* 2004 May;79(5):913S-920S.

6. Blumenthal JA, Babyak MA, Doraiswamy PM, et al. Exercise and pharmacotherapy in the treatment of major depressive disorder. *Psychosom Med.* 2007;69(7):587-596.

7. Buckworth J, Dishman RK, O'Connor PJ, Tomporowski PD, eds. Depression. In: *Exercise Psychology,* 2nd ed. Champaign, (IL): Human Kinetics; 2013. 544 p.

8. Cameron C, Habert J, Anand L, Furtado M. Optimizing the management of depression: primary care experience. *Psychiatry Res.* 2014 Dec;220 suppl 1:S45-S57.

9. Chambliss HO, Martin SB, Greenleaf C. Principles of behavior change: Skill building to promote physical activity. In: *ACSM's Resource Manual for Guidelines for Exercise Testing and Prescription,* 7th ed. Philadelphia (PA): Lippincott Williams & Wilkins; 2013. p. 745-760.

10. Chambliss HO, Van Hoomisen JD, Holmes PV, Bunnell BN, Dishman RK. Effects of chronic activity wheel running and imipramine on masculine copulatory behavior after olfactory bulbectomy. *Physiol Behav.* 2004;82(4):593-600.

11. Craft LL, Vaniterson EH, Helenowski IB, Rademaker AW, Courneya KS. Exercise effects on depressive symptoms in cancer survivors: a systematic review and meta-analysis. *Cancer Epidemiol Biomarkers Prev.* 2012 Jan;21(1):3-19.

12. Cramer H, Lauche R, Langhorst J, Dobos G. Yoga for depression: a systematic review and meta-analysis. *Depress Anxiety.* 2013 Nov;30(11):1068-1083.

13. Dishman RK. Brain monoamines, exercise and behavioral stress: animal models. *Med Sci Sports Exerc.* 1997;29:63-74.

14. Dishman RK, Berthoud HR, Booth FW, et al. Neurobiology of exercise. *Obesity (Silver Spring).* 2006;14(3):345-356.

15. Dishman RK, Sui X, Church TS, Hand GA, Trivedi MH, Blair SN. Decline in cardiorespiratory fitness and odds of incident depression. *Am J Prev Med.* 2012;43:361-368.

16. Dishman RK, Thom NJ, Puetz TW, O'Connor PJ, Clementz BA. Effects of cycling exercise on vigor, fatigue, and electroencephalographic activity among young adults who report persistent fatigue. *Psychophysiology.* 2010 Nov;47(6):1066-1074.

17. Dunn AL, Reigle TG, Youngstedt SD, Armstrong RB, Dishman RK. Brain norepinephrine and metabolites after treadmill training and wheel running in rats. *Med Sci Sports Exerc.* 1996;28:204-209.

18. Dunn AL, Trivedi MH, Kampert JB, Clark CG, Chambliss HO. Exercise treatment for depression efficacy and dose response. *Am J Prev Med.* 2005;28:1-8.

19. Galper DI, Trivedi MH, Barlow CE, Dunn AL, Kampert JB. Inverse association between physical inactivity and mental health in men and women. *Med Sci Sports Exerc.* 2006 Jan;38(1):173-178.

20. Greenwood BN, Fleshner M. Exercise, stress resistance, and central serotonergic systems. *Exerc Sport Sci Rev.* 2011 Jul;39(3):140-149.

21. Greer TL, Grannemann BD, Chansard M, Karim AI, Trivedi MH. Dose-dependent changes in cognitive function with exercise augmentation for major depression: results from the TREAD study. *Eur Neuropsychopharmacol.* 2015 Feb;25(2):248-256.

22. Greer TL, Kurian BT, Trivedi MH. Defining and measuring functional recovery from depression. *CNS Drugs.* 2010;24(4):267-284.

23. Helgadóttir B, Forsell Y, Ekblom Ö. Physical activity patterns of people affected by depressive and anxiety disorders as measured by accelerometers: a cross-sectional study. *PLoS One.* 2015 Jan 13;10(1):e0115894.

24. Hunsberger JG, Newton SS, Bennett AH, Duman CH, Russell DS, Salton SR, Duman RS. Antidepressant actions of the exercise-regulated gene VGF. *Nat Med.* 2007;13(12):1476-1482.

25. Janakiramaiah N, Gangadhar BN, Naga Venkatesha Murthy PJ, Harish MG, Subbakrishna DK, Vedamurthachar A. Antidepressant efficacy of Sudarshan Kriya Yoga (SKY) in melancholia: a randomized comparison with electroconvulsive therapy (ECT) and imipramine. *J Affect Disord.* 2000 Jan-Mar;57(1-3):255-259.

26. Katon WJ. Clinical and health services relationships between major depression, depressive symptoms, and general medical illness. *Biol Psychiatry.* 2003 Aug 1;54(3):216-226.

27. Katon WJ. Epidemiology and treatment of depression in patients with chronic medical illness. *Dialogues Clin Neurosci.* 2011;13(1):7-23.

28. Katon W, Lin EH, Kroenke K. The association of depression and anxiety with medical symptom burden in patients with chronic medical illness. *Gen Hosp Psychiatry.* 2007;29:147-155.

29. Kessler RC, Berglund P, Demler O, Jin R, Merikangas KR, Walters EE. Lifetime prevalence and age-of-onset distributions of DSM-IV disorders in the National Comorbidity Survey Replication. *Arch Gen Psychiatry.* 2005 Jun;62(6):593-602.

30. Kessler RC, Chiu WT, Demler O, Merikangas KR, Walters EE. Prevalence, severity, and comorbidity of 12-month DSM-IV disorders in the National Comorbidity Survey Replication. *Arch Gen Psychiatry.* 2005 Jun;62(6):617-627.

31. Krogh J, Nordentoft M, Sterne JA, Lawlor DA. The effect of exercise in clinically depressed adults: systematic review and meta-analysis of randomized controlled trials. *J Clin Psychiatry.* 2011 Apr;72(4):529-538.

32. Lampe L, Coulston CM, Berk L. Psychological management of unipolar depression. *Acta Psychiatr Scand.* 2013;127(suppl 443):24-37.

33. Lawlor DA, Hopker SW. The effectiveness of exercise as an intervention in the management of depression: systematic review and meta-regression analysis of randomized trials. *BMJ.* 2001;322:1-8.

34. Ludwig DS, Kabat-Zinn J. Mindfulness in medicine. *JAMA.* 2008;300(11):1350-1352.

35. Mammen G, Faulkner G. Physical activity and the prevention of depression: a systematic review of prospective studies. *Am J Prev Med.* 2013 Nov;45(5):649-657.

36. Marcus M, Yasamy MT, van Ommeren M, Chisholm D, Saxena S. Depression: a global public health concern. Available from: www.who.int/mental_health/management/depression/who_paper_depression_wfmh_2012.pdf?ua=1.

37. Mead GE, Morley W, Campbell P, Greig CA, McMurdo M, Lawlor DA. Exercise for depression. *Cochrane Database Syst Rev.* 2009 Jul 8;(3):CD004366.

38. Morris DW, Trivedi MH. Measurement-based care for unipolar depression. *Curr Psychiatry Rep.* 2011 Dec;13(6):446-458.

39. Motl RW, Konopack JF, McAuley E, Elavsky S, Jerome GJ, Marquez DX. Depressive symptoms among older adults: long-term reduction after a physical activity intervention. *J Behav Med.* 2005;28:385-394.

40. National Institute of Mental Health Web site [Internet]. What is depression? U.S. Department of Health and Human Services; Washington, DC [cited 2015 September 24]. Available from: www.nimh.nih.gov/health/topics/depression/index.shtml.

41. Passos GS, Poyares D, Santana MG, Garbuio SA, Tufik S, Mello MT. Effect of acute physical exercise on patients with chronic primary insomnia. *J Clin Sleep Med.* 2010 Jun 15;6(3):270-275.

42. Peterson JC, Charlson ME, Wells MT, Altemus M. Depression, coronary artery disease, and physical activity: how much exercise is enough? *Clin Ther.* 2014 Nov 1;36(11):1518-1530.

43. Physical Activity Guidelines Advisory Committee. *Physical Activity Guidelines Advisory Committee Report, 2008.* Washington, DC: USDHHS; 2008.

44. Pinchasov BB, Shurgaja AM, Grischin OV, Putilov AA. Mood and energy regulation in seasonal and non-seasonal depression before and after midday treatment with physical exercise or bright light. *Psychiatry Res.* 2000;94(1):29-42.

45. Puetz TW, O'Connor PJ, Dishman RK. Effects of chronic exercise on feelings of energy and fatigue: a quantitative synthesis. *Psychol Bull.* 2006 Nov;132(6):866-876.

46. Rethorst CD, Sunderajan P, Greer TL, Grannemann BD, Nakonezny PA, Carmody TJ, Trivedi MH. Does exercise improve self-reported sleep quality in non-remitted major depressive disorder? *Psychol Med.* 2013 Apr;43(4):699-709.

47. Russo-Neustadt A. Brain-derived neurotrophic factor, behavior, and new directions for the treatment of mental disorders. *Semin Clin Neuropsychiatry.* 2003;8:109-118.

48. Sathyanarayana Rao TS, Asha MR, Ramesh BN, Jagannatha Rao KS. Understanding nutrition, depression and mental illnesses. *Indian J Psychiatry.* 2008 Apr-Jun;50(2):77-82.

49. Schatzberg AF. Development of new psychopharmacological agents for depression and anxiety. *Psychiatr Clin North Am.* 2015 Sep;38(3):379-393.

50. Silveira H, Moraes H, Oliveira N, Coutinho ES, Laks J, Deslandes A. Physical exercise and clinically depressed patients: a systematic review and meta-analysis. *Neuropsychobiology.* 2013;67(2):61-68.

51. Singh NA, Stavrinos TM, Scarbek Y, Galambos G, Liber C, Singh MA. A randomized controlled trial of high versus low intensity weight training versus general practitioner care for clinical depression in older adults. *J Gerontol A Biol Med Sci.* 2005;60(6):768-776.

52. Stanton R, Reaburn P. Exercise and the treatment of depression: a review of the exercise program variables. *J Sci Med Sport.* 2014 Mar;17(2):177-182.

53. Stewart WF, Ricci JA, Chee E, Hahn SR, Morganstein D. Cost of lost productive work time among US workers with depression. *JAMA.* 2003;289:3135-3144.

54. Trivedi MH. Treating depression to full remission. *J Clin Psychiatry.* 2009 Jan;70(1):e01.

55. Trivedi MH, Greer TL, Grannemann BD, Church TS, Galper DI, Sunderajan P, Wisniewski SR, Chambliss HO, Jordan AN, Finley C, Carmody TI. Exercise as an augmentation strategy for treatment of major depression. *J Psychiatr Pract.* 2006 Jul;12(4):205-213.

56. U.S. Department of Health and Human Services and U.S. Department of Agriculture website. Dietary Guidelines for Americans. USDHHS; Washington, DC [cited 2015 November 5]. Available at http://health.gov/dietaryguidelines/.

57. Waelde LC, Thompson L, Gallagher-Thompson D. A pilot study of a yoga and meditation intervention for dementia caregiver stress. *J Clin Psychol.* 2004 Jun;60(6):677-687.

58. Wang F, Lee EK, Wu T, Benson H, Fricchione G, Wang W, Yeung AS. The effects of tai chi on depression, anxiety, and psychological well-being: a systematic review and meta-analysis. *Int J Behav Med.* 2014 Aug;21(4):605-617.

INDEX

ABOUT THE ACSM

The **American College of Sports Medicine (ACSM)**, founded in 1954 is the largest sports medicine and exercise science organization in the world. With more than 50,000 members and certified professionals worldwide, ACSM is dedicated to improving health through science, education, and medicine. ACSM members work in a wide range of medical specialties, allied health professions, and scientific disciplines. Members are committed to the diagnosis, treatment, and prevention of sport-related injuries and the advancement of the science of exercise. The ACSM promotes and integrates scientific research, education, and practical applications of sports medicine and exercise science to maintain and enhance physical performance, fitness, health, and quality of life.

ABOUT THE EDITOR

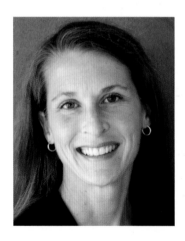

Barbara A. Bushman, PhD, is a professor at Missouri State University and is an American College of Sports Medicine (ACSM) Certified Program Director and Clinical Exercise Physiologist. She received her PhD in exercise physiology from the University of Toledo and has teaching experience in identification of health risks, exercise testing and prescription, anatomy, and physiology. Bushman served as senior editor of *ACSM's Resources for the Personal Trainer, Fourth Edition,* and as a reviewer for ACSM's *Medicine & Science in Sports & Exercise, Women & Health,* and *ACSM's Health & Fitness Journal.* She has been a fellow of ACSM since 1999, serving on the ACSM Media Referral Network. As an associate editor of *ACSM's Health & Fitness Journal,* Bushman writes the "Wouldn't You Like to Know" column, which covers a variety of topics in health and fitness.

Bushman is the lead author of *Action Plan for Menopause* as well as numerous research articles. She maintains a Facebook page focused on health and fitness (www.Facebook.com/FitnessID). She resides in Strafford, Missouri, with her husband, Tobin. She enjoys walks with her husband and German Shepherds, Kiddoo and Teddee. She participates in numerous activities in her leisure time, including running, cycling, hiking, weightlifting, kayaking, and scuba diving.

ABOUT THE CONTRIBUTORS

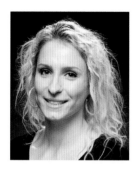

Michelle Kulovitz Alencar, PhD, CCN, currently an assistant professor of kinesiology at California State University, Long Beach, is a Certified Clinical Nutritionist and ACSM Certified Exercise Physiologist. Her research interests are in obesity treatment, assessments, and management through fitness and nutrition.

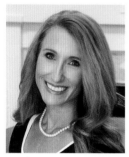

Heather Chambliss, PhD, is a consultant in health research and programming. She has a master's degree in counseling from Louisiana Tech University and a doctorate in exercise science (exercise psychology) from the University of Georgia. After receiving her degree, she completed a postdoctoral fellowship at The Cooper Institute in Dallas, Texas. Chambliss is a fellow of ACSM and serves on the ACSM board of trustees. Her interests include physical activity promotion, health behavior change, and exercise and mental health. Chambliss and her husband Donnie live in Southaven, Mississippi, with their daughters, Karis and Clare.

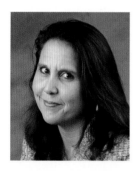

Sheri R. Colberg, PhD, is a professor emerita of exercise science at Old Dominion University. She has authored 10 books, 17 book chapters, and close to 300 articles on exercise and diabetes. With almost 50 years of practical experience as a (type 1) diabetic exerciser, she provides professional expertise on physical activity to the American Diabetes Association and is a fellow of ACSM.

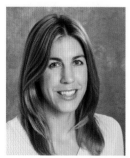

Shannon Lennon-Edwards, PhD, RD, is an associate professor in the Department of Kinesiology and Applied Physiology at the University of Delaware. Lennon-Edwards completed her bachelor's and master's degrees from the University of Connecticut in nutritional sciences, a doctoral degree in exercise physiology from the University of Florida, and her postdoctoral training at the Whitaker Cardiovascular Institute at Boston University Medical Center. She is also a Registered Dietitian. Lennon-Edwards' current research focuses on the effect of diet on cardiovascular health. Her research is funded by the National Institutes of Health, and she publishes regularly in peer-reviewed journals.

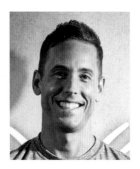

Nicholas H. Evans, MHS, is a member of the ACSM and the American Congress of Rehabilitation Medicine. He is an ACSM Certified Clinical Exercise Physiologist and a research coordinator working in neurorehabilitation and neurophysiology in the Beyond Therapy program and Hulse Spinal Cord Injury Laboratory at the Shepherd Center in Atlanta, Georgia. In addition, Evans is a graduate student in the Department of Applied Physiology at the Georgia Institute of Technology. His clinical and research interests include the effects of exercise and therapeutic interventions on neuromuscular function and neural plasticity following neurological injury and disease.

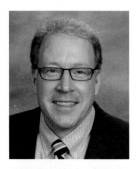

Avery D. Faigenbaum, PhD, is a full professor in the Department of Health and Exercise Science at the College of New Jersey. His research interests focus on pediatric exercise science, resistance exercise, and preventive medicine. He has coauthored over 200 peer-reviewed publications, 40 book chapters, and 9 books and has been an invited speaker at more than 300 regional, national, and international conferences. Faigenbaum is a fellow of ACSM and of the National Strength and Conditioning Association.

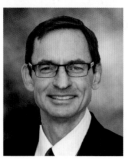

William B. Farquhar, PhD, is a professor and chair of the Department of Kinesiology and Applied Physiology at the University of Delaware. He completed his bachelor's and master's degrees at East Stroudsburg University and his PhD at Penn State University. His postdoctoral training was completed at Beth Israel Deaconess Medical Center and the Hebrew Rehabilitation Center. He is trained as an exercise physiologist, and his recent work focuses on the effect of diet and exercise on physiological function. His research is funded by the National Institutes of Health, and he regularly publishes in peer-reviewed journals. He previously served as president of the Mid-Atlantic regional chapter of ACSM.

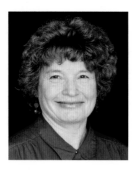

Linda Fredenberg, RD, LN, is a native Montanan who received her bachelor of science degree from Montana State University. She completed a dietetic internship at Brigham and Women's Hospital in Boston, Massachusetts, a teaching affiliate of Harvard Medical School. In her present role as an outpatient nutrition educator at Summit Medical Fitness Center, Kalispell Regional Health, she provides medical nutrition therapy for a wide range of conditions. Fredenberg serves on the board of directors of the Montana Dietetic Association.

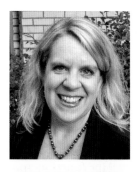

Tracy L. Greer, PhD, MSCS, is an associate professor of psychiatry in the Center for Depression Research and Clinical Care at the University of Texas Southwestern Medical Center. Greer's primary research interests include exercise as a treatment for psychiatric conditions and the examination of targeted treatments for cognitive impairments associated with psychiatric conditions, with a primary focus on depressive and stimulant use disorders.

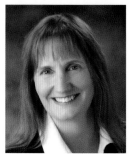

Jean M. Kerver, PhD, MSc, RD, is an assistant professor in the College of Human Medicine at Michigan State University, serving in the Departments of Epidemiology & Biostatistics and Pediatrics & Human Development. As a nutritional epidemiologist and a Registered Dietitian, Kerver has spent her career studying details on what a woman eats during pregnancy that affects not only her health but also the long-term development of her child.

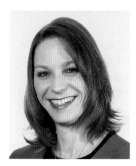

Laura J. Kruskall, PhD, RDN, CSSD, LD, received her master's degree in human nutrition from Columbia University and her PhD in nutrition from Penn State University. She is a fellow of both ACSM and the Academy of Nutrition and Dietetics (AND). In addition, she is a Registered Dietitian and a Board Certified Specialist in Sports Dietetics and holds a certification in Adult Weight Management, Level 2, from AND. She is currently director of Nutrition Sciences and the Nutrition Center at the University of Nevada, Las Vegas. Her areas of expertise are sports nutrition, weight management, and medical nutrition therapy. Kruskall is a member of the editorial board for ACSM's *Health & Fitness Journal* and is an ACSM Certified Exercise Physiologist.

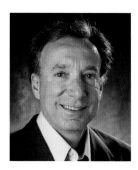

Robert S. Mazzeo, PhD, received his doctoral degree from the University of California at Berkeley and postdoctoral training at the University of California at Santa Barbara. He has been at the University of Colorado at Boulder since 1985 in the Department of Integrative Physiology. His research has focused on the metabolic and physiological adaptations made by the body in response to a single bout of exercise as well as after chronic endurance training in aging populations. He has appeared on the *Today Show* discussing the benefits of regular exercise for older individuals.

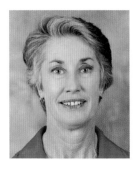

A. Lynn Millar, PhD, is a professor of physical therapy at Winston-Salem State University. She received her PhD in exercise physiology from Arizona State University and her physical therapy degree from Andrews University. Her research has been diverse, addressing special populations and exercise as well as physical therapy-related topics. She has authored several book chapters related to arthritis and one book, *Action Plan for Arthritis.* Her current areas of research include arthritis and response to various exercise therapy routines. Millar is a fellow of ACSM and is active in both ACSM and the American Physical Therapy Association.

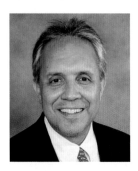

Don W. Morgan, PhD, is a professor in the Department of Health and Human Performance at Middle Tennessee State University and director of the Center for Physical Activity and Health in Youth, a university–community partnership aimed at increasing the activity and fitness levels of Tennessee youth. An exercise physiologist and past president of the North American Society for Pediatric Exercise Medicine, Morgan is a fellow of the ACSM, the National Academy of Kinesiology, and the American Academy for Cerebral Palsy and Developmental Medicine.

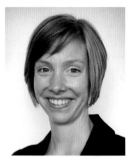

Lanay M. Mudd, PhD, holds a dual-major doctoral degree in kinesiology and epidemiology from Michigan State University. She has given invited presentations and published several review papers and original research articles on the health benefits of physical activity during pregnancy. Mudd has held faculty positions at Appalachian State University and Michigan State University.

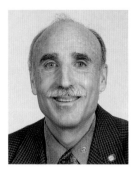

Brad A. Roy, PhD, is the administrator at the Summit Medical Fitness Center and is part of the executive team for Kalispell Regional Medical Center in Kalispell, Montana. Roy has 35 years of experience in health care and the fitness industry and oversees a number of hospital services including the 114,800-square-foot medically integrated fitness center. He serves as editor in chief for ACSM's *Health & Fitness Journal* and is also a fellow in ACSM, the American College of Healthcare Executives, and the Medical Fitness Association.

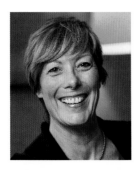

Kathryn H. Schmitz, PhD, MPH, is a professor in the Department of Biostatistics and Epidemiology at the University of Pennsylvania. She currently serves as vice president for ACSM. She was the lead author on ACSM's roundtable guidelines for exercise after cancer, published in 2010. Her research focuses on developing effective, broadly disseminable interventions to improve function, symptoms, and other outcomes among persons who have had a cancer diagnosis.

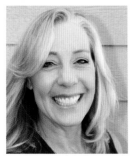

Jan Schroeder, PhD, is a professor and chair of Kinesiology at California State University, Long Beach. She is director of the bachelor of science in fitness, which specializes in preparing students for careers in the fitness industry. She is a Certified Personal Trainer and group exercise instructor who teaches weekly in the private sector. Schroeder has authored over 50 research and applied articles in the area of exercise physiology and fitness. Her current line of research specializes in trends within the fitness industry such as programming, equipment, and compensation for fitness professionals.

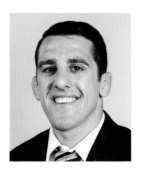

Joseph R. Stanzione, MS, is a graduate of Drexel University, Department of Nutrition Sciences. Stanzione is an aspiring dietitian interested in the field of sports nutrition. Currently he is an assistant wrestling coach at Drexel University. He completed his undergraduate degree at Cornell University, where he received his bachelor's in sociology and nutrition. While attending he was a member of the wrestling team as well as the team captain for the 2012 to 2013 season.

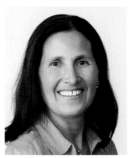

Stella Lucia Volpe, PhD, RD, LDN is professor and chair of the Department of Nutrition Sciences at Drexel University. Volpe is a nutritionist and exercise physiologist who focuses her research on obesity and diabetes prevention, as well as sports nutrition. She is a Certified Clinical Exercise Physiologist (ACSM) and a Registered Dietitian. She is a fellow of ACSM and a past vice president of the ACSM. Volpe competes in field hockey, rowing, and ice hockey. She enjoys being active with her husband, Gary, and their German Shepherds, Sasha and Bear.

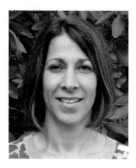

Kerri M. Winters-Stone, PhD, is an exercise scientist and research professor in the Oregon Health & Science University School of Nursing and co-program leader of the Cancer Prevention and Control Program for the OHSU Knight Cancer Institute. Her research focuses on the effects of cancer treatment on fracture, frailty, and cancer recurrence risk and the ability of exercise to improve health and longevity in cancer survivors, including loved ones affected by cancer. The long-term goal of her research is to develop prescriptive exercise programs for cancer survivors that meet their needs and preferences and optimize their health outcomes. Winters-Stone is author of *Action Plan for Osteoporosis,* which is part of ACSM's *Action Plan* series of evidence-based exercise guides for health.

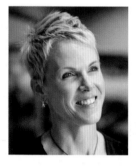

Kara A. Witzke, PhD, is the program lead for kinesiology at Oregon State University, Cascades, in Bend, Oregon. Her passion is in the classroom and in inspiring undergraduate students to answer questions using inquiry-based research. Her primary research focus is the use of high-impact exercise to improve bone health in younger women. Recently she has studied the benefits of functional, high-intensity exercise for apparently healthy individuals as well as those with chronic disease.